T0294794

Body Contouring

Editors

DENNIS J. HURWITZ
DANI KRUCHEVSKY
ARMANDO A. DAVILA

CLINICS IN PLASTIC SURGERY

www.plasticsurgery.theclinics.com

January 2024 • Volume 51 • Number 1

ELSEVIER

1600 John F. Kennedy Boulevard • Suite 1800 • Philadelphia, Pennsylvania, 19103-2899

http://www.theclinics.com

CLINICS IN PLASTIC SURGERY Volume 51, Number 1
January 2024 ISSN 0094-1298, ISBN-13: 978-0-443-13095-3

Editor: Stacy Eastman
Developmental Editor: Anita Chamoli

Clinics in Plastic Surgery (ISSN 0094-1298) is published quarterly by Elsevier Inc., 360 Park Avenue South, New York, NY 10010-1710. Months of issue are January, April, July, and October. Business and Editorial Offices: 1600 John F. Kennedy Blvd., Suite 1800, Philadelphia, PA 19103-2899. Periodicals postage paid at New York, NY and additional mailing offices. Subscription prices are $576.00 per year for US individuals, $100.00 per year for US students/residents, $631.00 per year for Canadian individuals, $703.00 per year for international individuals, $100.00 per year for Canadian students/residents, and $305.00 per year for international students/residents. For institutional access pricing please contact Customer Service via the contact information below. To receive student/resident rate, orders must be accompanied by name of affiliated institution, date of term, and the *signature* of program/residency coordinator on institution letterhead. Orders will be billed at individual rate until proof of status is received. Foreign air speed delivery is included in all *Clinics* subscription prices. All prices are subject to change without notice. **POSTMASTER:** Send address changes to *Clinics in Plastic Surgery*, Elsevier Health Sciences Division, Subscription Customer Service, 3251 Riverport Lane, Maryland Heights, MO 63043. **Customer Service: 1-800-654-2452 (US and Canada). From outside of the United States and Canada, call 314-447-8871. Fax: 314-447-8029. E-mail: JournalsCustomerService-usa@elsevier.com (for print support); JournalsOnlineSupport-usa@elsevier.com (for online support).**

Reprints. For copies of 100 or more of articles in this publication, please contact the Commercial Reprints Department, Elsevier Inc., 360 Park Avenue South, New York, New York 10010-1710. Tel.: +1-212-633-3874; Fax: +1-212-633-3820; E-mail: reprints@elsevier.com.

Clinics in Plastic Surgery is covered in *Current Contents, EMBASE/Excerpta Medica, Science Citation Index, MEDLINE/PubMed (Index Medicus), ASCA, and ISI/BIOMED.*

Contributors

EDITORS

DENNIS J. HURWITZ, MD
Hurwitz Center for Plastic Surgery, Clinical Professor of Plastic Surgery, University of Pittsburgh, Pittsburgh, Pennsylvania, USA

DANI KRUCHEVSKY, MD
Aesthetic and Body Contouring Fellow, Hurwitz Center for Plastic Surgery, Pittsburgh, Pennsylvania, USA

ARMANDO A. DAVILA, MD
Hurwitz Center for Plastic Surgery, Pittsburgh Center for Plastic Surgery, Assistant Clinical Professor of Plastic Surgery, University of Pittsburgh, Pittsburgh, Pennsylvania, USA

AUTHORS

AHMED M. AFIFI, MD
Professor of Surgery, Division of Plastic and Reconstructive Surgery, University of Wisconsin-Madison School of Medicine and Public Health, University of Wisconsin-Madison, Madison, Wisconsin, USA

BROOKE E. BARROW, MD, MEng
Division of Plastic, Maxillofacial, and Oral Surgery, Department of Surgery, Duke University, Durham, North Carolina, USA

JENNIFER CAPLA, MD
Department of Plastic Surgery, Lenox Hill Hospital, Northwell Health System, New York, New York, USA

JOSHUA A. DAVID, MD
Department of Plastic Surgery, University of Pittsburgh Medical Center, Pittsburgh, Pennsylvania, USA

ARMANDO A. DAVILA, MD
Hurwitz Center for Plastic Surgery, Pittsburgh Center for Plastic Surgery, Assistant Clinical Professor of Plastic Surgery, University of Pittsburgh, Pittsburgh, Pennsylvania, USA

EMMANUEL DE LA CRUZ, MD, PLLC
Diplomate, American Board of Plastic Surgery; Diplomate, American Board of Surgery; Houston, Texas, USA

LYDIA MASAKO FERREIRA, MD, PhD, MBA
Head and Full Professor, Federal University of São Paulo, UNIFESP, EPM, São Paulo, São Paulo, Brazil

ONELIO GARCIA Jr, MD
Vol. A. Professor, Division of Plastic Surgery, University of Miami, Miller School of Medicine, Miami, Florida, USA

JEFFREY A. GUSENOFF, MD
Department of Plastic Surgery, University of Pittsburgh Medical Center, Pittsburgh, Pennsylvania, USA

STEVEN A. HANNA, MD, FRCSC
Department of Plastic Surgery, Manhattan Eye, Ear & Throat Hospital, New York, New York, USA

POOJA HUMAR, BS
Department of Plastic Surgery, Medical Student, University of Pittsburgh, Pittsburgh, Pennsylvania, USA

DENNIS J. HURWITZ, MD
Hurwitz Center for Plastic Surgery, Clinical Professor of Plastic Surgery, University of Pittsburgh, Pittsburgh, Pennsylvania, USA

MILIND D. KACHARE, MD
Private Practice, El Paso Cosmetic Surgery, El Paso, Texas, USA

DANI KRUCHEVSKY, MD
Aesthetic and Body Contouring Fellow, Hurwitz Center for Plastic Surgery, Pittsburgh, Pennsylvania, USA

ALINE CURADO MACHADO BORGES, MD
Residents of the Osvaldo Saldanha Plastic Surgery Service, Santos, São Paulo, Brazil

FLAVIO HENRIQUE MENDES, MD, PhD
Professor of the Plastic Surgery Division, Botucatu Medical School, Paulista State University, São Paulo, Brazil

KARIN LUIZA MOKARZEL, MD
Residents of the Osvaldo Saldanha Plastic Surgery Service, Santos, São Paulo, Brazil

WEBER RIBOLLI MORAGAS, MD
Resident at the Plastic Surgery Division, Botucatu Medical School, Paulista State University, São Paulo, Brazil

EDUAR ARNALDO MURCIA BONILLA, MD
Resident of the Osvaldo Saldanha Plastic Surgery Service, Santos, São Paulo, Brazil

FABIO XERFAN NAHAS, MD, PhD, MBA, FACS
Adjunct Professor of Plastic Surgery, Federal University of São Paulo, UNIFESP, EPM, São Paulo, São Paulo, Brazil

BRENT ROBINSON, MD
Chief Resident, Department of Plastic Surgery, University of Pittsburgh, Pittsburgh, Pennsylvania, USA

CRISTIANNA BONETTO SALDANHA, MD
Staff of Osvaldo Saldanha Plastic Surgery Service, Body Sculping Course Coordinator, Santos, São Paulo, Brazil

OSVALDO SALDANHA FILHO, MD
Staff of Osvaldo Saldanha Plastic Surgery Service, Body Sculping Course Coordinator, Santos, São Paulo, Brazil

OSVALDO SALDANHA, PhD
Chair of Osvaldo Saldanha Plastic Surgery Service, Former President of SBCP (Brazilian Society of Plastic Surgery), Body Sculping Course Coordinator, Santos, São Paulo, Brazil

EVGENI VANYOV SHARKOV, MD
Owner and Plastic Surgeon, VDerm Clinic Private Practice, Sofia, Bulgaria

SADRI OZAN SOZER, MD
Private Practice, El Paso Cosmetic Surgery, El Paso, Texas, USA

FAUSTO VITERBO, MD, PhD
Full Professor of the Plastic Surgery Division, Botucatu Medical School, Paulista State University, São Paulo, Brazil

PETER WIRTH, MD
Resident Physician, Division of Plastic and Reconstructive Surgery, University of Wisconsin-Madison School of Medicine and Public Health, University of Wisconsin-Madison, Madison, Wisconsin, USA

LUCCIE M. WO, MD, MSE
Chief Resident, Division of Plastic Surgery, University of Miami, Miller School of Medicine, Miami, Florida, USA

Contents

The practice of large volume liposuction, when executed by board-certified plastic surgeons using a variety of energy-assisted liposuction devices, has been substantiated as a secure procedure, yielding enhanced aesthetic results and minimal complications. Techniques including the superwet technique and ultrasonic-assisted liposuction are utilized to diminish blood loss, while also maintaining a keen awareness of the maximum volume of infiltration fluid permissible for safe infusion. Adherence to evidence-based protocols is of paramount importance to reduce the risk of postoperative complications. These protocols encompass hypothermia prevention, deep vein thrombosis (DVT) prophylaxis, and perioperative antibiotic prophylaxis. To ensure the highest quality of care, it is recommended that large volume liposuction procedures be performed in accredited hospitals or certified ambulatory surgery centers. Postoperative procedures should include overnight admission of patients to facilitate proper hemodynamic monitoring. While the employment of multiple devices such as VASERLipo and Renuvion has been noted to augment skin and soft tissue contraction, it is worth noting that there may be a heightened risk of seroma formation (at 2.27%) and subcutaneous emphysema (at 1.47%). Consequently, prudent use of these advanced medical devices is essential to avoid any potential adverse events.

There is a continuous search for better technical alternatives for the treatment of abdominal contour deformities in the practice of plastic surgeons. LADE—lipoabdominoplasty (LAP) with anatomical definition—is a step ahead of the traditional LAP technique. This technique incorporated the principles of highlighting the definition of the abdominal musculature, achieving more natural results with fewer reminders of a surgical intervention. The esthetic results are much harmonious, with a true abdominal rejuvenated appearance. We can reduce morbidity by the preservation of perforating blood vessels and suspension of Scarpa's fascia. The correct selection of the patient makes the procedure safe and reproducible.

Abdominoplasty has evolved in the last few decades, especially the treatment of the myoaponeurotic deformities. Bulging, lack of definition of the abdominal contour, should be understood and treated according to the individual deformity. Many types of deformities have been recognized and treatment respects the local anatomy in most cases. Scientific basis that consolidate these treatments are discussed as well as possible recurrences and pitfalls of these techniques. The histological composition of muscles and fascia are also discussed and anatomical details help to enrich the knowledge of the correction of this layer. Specific types of sutures are suggested for both plications and muscle advancement.

TULUA is an effective non-undermined lipoabdominoplasty with a low transverse wide plication of the rectus fascia that allows aggressive liposuction. For an esthetic 360° torso reshaping, oblique flankplasty, also without undermining, is added to correct

CLINICS IN PLASTIC SURGERY

FORTHCOMING ISSUES

April 2024
Acute and Reconstructive Burn Care, Part I
Francesco M. Egro and C. Scott Hultman, *Editors*

July 2024
Acute and Reconstructive Burn Care, Part II
Francesco M. Egro and C. Scott Hultman, *Editors*

October 2024
Hand and Upper Extremity Surgery
Kevin C. Chung and Brian Starr, *Editors*

RECENT ISSUES

October 2023
Gluteal Augmentation
Ashkan Ghavami, Pat Pazmiño, and Neil M. Vranis, *Editors*

July 2023
Injectables and Nonsurgical Rejuvenation
Jessyka G. Lightall, *Editor*

April 2023
Breast Reconstruction
Neil Tanna, *Editor*

SERIES OF RELATED INTEREST

Facial Plastic Surgery Clinics
https://www.facialplastic.theclinics.com/
Otolaryngologic Clinics
https://www.oto.theclinics.com/
Advances in Cosmetic Surgery
www.advancesincosmeticsurgery.com/

Preface

State-of-the-Art in Body-Contouring Surgery

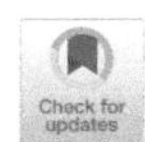

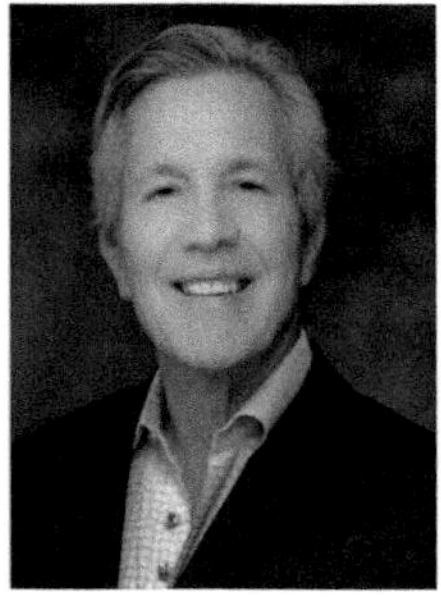

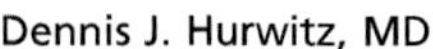

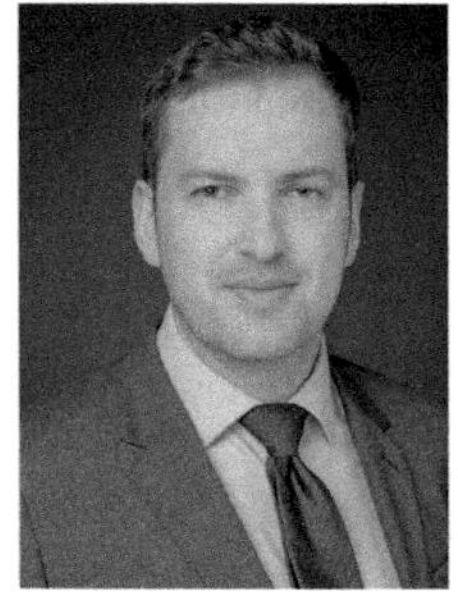

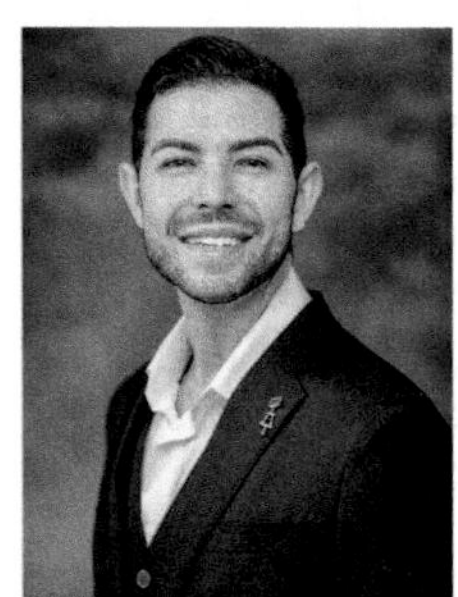

Dennis J. Hurwitz, MD Dani Kruchevsky, MD Armando A. Davila, MD
Editors

As a relatively new subspecialty of Plastic Surgery, Body Contouring is understandably rapidly evolving. This 15-article *Clinics in Plastic Surgery*, authored by recognized experts, covers advances in traditional approaches as well as unconventional new skin excision patterns and minimally invasive technology. Our comprehension, approaches, and outcomes have dramatically improved since the last *Clinics in Plastic Surgery* devoted to Body Contouring in January 2014.

All articles cover patient selection, technique, aesthetics, and safety. In the first two articles, patient preparation, evaluation, and staging are thoroughly discussed as well as setting expectations and anticipating risks. Better preparation reduces dissatisfaction and increases acceptance of revisions. The nuances of treating skin laxity after new medication-induced weight loss are presented. The next two articles cover the use of the most recent ultrasonic-assisted lipoplasty and radiofrequency skin-tightening technology in normal and oversized patients. Properly used, VASER reduces collateral damage, and fat can be harvested for lipoaugmentation. In obese patients, dramatic reduction in size with curvaceous or muscular contours can be achieved after VASER with radiofrequency skin tightening.

In "Lipoabdominoplasty with Anatomical Definition—Update," by Osvaldo Saldanha and colleagues, sophisticated integration of multilayered liposuction with abdominoplasty defines superficial muscles without increasing complications. A variety of plication techniques are advised for the most common patterns of musculoaponeurotic weakness by the world's authority in "Management of the Musculoaponeurotic Layer in Abdominoplasty," by Nahas and Masako Ferreira, followed by an understanding of recurrence based on collagen deficiency, materials, and technique. The next article introduces TULUA lipoabdominoplasty combined with an alternative posterior lower body lift called Oblique Flankplasty for an aesthetic 360° skintight torsoplasty. In "Finesse in Fleur De Lys Abdominoplasty" by Mendes, the master of Fleur de Lys abdominoplasty shares his updated technique, including neo umbilicoplasty. "Surgical Circumferential Contouring: Lower Body, Upper Body" by Gusenoff and David, presents the state-of-the-art transverse upper and lower body lifts with management of the breasts and extremities. A variety of staging strategies are expounded with cautionary pitfalls.

The next three articles focus on Oblique Flankplasty. An enthusiastic recent adopter describes his version on smooth reduction of the waist through direct excision of sagging and oversized flanks. In "Spiral Flap Breast Reshaping with J Torsoplasty" by Hurwitz and Kruchevsky, Oblique Flankplasty is presented as an adjunct to J Torsoplasty to sculpt the entire torso through oblique excisions. Finally, optimal aesthetics can be achieved with holistic contouring of the lower buttocks, mons pubis, and thighs through Oblique Flankplasty and lipoabdominoplasty with Vertical medial thighplasty.

The manner of artful integration of radiofrequency nonsurgical skin tightening with excisional body contouring is the objective of "The Role of Noninvasive and Minimally Invasive Techniques in

Clin Plastic Surg 51 (2024) xi–xii
https://doi.org/10.1016/j.cps.2023.07.009
0094-1298/24/© 2023 Published by Elsevier Inc.

Open Surgical Interventions for the Purpose of Body Contouring" by Sharkov. Residual skin laxity after excisional surgery may be best treated with this technology. "Emerging Approaches to Augmentation Mastopexy in the Nontraditional Weight Loss Patient" by Davila takes a systematic look at combining body contouring with breast enhancement, including the use of silicone implants, supporting sutures, and synthetic meshes. These approaches are necessary when neighboring tissue is not available for breast augmentation, or the patient refuses the risks of flap reconstruction. The final article, devoted to secondary surgery, insightfully prepares patients for revision surgery, starting with setting realistic expectations. From malpositioned closures, subcutaneous scarring, to deformity due to skin loss, correction through revision surgery tends to be more difficult than primary and often requires reconstructive plastic surgery.

Assisting with this reflective coda to the Hurwitz Center for Plastic Surgery are my coeditors, President and owner of the now named Pittsburgh Center for Plastic Surgery, Armando A. Davila, MD, and my Aesthetic and Body Contouring fellow, Dani Kruchevsky, MD. They have guided the progress of this publication at every step, as well as contributed to multiple articles. Moreover, their enthusiastic acceptance and creative modification of my innovations have been exhilarating. They enduringly enhance my legacy in body-contouring surgery. I am proud of the symbiotic relationship I have with the University of Pittsburgh surgeon contributors, who are both supportive friends and worthy competitors. The remaining esteemed creative authors are either long-term or recent colleagues, who are adept at sharing wisdom and extending friendship on every occasion that we meet. Please accept my gratitude as well as the appreciation of the thousands of patients we all indirectly improve by contributing to this cohesive update in *Clinics in Plastic Surgery*.

Dennis J. Hurwitz, MD
Pittsburgh Center for Plastic Surgery
University of Pittsburgh
3109 Forbes Avenue, #500
Pittsburgh, PA 15213, USA

Dani Kruchevsky, MD
Pittsburgh Center for Plastic Surgery
3109 Forbes Avenue, #500
Pittsburgh, PA 15213, USA

Armando A. Davila, MD
Pittsburgh Center for Plastic Surgery
University of Pittsburgh
3109 Forbes Avenue, #500
Pittsburgh, PA 15213, USA

E-mail addresses:
drhurwitz@pghplasticsurgery.com (D.J. Hurwitz)
dkruchevsky@gmail.com (D. Kruchevsky)
drdavila@pghplasticsurgery.com (A.A. Davila)

Preparing Patients for Body Contouring Surgery and Postoperative Surveillance for Deep Venous Thrombosis

Pooja Humar, BS, Brent Robinson, MD*

KEYWORDS

• Body contouring • DVT • Preoperative nutrition • Postoperative surveillance

KEY POINTS

- Preoperative evaluation is essential to ensure patient safety and optimize outcomes in body contouring surgery after massive weight loss. Evaluation includes assessing BMI, weight stabilization, and potential for further weight loss.
- Medical comorbidities should be carefully assessed before surgery to manage risks and optimize surgical outcomes. Such conditions as diabetes, hypertension, and sleep apnea may improve after weight loss, but ongoing management is important.
- Nutritional optimization is crucial for preparing patients for body contouring surgery. Deficiencies in essential minerals and vitamins are common after weight loss surgery and should be addressed with supplements and dietary counseling.
- Psychosocial factors play a significant role in patient satisfaction and outcomes. Understanding patient expectations, evaluating psychiatric well-being, and assessing social support are important aspects of preoperative evaluation.
- Thromboembolic risk is a concern in body contouring surgery, and appropriate prophylactic measures should be taken. Risk stratification, including Caprini score assessment, can guide the use of chemoprophylaxis, whereas postoperative surveillance for deep vein thrombosis is essential.

INTRODUCTION

With the number of overweight and obese individuals rising in America, massive weight loss (MWL) through bariatric surgery or even major lifestyle modifications is becoming increasingly common. Despite successful weight loss, patients are often left with whole body deformities that can contribute to potential problems including skin infections and persistent poor body image.[1] The excess skin left after MWL can be addressed by body contouring surgery, and thus the increase in these procedures has paralleled the increase in bariatric surgery cases. According to the American Society of Plastic Surgery, in 2019, more than 49,000 patients underwent body contouring after an MWL procedure. Many patients are now electing to have multiple body contouring procedures, to address various areas of deformities.

The life after weight loss patient population presents with unique surgical challenges and assessment of the patient's risk along with patient expectations, is crucial before undergoing elective surgery.[2] Obesity is associated with a plethora of medical comorbidities, and although many patients see improvements in overall health after undergoing significant weight loss, past and current medical conditions can affect surgical outcomes. After MWL patients are also subject to significant

Department of Plastic Surgery, University of Pittsburgh, 3550 Terrace Street, 6B Scaife Hall, Pittsburgh, PA 15261, USA
* Corresponding author. 5292 South College Drive #302, Murray, UT 84123
E-mail address: brentr01@gmail.com

Clin Plastic Surg 51 (2024) 1–6
https://doi.org/10.1016/j.cps.2023.06.007

nutritional deficiencies and psychosocial issues.[3] Additionally, body contouring surgery can pose significant stress on the body with risk of complications including bleeding, skin necrosis, and infection. Given these factors, a thorough preoperative evaluation is required for patient safety, optimal aesthetic outcome, and satisfaction. Therefore, we describe the key considerations in preparation and aftercare of patients for body contouring surgery.

PREOPERATIVE EVALUATION

Evaluation of Body Mass Index and Stabilization

When evaluating patients after MWL, weight stability, along with current and maximum body mass index (BMI) must be factored into risk evaluation and surgical planning. For patients to be considered eligible for body contouring procedures, they must typically wait until they have no more than a 1 to 2 lb per month weight fluctuation for 3 to 6 months.[4] This weight stabilization occurs in patients anywhere from 18 to 24 months after bariatric surgery. Performing body contouring on patients with ongoing weight loss can put patients at risk for poor wound healing and recurrence in tissue laxity,[5] and therefore result in an increased risk of postoperative complications and poor aesthetic outcomes.

On stabilization, the ideal candidates for body contouring surgery typically have a BMI between 25 and 30.[4] These patients can often undergo a variety of procedure combinations, with excellent aesthetic outcomes. For patients with BMI greater than 30, body shape, fat distribution, and likelihood of additional weight loss must all be considered. Current literature has shown that high preoperative BMI is associated with an increased risk of postoperative complications.[5–7] This is partly affected by the fact that patients with high BMI have been found to have increased operative times, hospital stays, and duration of drain placement.[8] Patients who present with a BMI at or higher than 40 are at increased risk for any surgical procedure and are encouraged to undergo further weight loss before body contouring surgery.

Although bariatric surgery has been proven effective in assisting patients with undergoing MWL, having inadequate weight loss or weight regain is not uncommon. In this setting, for patients aiming to undergo additional weight loss before body contouring surgery, diet modifications and medications are a potential option. Most commonly, existing diabetes, antiseizure, and antidepressant medications can also be use as pharmacotherapy for promoting weight loss, including metformin, topiramate, or bupropion.[9] Appetite suppressing drugs, such as phentermine, have also been used by patients. Previous studies looking at the use of these medications in the MWL population have shown that patients, on average, underwent an additional 15 to 20 lb weight loss with the added pharmacotherapy.[9] However, patients undergoing bariatric surgery are at high risk for nutritional deficits and therefore should continue to undergo nutritional counseling while undergoing continued weight loss.[10]

Medical Comorbidities

Significant weight loss after bariatric surgery or lifestyle modifications can result in improvements in medical conditions, such as hypertension, diabetes, hyperlipidemia, and sleep apnea. Previous literature estimates resolution of diabetes in 75% of patients, hypertension in 50% to 60% of patients, and sleep apnea in up to 85% of patients.[11,12] Any amount of weight loss can result in improvements in comorbid conditions; however, complete resolution may not occur. Given this, it is crucial for plastic surgeons to understand the status of a patient's comorbid conditions before operating and manage them accordingly throughout the perioperative period.

Many patients have resolution of diabetes after weight loss, defined as discontinuing all diabetes medications and maintaining blood glucose levels within a normal range postoperatively.[13,14] However, even after MWL, patients can continue to have insulin resistance and therefore patients should have a hemoglobin A_{1c} checked alongside other preoperative laboratory studies. For patients who have persistent diabetes after weight loss, medication adjustments are required, similar to other surgical procedures. In the 24 hours before surgery, oral hypoglycemics are paused and insulin dose is decreased by 20% to 25% to account for fasting before and during surgery.

Even after MWL, patients with a history of obesity can have long lasting cardiovascular damage. Although up to 60% of patients become normotensive after bariatric surgery, hypertension in the perioperative period can increase the risk of complications, such as bleeding events, stroke, or myocardial infarction.[12,15] Therefore, blood pressure should be monitored routinely, starting before surgical intervention. Method of weight loss can have significant effects on cardiac health, where weight loss through diet and exercise strengthens the heart in a way that bariatric surgery does not. Given this, the method of weight loss can be factored into a preoperative cardiovascular workup.

Surgeons must also have an understanding of patients' smoking status. Patients with a recent or active history of smoking are subject to poor wound healing and are at risk for complications potentially resulting in poor aesthetic outcomes. Given this, patients must quit smoking 4 to 6 months before operation.[4] Patients who have not ceased use of tobacco products are rescheduled given the elective nature of body contouring procedures.

Nutritional Optimization

In anticipation of body contouring surgery preoperative nutritional optimization plays a crucial role in preparing patients for the physiologic stress of surgery into the recovery period. By ensuring adequate nutrition before the procedure, patients can enhance their overall health, optimize wound healing, and promote better surgical outcomes. In a prospective analysis of bariatric surgery patients presenting for plastic surgery it was noted that there was a 25% increase in protein-calorie requirements in the period after major surgery.[3] Even modest protein-calorie malnutrition may lead to decreased fibroplasia and impaired wound healing and therefore the authors recommended a target a goal of at least 1 g/kg/d of protein intake.[3]

Furthermore, a comprehensive assessment of the patient's nutritional status, including such factors as BMI, micronutrient deficiencies, and overall dietary habits, must be thoroughly assessed. Through proper nutrition, including a balanced diet rich in vitamins, minerals, and proteins, patients can improve their immune function, reduce the risk of postoperative complications, and promote tissue regeneration. Nutritional optimization helps patients maintain optimal body composition, enabling surgeons to achieve better aesthetic results.

Weight loss surgery can result in deficiencies in the absorption and metabolism of essential minerals and vitamins in the body. These procedures alter the gastrointestinal anatomy, leading to changes in nutrient absorption thereby potentially causing deficiencies. Common mineral and vitamin deficiencies following bariatric surgery include the following:

1. Iron deficiency: Impaired iron absorption caused by the reduction in stomach acid and changes in the digestive tract. Iron deficiency anemia may occur, leading to such symptoms as fatigue, weakness, and decreased exercise tolerance.
2. Vitamin B_{12} deficiency: B_{12} is primarily absorbed in the stomach, and alterations in the anatomy of the gastrointestinal tract can hinder its absorption. Vitamin B_{12} deficiency can result in such symptoms as fatigue, nerve damage, and megaloblastic anemia.
3. Calcium deficiency: Calcium absorption is affected by bariatric surgery, especially in procedures involving malabsorptive components. Inadequate calcium levels can lead to bone loss, increased risk of fractures, and the development of osteoporosis.
4. Vitamin D deficiency: Bariatric surgery can impact the absorption of vitamin D, which is crucial for calcium metabolism and bone health. Vitamin D deficiency can lead to decreased bone mineral density, increased fracture risk, and potential muscle weakness.
5. Vitamin A deficiency: Some bariatric procedures may affect the absorption of fat-soluble vitamins, such as vitamin A. Inadequate vitamin A levels can cause visual problems, dry skin, and impaired immune function.
6. Thiamine (vitamin B_1) deficiency: Certain bariatric procedures can interfere with thiamine absorption, potentially leading to thiamine deficiency. Thiamine deficiency can cause neurologic symptoms, including confusion, memory problems, and muscle weakness.

To prevent these deficiencies, patients who undergo bariatric surgery should be advised to take lifelong nutritional supplements, including a multivitamin, iron, calcium, vitamin D, and other specific supplements as needed. Close monitoring in anticipation of body contouring surgery is essential to identify and address deficiencies promptly. Nutritional counseling and follow-up with health care professionals experienced in bariatric surgery are crucial for optimizing postoperative outcomes and maintaining adequate nutrient status.

Nutritional optimization is further quantified with laboratory markers in anticipation of body contouring surgery. In the preoperative phase of post-bariatric body contouring plastic surgery for patients who have previously undergone bariatric surgery, several essential laboratory tests are typically performed to ensure patient safety and optimize surgical outcomes. These preoperative laboratory studies serve as important diagnostic tools to assess the patient's overall health status and identify any potential risk factors or underlying medical conditions that may impact the surgery. Common preoperative laboratory tests in this context include a complete blood count to evaluate red and white blood cell counts, hemoglobin levels, and platelet count; and a comprehensive metabolic panel to assess liver and kidney function, electrolyte levels, and blood glucose levels. Additionally, coagulation studies, such as prothrombin time and activated partial thromboplastin time, are often performed to evaluate the patient's blood clotting abilities. These preoperative laboratory studies play a crucial role in ensuring the patient's readiness for surgery and enabling the surgical team to make informed decisions regarding anesthesia, intraoperative management, and postoperative care.

Postbariatric patients are not prescribed a specific diet per se, but rather an emphasis on eating slowly, chewing well, and eating three to five small meals per day.[16] Patients are also advised to consume protein-containing foods at every meal and to take nutritional supplements to reduce the risk of developing nutritional deficiencies.[16] With a focus on preoperative nutritional optimization, patients can significantly enhance their surgical experience and achieve more satisfactory outcomes in body contouring plastic surgery.

Social Factors

Psychiatric comorbidities are common among obese patients, which often persist even after MWL. Although a formal psychosocial evaluation is not required before undergoing body contouring surgery, it is important for the surgeon to understand these factors. The Body-Q is a validated survey of patient-reported outcomes, which is used to identify a variety of preoperative psychosocial factors that could potentially influence postoperative outcomes including perceptions of self-image, diagnosis and management of psychiatric conditions, and social support.[17]

The Body-Q also helps to evaluate areas of concern to the patient. As part of the preoperative evaluation, the surgeon must understand and manage patient expectations. The surgeon must understand why the patient is interested in body contouring surgery, including functional and physical factors. To manage patient expectations, conduct a thorough preoperative evaluation with discussion of anticipated improvements in shape and contour, scar location, recovery timeline, and potential risk of postoperative complications. As part of preoperative surgical planning, it is crucial for the surgeon to take photographs. These can help the surgeon and patient track improvements at postoperative follow-up visits.

It is well known that depression and anxiety can increase the risk of subsequent obesity development. However, previous longitudinal studies have shown that successful weight loss is associated with decreased anxiety and depression, whereas active, uncontrolled depression can predict poorer success in weight loss.[18,19] Previous studies have shown that patients with generalized anxiety disorder or depression are less likely to report positive postoperative body image and are less likely to maintain weight loss than patients without these comorbid diagnoses.[20] Given these findings, it is valuable for the surgeon to assess a patient's psychiatric well-being, and current management of underlying comorbidities.

Psychosocial support is an important factor affecting patients' management and outcomes in a wide range of medical and surgical procedures. However, given that body contouring surgery has drastic impact on patient appearance, patients commonly require strong mental and emotional support. This is where evaluation of the patient's social support system preoperatively can help with the postoperative recovery. Social support from a spouse or friends has been associated with increased satisfaction with body image postoperatively. Additionally, patients with spousal support were more likely to maintain their weight loss following body contouring procedures.

DEEP VENOUS THROMBOSIS PROPHYLAXIS AND POSTOPERATIVE SURVEILLANCE

As with any surgical intervention, body contouring surgery puts patients at risk for venous thromboembolic (VTE) events. Risk factors in this population often include obesity, multiple site surgery, long operative times, and difficulty ambulating after surgery.[21] The estimated risk of VTE in this patient population is reported to be between 1% and 3%; however, this risk can increase to 5% to 10% in patients with BMI greater than 35.[21,22]

Prophylactic measurements including the use of intraoperative compression devices and chemoprophylaxis, most commonly unfractionated heparin or low-molecular-weight heparin, are used to minimize the risk of postoperative VTE. However, many surgeons have noted an increased risk of bleeding in the MWL population, and therefore choose to use anticoagulation medications sparingly in this population.[23] In a 2016 systematic review of the risks and benefits of deep venous thrombosis prophylaxis among all plastic surgery patients, the recommendations stated that patients should be risk-stratified for postoperative VTE risk using Caprini score and only patients with a score greater than eight should be considered to received chemoprophylaxis.[24] Although these are robust guidelines for all plastic surgery cases, there is a lack of evidence-based guidelines on the use and optimal timing for chemoprophylaxis in the MWL patient undergoing body contouring.

Postoperative surveillance for VTE typically involves a routine assessment of clinical signs of symptoms including leg swelling, pain, warmth, and redness, along with vital signs.[25] For patients that clinically show signs indicative of a deep venous thrombosis, imaging studies, such as a Doppler ultrasound, are used to detect a blood clot. Given the ease of performing these studies and importance of early detection and treatment, the threshold to check for a deep venous thrombosis is typically low.

SUMMARY

The increasing prevalence of overweight and obesity in America has led to a rise in MWL procedures, such as bariatric surgery, to combat these conditions. However, although successful weight loss is achieved, patients often face the challenge of excess skin and body deformities. Body contouring surgery has emerged as a solution to address these issues, leading to a parallel increase in the number of these procedures. The population of patients who undergo MWL presents unique surgical challenges, and it is essential to assess their risks and manage their expectations before elective surgery. Obesity is associated with various medical comorbidities that can impact surgical outcomes, and the stress imposed by body contouring surgery increases the risk of complications. Therefore, a comprehensive preoperative evaluation is crucial to prioritize patient safety and achieve desirable aesthetic outcomes. By understanding and addressing key considerations, plastic surgeons can effectively prepare patients for body contouring surgery, improving their overall well-being and quality of life.

CLINICS CARE POINTS

- Patients should undergo a thorough preoperative evaluation before body contouring surgery, taking into account weight stability, BMI, and risk of complications to optimize postoperative outcomes.
- Weight stabilization is important before body contouring surgery to reduce the risk of poor wound healing and recurrence of tissue laxity.
- Patients with a BMI at or greater than 40 are at high risk for surgical procedures and are encouraged to undergo further weight loss before body contouring surgery.
- Assessment of medical comorbidities is crucial before surgery to manage conditions, such as diabetes, hypertension, and sleep apnea, which can impact surgical outcomes.
- Nutritional optimization plays a significant role in preparing patients for body contouring surgery, including ensuring adequate protein intake and addressing deficiencies in essential minerals and vitamins.
- Preoperative laboratory studies, including a complete blood count, comprehensive metabolic panel, and coagulation studies, help assess the patient's overall health status and identify potential risk factors.
- Understanding and addressing psychosocial factors, including patient expectations, psychiatric comorbidities, and social support, are important for successful outcomes in body contouring surgery.
- Thromboembolic prophylaxis should be considered based on risk stratification, and postoperative surveillance for deep vein thrombosis is crucial because this population is at an elevated risk for DVT.

DISCLOSURE

The authors have nothing to disclose.

REFERENCES

1. Hurwitz DJ, Ayeni O. Body contouring surgery in the massive weight loss patient. Surg Clin North Am 2016;96(4):875–85.
2. Gusenoff JA. Prevention and management of complications in body contouring surgery. Clin Plast Surg 2014;41(4):805–18.
3. Naghshineh N, et al. Nutritional assessment of bariatric surgery patients presenting for plastic surgery: a prospective analysis. Plast Reconstr Surg 2010; 126(2):602–10.
4. Naghshineh N, Rubin JP. Preoperative evaluation of the body contouring patient: the cornerstone of patient safety. Clin Plast Surg 2014;41(4):637–43.
5. Coon D, et al. Body mass and surgical complications in the postbariatric reconstructive patient: analysis of 511 cases. Ann Surg 2009;249(3): 397–401.
6. Marouf A, Mortada H. Complications of body contouring surgery in postbariatric patients: a systematic review and meta-analysis. Aesthetic Plast Surg 2021;45(6):2810–20.
7. Chetta MD, et al. Complications in body contouring stratified according to weight loss method. Plast Surg (Oakv) 2016;24(2):103–6.
8. Ghnnam W, Elrahawy A, Moghazy ME. The effect of body mass index on outcome of abdominoplasty operations. World J Plast Surg 2016;5(3):244–51.
9. Stanford FC, et al. The utility of weight loss medications after bariatric surgery for weight regain or inadequate weight loss: a multi-center study. Surg Obes Relat Dis 2017;13(3):491–500.

10. Bettini S, et al. Diet approach before and after bariatric surgery. Rev Endocr Metab Disord 2020; 21(3):297–306.
11. Carson JL, et al. The effect of gastric bypass surgery on hypertension in morbidly obese patients. Arch Intern Med 1994;154(2):193–200.
12. Liang Z, et al. Effect of laparoscopic Roux-en-Y gastric bypass surgery on type 2 diabetes mellitus with hypertension: a randomized controlled trial. Diabetes Res Clin Pract 2013;101(1):50–6.
13. Nandagopal R, Brown RJ, Rother KI. Resolution of type 2 diabetes following bariatric surgery: implications for adults and adolescents. Diabetes Technol Ther 2010;12(8):671–7.
14. Affinati AH, et al. Bariatric surgery in the treatment of type 2 diabetes. Curr Diab Rep 2019;19(12):156.
15. Aronow WS. Management of hypertension in patients undergoing surgery. Ann Transl Med 2017; 5(10):227.
16. Agha-Mohammadi, Siamak MB, Chir B, et al. Potential impacts of nutritional deficiency of postbariatric patients on body contouring surgery. Plast Reconstr Surg 2008;122(6):1901–14.
17. Poulsen L, et al. Patient-reported outcome measures: body-Q. Clin Plast Surg 2019;46(1):15–24.
18. Fu R, et al. Bariatric surgery alleviates depression in obese patients: a systematic review and meta-analysis. Obes Res Clin Pract 2022;16(1):10–6.
19. Sarwer DB, Fabricatore AN. Psychiatric considerations of the massive weight loss patient. Clin Plast Surg 2008;35(1):1–10.
20. Sarwer DB, Polonsky HM. Body image and body contouring procedures. Aesthet Surg J 2016;36(9): 1039–47.
21. Shermak MA, Chang DC, Heller J. Factors impacting thromboembolism after bariatric body contouring surgery. Plast Reconstr Surg 2007;119(5): 1590–6.
22. Newall G, et al. A retrospective study on the use of a low-molecular-weight heparin for thromboembolism prophylaxis in large-volume liposuction and body contouring procedures. Aesthetic Plast Surg 2006; 30(1):86–95 [discussion: 96–7].
23. Yin C, et al. Body contouring in massive weight loss patients receiving venous thromboembolism chemoprophylaxis: a systematic review. Plast Reconstr Surg Glob Open 2021;9(8):e3746.
24. Pannucci CJ, et al. Benefits and risks of prophylaxis for deep venous thrombosis and pulmonary embolus in plastic surgery: a systematic review and meta-analysis of controlled trials and consensus conference. Plast Reconstr Surg 2016;137(2): 709–30.
25. Nelson RE, et al. Using multiple sources of data for surveillance of postoperative venous thromboembolism among surgical patients treated in Department of Veterans Affairs hospitals, 2005-2010. Thromb Res 2015;135(4):636–42.

Patient Evaluation and Surgical Staging

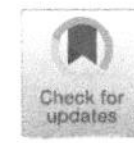

Jennifer Capla, MD[a,*], Steven A. Hanna, MD, FRCSC[b]

KEYWORDS

- Massive weight loss • Moderate medication-assisted weight loss • Post-bariatric • BMI • Body contouring • Staging • Ozempic • Ozempic face

KEY POINTS

- Weight loss patients require a thorough preoperative evaluation including a complete medical workup focused on comorbidities, weight history, and nutritional status.
- Planning procedures requires the consideration of the patient's goals, setting realistic expectations, and staging surgery appropriately.
- Recent increases in the use of incretin mimetic medications have created an emerging group of weight loss patients who have undergone what we have termed "Moderate Medication Assisted Weight Loss." While some of the concepts regarding the management of massive weight loss patients apply to this group, they do require specific considerations.

INTRODUCTION

Success in body contouring after massive weight loss requires careful planning with a clear understanding of the patient's goals, medical comorbidities and fitness for surgery in mind. Surgeons must balance patients' demand for convenient combination procedures against what is safe and what is most likely to achieve an optimal aesthetic outcome. It is critical to stage these procedures appropriately to minimize operative time, decrease complications, and avoid undue tension on operative sites.

With the recent popularity of medications such as Ozempic and Mounjaro, these concepts are becoming increasingly relevant outside the massive weight loss population. This article will discuss the evaluation and staging of the Massive Weight Loss (MWL) population as well as define and discuss the management of the Moderate Medication-Assisted Weight Loss (MMA) population.

PATIENT EVALUATION

Patient evaluation begins with a thorough history from the patient which includes their complete medical and surgical history. Specific elements critical for the evaluation of weight loss patients are detailed later in discussion.

Mechanism and sequelae of weight loss

The mechanism of weight loss is a critical component in the evaluation of a weight loss patient. If surgery is the etiology of weight loss, then delineating between restrictive and malabsorptive techniques is important in order to assess nutritional deficiencies. Of note, iron deficiency is noted in up to half of the post-bariatric surgical population, which may lead to anemia. Other nutrients impacted in this patient population include calcium, vitamin B12, and thiamine. Protein deficiency is another issue, the cause of which may be multifactorial following bariatric surgery. Protein deficiency can lead to protracted recovery and suboptimal wound healing. Weight loss patients should be nutritionally optimized preoperatively.[1]

Recently, patients who do not have type 2 diabetes have increasingly been using incretin mimetic medications to assist with weight loss. Patients who have lost weight through the use of

[a] Department of Plastic Surgery, Lenox Hill Hospital, Northwell Health System, 125 East 63rd Street, New York, NY 10065, USA; [b] Department of Plastic Surgery, Manhattan Eye, Ear & Throat Hospital, 210 East 64th Street, New York, NY, USA
* Corresponding author.
E-mail address: jennifer.capla@gmail.com

Clin Plastic Surg 51 (2024) 7–12
https://doi.org/10.1016/j.cps.2023.07.004
0094-1298/24/

these medications present an interesting and emerging population of weight loss patients which we have termed Moderate Medication-Assisted Weight Loss (MMA). In our experience, MMA patients will typically lose no more than 25% of their total body weight and therefore are not true massive weight loss patients. Furthermore, these patients tend to have fewer comorbidities typically associated with massive weight loss. Despite that, many of the sequelae of massive weight loss are present in this patient population but to less of an extent. In particular, their tissue tends to be of better quality and has retained some of its inherent elasticity.

For MMA patients, surgeons should note which medication was used, for how long the medication has been taken and the current dose. In our experience, the most common medications used for weight loss at the time of writing have been semaglutide (Ozempic) and tirzepatide (Mounjaro). Briefly, semaglutide increases insulin release in response to glucose by activating glucagon-like peptide-1 receptors (GLP-1). This also inhibits glucagon secretion which decreases hepatic glucose production.[2,3] Similarly, tirzepatide is a GLP-1 agonist and additionally acts as a glucose-dependent insulinotropic polypeptide (GIP) agonist. Both of these medications have been associated with delayed gastric emptying, particularly early in the course of their use.[4,5] This has relevance to the perioperative management of these patients which is discussed later in discussion.

Body mass index, weight change, and stability

It is well described that patients with a high BMI (>30) are at a greater risk for postoperative complications. Patients who have had larger amounts of weight loss and greater changes in their BMI are also at elevated risk. In general, we would consider a current BMI of 30 kg/m2 or less to be a safe threshold for a patient to undergo body contouring procedures.[6,7] It follows that weight stability is also critical in assessing operative candidates. In our practice, in order to undergo body contouring surgery patients must have achieved weight stability for at least three months. We define weight stability as no more than 5 lbs of weight loss over 3 consecutive months. While we, along with our colleagues, may prefer a 6 month period of weight stability, 3 months is the absolute minimum. This period of stability allows time for medical comorbidities to resolve and physiologic homeostasis to be achieved. Furthermore, weight stability makes it possible from a technical perspective to achieve optimal results from body contouring.

Both MMA and MWL patients are more likely to have medical comorbidities by virtue of being overweight to obese. These patients experience a higher incidence of diabetes mellitus, cardiac disease, hypertension, sleep apnea, osteoarthritis, and other medical issues. Weight loss may ameliorate but not entirely alleviate some of these concerns and a full workup is required. All medical issues should be optimized prior to body contouring surgery. Excess skin and intertriginous folds may create additional concerns such as infections and rashes, difficulty with physical activity, and psychiatric concerns such as depression.[8] As above, these issues must be addressed prior to body contouring surgery.

Smoking and social support

Additional factors to be considered in the weight loss population include smoking status and social support. It is well known that smoking negatively affects surgical outcomes. We recommend deferring surgery on active smokers, and requiring that patients with a history of smoking abstain for at least 4 weeks before and after surgery. With respect to social support, body contouring surgery may result in some physical limitation postoperatively and having assistance during convalescence is advantageous for patients —especially those who have undergone extremity procedures.

PHYSICAL EXAMINATION

Physical examination for weight loss patients should include a general inspect for body shape and habitus, routine vital signs, height, weight, and a calculation of the patient's BMI. The areas in question should be evaluated for skin or fat excess or a combination of the two. Any striae, intertriginous rashes or infections, prior surgical or traumatic scars should be noted. The quality of the patient's skin and the associated elasticity should be assessed. The examiner should note the locations of any rolls. Specific to the abdomen, it should be determined if there is a significant component of intra-abdominal fat, and a thorough examination should be performed to determine if there are any hernias present and if there is a rectus diastasis (**Table 1**).

SURGICAL PLANNING

Even with appropriate operative candidate selection, management of patient expectations is crucial in body contouring surgery. These patients often have multiple areas to be addressed and the rationale for staging must be explained. Results can be simulated for the patient to appreciate by

Table 1
Weight Loss Patient Classification

	Moderate Medication-Assisted (MMA) Weight Loss	Massive Weight Loss (MWL)
Extent of Weight Loss	No more than 25% of total body weight	Weight loss of at least 100 lbs
Nutritional Deficits	None appreciable at the time of writing	With malabsorptive surgery: iron, calcium, vitamin B12, thiamine, and protein deficiencies are all possible
Tissue Quality	Moderate tissue elasticity and skin excess	Poor elasticity, significant skin excess
Preoperative Concerns	Delayed gastric emptying	For patients who have had gastric band surgery, surgeons may consider deflating the band to decrease the risk of aspiration
Excisional Surgery	• Very likely to combine multiple procedures to minimize the number of surgeries • Limited skin excisions	• Conservative combination procedures performed over multiple surgeries • Larger skin excisions to address significant skin excess
Debulking Liposuction	Often performed in the same stage as excisional surgery	When indicated, performed in a stage prior to excisional surgery
Energy Devices	May be used in the same stage as excisional surgery	Reserved for use in a stage following excisional surgery to address recurrent skin laxity

pinching or displacing skin in front of a mirror. The expected extent and locations of scars should be pointed out to the patient. Lastly, the limitations of the procedures must be made clear. Patients must understand that as with all forms of plastic surgery, body contouring involves a compromise —exchanging extensive scarring for better contour of the affected areas. Staging should be guided by the patient's goals when possible; their top priority should be addressed in the first stage when appropriate.

Patient safety

It is our practice to limit the duration of anesthesia for aesthetic surgery to 6 hours as it has been demonstrated that the duration of surgery is an independent risk factor for postoperative complications.[9] This is of particular importance when body contouring procedures are performed in outpatient ambulatory surgical centers. These procedures are increasingly being performed outside the hospital in ambulatory surgical centers where there is less support should an issue arise. In surgical centers, we ensure that patients are American Society of Anesthesiologists class 1 or 2, that the duration of anesthesia is less than 6 hours, and that liposuction volume is limited to 2 L when it is combined with other procedures. Certainly as more excisional procedures are combined, the risk for wound healing complications also increases proportionally.

Specific to the MMA weight loss population, the delayed gastric emptying caused by these medications may put patients at increased risk for intraoperative pulmonary aspiration.[10] It is our practice to stop these medications for two weeks preoperatively, though we look to our anesthesia colleagues for formal guidelines on this emerging issue —it is conceivable that stopping these medications may not be necessary in patients who have been on them for some time as the delayed gastric emptying has been shown to improve with time.[4] Further consideration should also be given to the length of time these patients are asked to avoid oral intake prior to surgery.

For all body contouring procedures, we recommend the involvement of an assistant surgeon when possible to limit operative time and fatigue. With combined procedures, this may allow for a 2-team approach. An engaged and experienced surgical team is critical; we routinely review the operative plan with the entire surgical team to ensure patient positioning, draping, placement of monitors and safety devices, and surgical sequence are well understood and efficiently executed.[11]

STAGING

There are several common options for combinations of body contouring procedures in massive weight loss patients and the ideal combination is surgeon-dependent. We review several common combinations for massive weight loss patients later in discussion.

Abdominoplasty/breast procedure

Combining breast and abdominal surgery is very common. A traditional abdominoplasty technique is performed and any hernias are repaired. In addition to this, a breast procedure appropriate to the situation is performed—mastopexy, augmentation, reduction, or gynecomastia excision are all possible. Should the patient have the characteristic massive weight loss breast deformity and require a dermal suspension mastopexy utilizing the lateral rolls, we would recommend addressing this in a separate surgery as this is technically challenging and time-consuming. Combination with an abdominal procedure may be considered if the surgeon is experienced with the correction of this deformity and the patient prefers this to be done in a single stage.

The advantages of this combination are that all procedures are performed in the supine position and thereby eliminate any time lost on turning the patient. It should be noted however that structures that surgeons may consider to be "fixed" in non-weight loss patients, such as the inframammary fold, may be loose and easily displaced in massive weight loss patients with poor tissue quality. This is important as the downward pull on the midsection may displace the IMF inferiorly. Also note, if a fleur-de-lis abdominoplasty is planned, it is necessary to account for the inward pull on the IMF.

Abdominoplasty/lower body lift ± brachioplasty

This combination of procedures allows the surgeon to contour the midsection in a circumferential fashion, as well as adding on a less time-consuming procedure such as the arms. Specific to the trunk, this combination addresses laxity of the abdomen, mons, lateral thighs, and buttocks. Furthermore, combining abdominoplasty with a lower body lift eliminates standing cone deformities and allows for greater excision of the lateral abdominal tissues.

Patients are initially positioned prone for this combination of procedures and repositioning increases operative time. Adjunct procedures such as gluteal autoaugmentation further increases operative time and should be considered carefully—we would recommend performing the brachioplasty in a separate stage in this case. Another consideration with this combination is the potential for a more challenging recovery. When rectus plication is performed, patients may have difficulty repositioning themselves and will rely on their arms for this; this should be discussed with patients preoperatively and reinforces the importance of social support in this patient population.

Breast procedure/upper body lift ± brachioplasty

Similar to the above, this combination allows for a circumferential procedure which eliminates standing cone deformities and improves aesthetic results by allowing excess skin excision. Again, this combination will need to be started prone and involves repositioning and an associated increase in operative time. If performing an autoaugmentation of the breast using a lateral chest roll, this should be planned and marked clearly in advance. If the upper body lift is planned for a subsequent stage, care should be taken to avoid violating this tissue otherwise the option of autoaugmentation may be compromised.

Medial thigh lift

This procedure is aimed at addressing laxity over the medial thighs and may be combined with any upper body procedure. For optimal aesthetic outcome and to minimize the risk of wound healing complications, it should never be combined with an abdominal contouring procedure. This is because the medial thigh lift exerts tension opposite to abdominal procedures which pull in an upward and lateral direction. Ideally contouring of the thighs is performed in a stage following the contouring of the abdomen. Positioning for this procedure is somewhat surgeon-dependent and may be done in the frog leg position, though some surgeons will choose to close the posterior extent of the excision in the prone position.

Debulking liposuction

In patients who have skin laxity combined with a significant amount of lipodystrophy, we recommend considering debulking liposuction in a stage prior to excisional surgery in the area. This allows for a better final contour of the area and gives time for any skin contracture to occur. This is of particular benefit in the arms and medial thighs. If performing liposuction in the same stage as excisional surgery, the volume should be more conservative to decrease the risk of swelling and likely return of some laxity postoperatively.

Facial aesthetic procedures

Weight gain can stretch the skin and soft tissue of the face. When large amounts of fat are lost, patients are left with sagging atrophic appearing faces with jowls and significant submental laxity—features that mimic the changes more commonly associated with advanced facial aging. There has been increasing awareness of this issue in the MMA population with much discussion in the media about "Ozempic Face," though this is in fact simply a feature of significant weight loss. These facial changes are best addressed with face and necklift surgery. Patients often have a greater skin excess than non-weight loss patients and thus wide skin undermining is necessary to better address the discrepancy between redundant skin and SMAS. In addition to skin laxity, many patients will have significant platysma bands which may be addressed through a submental incision and medial platysmaplasty. Facial fat grafting is often a beneficial adjunct to address the significant volume loss experienced by these patients. Typically, more volume is required in weight loss patients than typical facial rejuvenation patients.[12] With a two team approach, one may consider combining facial aesthetic surgery with body contouring or breast procedures in MMA patients.

STAGING FOR MODERATE MEDICATION-ASSISTED WEIGHT LOSS PATIENTS

Staging for MMA patients differs from massive weight loss patients. We are more inclined to perform more procedures in one stage, to utilize more limited excisions, and to potentially utilize energy devices such as ultrasound-assisted liposuction or radiofrequency energy-assisted skin tightening devices as adjuncts at the time of excisional surgery. In contrast, in massive weight loss patients with poor tissue quality, we do not combine any form of energy device with excisional surgery. Due to their tissue quality, massive weight loss patients are at risk for developing recurrent laxity despite excisional surgery. Energy devices are used as adjuncts to address this recurrent laxity after 6-12 months has passed from excisional surgery in the affected area.

SUMMARY

The present article describes an approach to the evaluation and surgical planning for weight loss patients. MWL patients require strict preoperative optimization directed towards addressing comorbidities, careful thought toward the staging of their multiple procedures, and efficient implementation in the operating room. While much of the discussion in this area is focused on MWL patients, we have identified an emerging group of weight loss patients in the MMA population. These patients often require multiple body contouring procedures which may generally be completed in fewer stages than MWL patients. Thought should be given to the perioperative management of incretin mimetic medications in this population and associated delayed gastric emptying. Lastly, we discuss the current interest in "Ozempic Face" and incorporation of facial rejuvenation in the surgical plan for both MWL and MMA patients.

CLINICS CARE POINTS

- When evaluating weight loss patients for body contouring procedures, surgeons must consider the mechanism and sequelae of weight loss, the patient's BMI, weight change, and weight stability, as well as their smoking status and degree of social support.
- With respect to the evaluation of MMA patients, surgeons are encouraged to consider the potential for delayed gastric emptying and to involve their anesthesia colleagues in the perioperative management of these medications.
- We recommend planning combination procedures such that anesthesia time is limited to 6 hours
- Staging should be guided by the patient's goals when possible -their top priority should be addressed in the first stage when appropriate.
- When planning combination procedures for MMA patients, surgeons may consider treating more areas as these excisions tend to be smaller and this population tends to have better tissue quality.

DISCLOSURE

None of the authors have disclosures related to this article.

REFERENCES

1. Bossert RP, Rubin JP. Evaluation of the weight loss patient presenting for plastic surgery consultation. Plast Reconstr Surg 2012;130:1361–9.
2. Ozempic® (semaglutide) injection 0.5 mg or 1 mg Mechanism of Action. novoMEDLINK. Available at: https://www.novomedlink.com/diabetes/products/

treatments/ozempic/about/mechanism-of-action. html. Accessed May 20, 2023.
3. Wilding JPH, Batterham RL, Calanna S, et al. Once-weekly semaglutide in adults with overweight or obesity. N Engl J Med 2021;384(11):989–1002.
4. Hulst AH, Polderman JAW, Siegelaar SE, et al. Preoperative considerations of new long-acting glucagon-like peptide-1 receptor agonists in diabetes mellitus. Br J Anaesth 2021;126(3):567–71.
5. Nauck MA, Kemmeries G, Holst JJ, et al. Rapid tachyphylaxis of the glucagon-like peptide 1–induced deceleration of gastric emptying in humans. Diabetes 2011;60(5):1561–5.
6. Almutairi K, Gusenoff JA, Rubin JP. Body contouring. Plast Reconstr Surg 2016;137:586e–602e.
7. Arthurs ZM, Cuadrado D, Sohn V, et al. Post-bariatric panniculectomy body mass index impacts the complication profile. Am J Surg 2007;193:567–70.
8. Rios LM, Khosla RK. Body contouring in the massive-weight-loss patient. In: Janis JE, editor. Essentials of plastic surgery. Boca Raton, FL: Thieme; 2017. p. 1285–99.
9. Hardy KL, Davis KE, Constantine RS, et al. The impact of operative time on complications after plastic surgery: a multivariate regression analysis of 1753 cases. Aesthetic Surg J 2014;34(4):614–22.
10. Klein SR, Hobai IA. Semaglutide, delayed gastric emptying, and intraoperative pulmonary aspiration: a case report. Can J Anesth/J Can Anesth 2023;. https://pubmed.ncbi.nlm.nih.gov/36977934/.
11. Czerniak S, Gusenoff JA, Rubin JP. Discussion: safety of outpatient circumferential body lift evidence from 42 consecutive cases. Plast Reconstr Surg 2017;139:1363–4.
12. Narasimhan K, Ramanadham S, Rohrich RJ. Face lifting in the massive weight loss patient: modifications of our technique for this population. Plast Reconstr Surg 2015;135(2):397–405.

Ultrasound-Assisted Lipoplasty

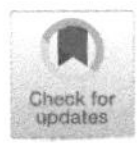

Luccie M. Wo, MD, MSE, Onelio Garcia Jr, MD*

KEYWORDS

• Liposuction • Ultrasound-assisted liposuction • UAL • VASER liposuction • VAL • Body contouring • Fat grafting • Gluteal fat grafting • Lipoplasty

KEY POINTS

- UAL is associated with less blood loss than traditional liposuction.
- UAL has a steeper learning curve than traditional liposuction.
- UAL is associated with less surgeon fatigue than traditional liposuction.

Over the past 40 years, liposuction has evolved into a highly sophisticated method of body contouring. The addition of ultrasound technology to traditional liposuction (SAL), has increased the efficacy of the procedure and expanded the indications for lipo-contouring in multiple anatomic regions. As UAL devices continue to evolve and improve, tissue fragmentation is maximized while energy delivery to the tissues is minimized. What was once considered large volume SAL, is now accepted as moderate volume for UAL since it is associated with less blood loss and decreased surgeon fatigue. Third-generation UAL, vibration amplification of sound energy at resonance (VASER) is currently considered the gold standard for contouring areas of fibrous fatty tissue, high-definition body sculpting, high volume cases, as a contouring adjunct to open procedures and for repeat or secondary liposuction. The volume of cases performed and its status as the most common aesthetic surgical procedure are a testament to the high patient satisfaction rate associated with liposuction.

INTRODUCTION

In 2021, liposuction was the most frequently performed cosmetic procedure in the United States of America with almost one-half million liposuction procedures reported.[1] Currently, ultrasound is employed in approximately 20% of the liposuction cases and this has remained consistent for the past decade.[2] At the present time, the great majority of ultrasound-assisted liposuction cases are performed using VASER-Lipo, which is considered the third-generation ultrasound device for body contouring procedures.

Historical perspectives

Ultrasonic instrumentation has been in use in dentistry and surgery since the 1950s.[3] Ultrasound energy was first employed in body contouring surgery in the late 1980s by Scuderi,[4] followed by Zocchi[5,6] who popularized the technique and introduced it to the United States in 1993.[7,8] A UAL task force was created 2 years later, composed of representatives from the American Society for Aesthetic Plastic Surgery, American Society of Plastic Surgeons, Lipoplasty Society of North America, Aesthetic Surgery Education and Research Foundation and Plastic Surgery Educational Foundation who collaborated with the Food and Drug Administration. The purpose of the task force consisted of evaluating the safety and efficacy of UAL in body contouring (**Box 1**), establishing appropriate indications, and designing the educational protocols necessary to train plastic

Division of Plastic Surgery, University of Miami, Miller School of Medicine, 7190 SW 87th Avenue, Suite 407, Miami, FL 33173, USA
* Corresponding author.
E-mail address: ogarciamd@aol.com

Clin Plastic Surg 51 (2024) 13–28
https://doi.org/10.1016/j.cps.2023.07.005

Box 1
Findings from Plastic Surgery UAL Task Force

- With proper training UAL is safe
- UAL should be performed in a wet environment (use wetting solutions).
- Use of incision site skin protectors is recommended to prevent thermal or friction burns.
- Compared to traditional suction-assisted liposuction (SAL), UAL cannula passage should be slower and more deliberate.
- Employing wetting solutions containing epinephrine decreases blood loss.
- The ultrasound probes should be in constant motion when in use, to avoid potential thermal injury to the tissues.
- UAL produces superior results in areas of fibrotic fat (ie, gynecomastia, back rolls) compared to SAL techniques.
- Surgeons can safely remove larger amounts of fat with less bleeding when employing UAL as opposed to SAL.
- UAL is typically associated with reduced surgeon fatigue as compared to SAL.
- UAL techniques have a steeper learning curve than SAL.
- UAL is a complement not a substitute for SAL

surgeons in the United States.[9] By 1997, the UAL Task Force offered comprehensive teaching courses that included didactic and practical, hands-on- training. During the first 2 years that the courses were offered, over 2000 plastic surgeons were trained in UAL, however, studies by Zukowswki and Ash suggested that surgeons would require a minimum of 30 cases to master the techniques.[10]

The SMEI Company in Italy, manufactured the original first-generation UAL device, which was relatively slow, taking 10 to 12 minutes to obtain a 250 to 300 mL of fat reduction.[11] The second-generation UAL devices were manufactured in the United States and were introduced in the mid-1990s. The two devices in this category consisted of the Mentor Contour Genesis (Mentor Corp., Santa Barbara, CA) which operated at a frequency of 27 kHz and the Lysonix 2000 (Lysonix Inc., Carpinteria, CA) with an operating frequency of 22.5 kHz. In 1999, Chang and Commons[12] published their experience comparing these two UAL devices in over 200 patients over a 2-year period and found both systems to be effective.

The VASER-Lipo system (Solta Medical, Inc., Bothell, WA), named for Vibration Amplification of Sound Energy at Resonance, was introduced in 2001 as a third-generation UAL device (**Fig. 1**). The system is highly efficient, operates at a frequency of 36 kHz and is capable of emulsifying fat rapidly while delivering lower amounts of energy to the tissues.[13] The VASER device employs a smaller diameter solid probe design, with grooves proximal to the tip (**Fig. 2**). VENTX suction cannulae (Solta Medical, Inc., Bothell, WA) are an integral component of the system (**Fig. 3**). The third generation VASER system is the UAL technology most frequently used at the present time. In 2002, Jewell et al.[14] published a multicentric, pilot clinical study using VASER Assisted Lipoplasty (VAL) and reported satisfactory results without complications in 77 patients. The senior author reported significantly lower quantities of blood in VAL aspirate in comparison to SAL aspirate in 57

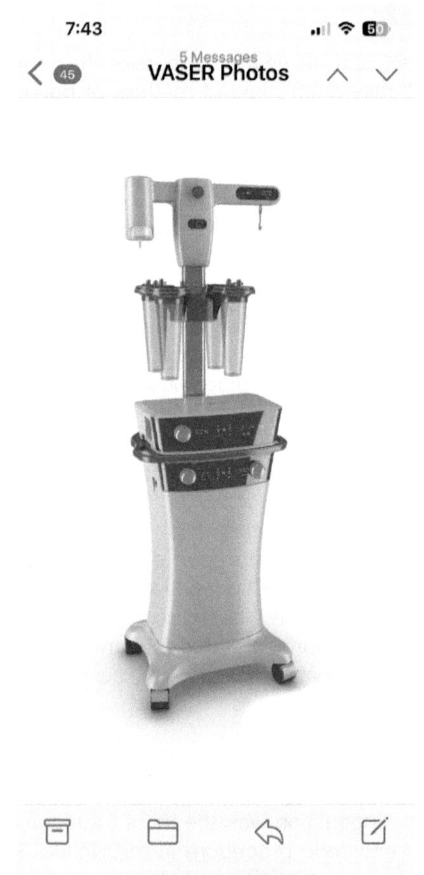

Fig. 1. VASER 2.0 Tower comprised of ultrasound generator, fluid infiltration pump and aspiration pump with aspirate reservoirs. (VASER 2.0. Courtesy of Solta Medical, Inc., Bothell, WA. VASER® is a trademark of Solta Medical Ireland Limited or its affiliates. The images and trademark do not imply endorsement or affiliation with the owner of the intellectual property rights.)

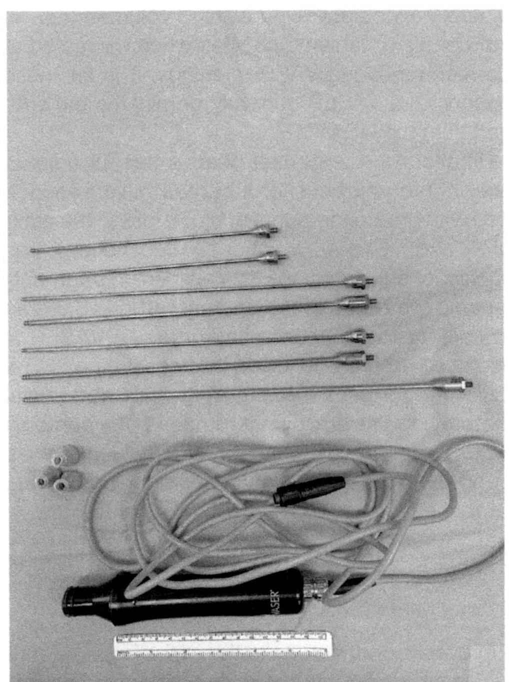

Fig. 2. VASER Ultrasonic Handpiece and an assortment of ultrasound probes. The greater the number of rings on the probe, the more circumferential dispersion of the ultrasound energy around the tip.

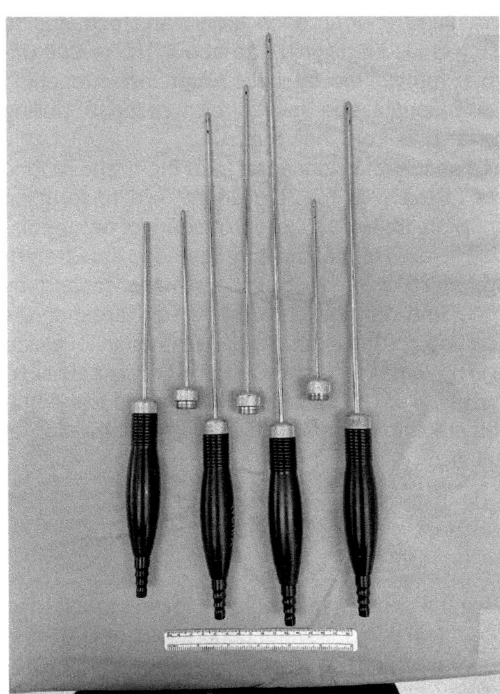

Fig. 3. VENTX cannulas with vented handles. These cannulas are designed to function more efficiently, even when aspirating viscous fat, by providing a small air bleed into the vacuum line at the handle, thus preventing "vacuum lock."

patients undergoing contouring of the posterior trunk.[15] A decrease in complications with third generation VAL when compared to early UAL technology was reported by de Souza Pinto.[16]

Mechanisms of action of UAL

Ultrasound is produced when matter vibrates at a frequency higher than 20 kHz. In medicine, low intensity (0.01-1 W/cm^2) and higher frequency ultrasound are used for diagnostic imaging and high intensity (>10 W/cm^2) and low frequency (20–100 kHz) ultrasounds are used for surgical application.[17] UAL employs frequencies of 20 to 36 kHz and can generate power of 90 W/cm^2.[18] The intricate physics of ultrasound is beyond the scope of this article which will focus on the interaction of UAL devices with adipose tissue.

Ultrasound technology can produce a wide range of clinical effects depending upon the choice of frequency, amplitude, mode of vibration, and/or probe design. The various mechanisms of action can be combined or adjusted to meet specific clinical requirements. The VASER is a third-generation UAL device that combines cavitation and acoustic streaming to create a safe and effective means of extracting adipocytes, with minimal effect on the surrounding tissue matrix.

Twenty-five years ago, earlier generations of UAL devices delivered large amounts of ultrasound energy to the tissues. Low-density media such as fat, easily undergo cavitation. The ultrasound energy caused adipocyte destruction by implosion. Currently, the third-generation devices such as the VASER, deliver approximately 50% of the ultrasound energy to the tissues than previous devices and create cavitation in the gas bubbles contained within the wetting solution that is interspersed within the fatty matrix. Cavitation involves the creation and action of air or gas bubbles in a liquid. In this case, the tumescent fluid which is introduced into the patient contains millions of microscopic bubbles. These bubbles occur naturally because the fluid is at equilibrium pressure with the air inside the IV bag Under the cyclic compression and rarefaction (squeezing and pulling) of the ultrasound field, the very small bubbles grow until they reach "resonant" size, at which point they collapse and the process repeats. The resonant size at which these air bubbles collapse is approximately 180 microns.

These millions of microscopic air bubbles are called cavitation nuclei and they are small enough to become interspersed among the fat cells. As mentioned before, when bubbles are exposed to ultrasound energy, each grows and expands to many times its original size about 180 to 200 microns forcing the fat cells apart. After reaching their resonant size, the bubbles collapse, pulling the fat cells from their matrix.[19]

Once the fat is loosened from the tissue matrix, it is mixed with the tumescent fluid to form an emulsion, that is, a thorough mixture of two immiscible fluids. This is done through Acoustic Streaming, which are powerful fluid forces caused by ultrasound energy. In the region around the vibrating tip, these forces cause intense localized swirling to further break up the fat into small clusters of cells. The cells contained within this emulsion are viable adipocytes and are suitable for fat grafting.[20–22]

Current technology in ultrasound-assisted liposuction

Since the conceptualization of ultrasound-assisted liposuction (UAL), several generations of UAL systems have been commercialized. The early UAL devices were poorly designed and associated with high complication rates, particularly seromas and thermal burns. Second-generation devices employed a 5 mm hollow cannula that delivered high amounts of ultrasound energy to the tissues however it was somewhat inefficient aspirating through a 2 mm internal lumen.[23] The great majority of the complications associated with this generation of devices were related to the thermal effects of high doses of ultrasound energy on the adipose layer and surrounding tissues.[24] In 2001 a third-generation device was introduced. The VASER system (Vibration, Amplification of Sound Energy at Resonance) is extremely efficient at fragmenting and aspirating adipose tissue while significantly reducing the amount of ultrasound energy delivered (less than 50% of what previous devices delivered) and this subsequently translates to a minimal thermal load on the tissues.[25] The system employs a solid probe and can deliver ultrasound energy in "pulsed" (VASER) mode. The VASER system, which operates at a frequency of 36 kHz, also uses a smaller diameter probe that allows for rapid fat fragmentation, while lowering the amount of energy delivered to the tissue. The probe diameters range from 2.9 to 3.7 mm and contain small grooves near the tip that enables transfer of the ultrasound vibrations from the tip to a region just proximal and circumferentially surrounding the tip. There are significant advantages to using this technology, including less blood loss,[26] less post-operative bruising, better skin retraction, decreased post-operative discomfort, and a low complication rate in experienced hands. The typical aspirate is generally bloodless even at high volumes (**Fig. 4**) and contains viable adipocytes when harvested at the recommended VASER settings. It is for these reasons that VASER currently dominates the UAL market in the USA.

Ultrasound energy has been a helpful adjunct when contouring tight fibrous areas that are associated with greater amounts of blood loss in the aspirate and where traditional liposuction has significant shortcomings. It is efficient in fragmenting adipose tissue in the posterior trunk,[27] and as an adjunct to gynecomastia surgery.[28] VASER is also used for high-definition body sculpting.[29] The senior author uses it to highlight male abdominal anatomy and as an adjunct to open body contouring procedures on the extremities.[30] Hurwitz has reported on the use of UAL during body contouring surgeries on massive weight loss patients.[31,32]

SURGICAL TECHNIQUES

Patient selection in UAL

Appropriate patient selection is of paramount importance in any type of body contouring procedure involving liposuction. A thorough medical history and physical exam should be performed. The physical exam should include a thorough assessment of skin quality and elasticity. The patient's history should place special emphasis on dietary habits, weight loss history, presence of autoimmune diseases, or history of hypercoagulability.

The ideal candidate for consistent, reproducible results, are healthy patients with good skin tone, who are close to their ideal body weight (within 20% of their ideal body weight as determined by insurance company statistics) and have limited,

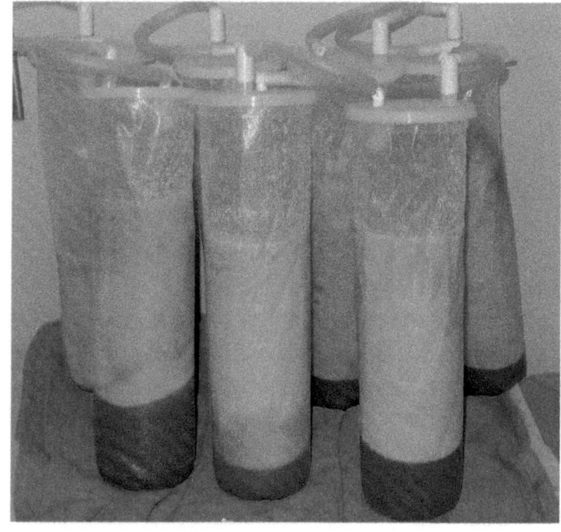

Fig. 4. VASER aspirate even following high volume extractions is relatively bloodless. Hematocrits on VASER aspirate measure approximately 1%.

well-defined areas of lipodystrophy.[33,34] The senior author has routinely performed high-volume UAL on patients with higher BMIs, however, expectations should be appropriately managed in this population.

The surgeon is responsible for determining whether the patient's expectations for the surgical outcome are realistic and attainable. Another cause for concern involves body dysmorphic disorder which has been under-recognized for years. Currently, it is estimated that 7% to 15% of aesthetic surgery patients are affected by this disorder.[35] These patients are obsessive about their appearance and tend to be difficult to satisfy, even with what would generally be considered an acceptable aesthetic result.

While reviewing before and after photographs of similar procedures is helpful for these patients, it is imperative that they realize that body frames and fat distribution varies greatly from patient to patient and has a significant effect on the outcome of the surgery.

Standardized medical photography is also essential for surgical planning. The photography should include anterior, anterior oblique, lateral, posterior, and posterior oblique views. For facial UAL, one should include anterior, oblique, and lateral views. Extremities should also be photographed separately.[36]

Wetting solutions

The French surgeons Illouz and Fournier are credited with being the first to employ a wetting solution infiltrate during liposuction.[37] During the late seventies, they injected saline in minimal amounts (less than 300 mL) per liposuction case and reported a favorable effect on decreasing the bleeding associated with the procedure. Jeffrey Klein, a dermatologist from California, began performing liposuction procedures using a tumescent local anesthesia formula in 1985. Initially, Klein used 35 mg/kg of bodyweight as the maximum dose for lidocaine.[38] Since then, several authors have published formulas that employ higher total doses of lidocaine which exceed 50 mg/kg of bodyweight.[39] Even lidocaine that is administered within the accepted maximum limits may result in toxicity.[40] Commonly encountered factors such as cigarette smoking, oral contraceptives, obesity, impaired renal function, impaired hepatic function, or cardiac disease can affect the protein binding of lidocaine. Certain medications such as tricyclic antidepressants, anorexiants, beta-blockers, and histamine-2-blockers also affect the protein binding of lidocaine. Taking cytochrome p450 inhibitors may result in lidocaine toxicity even when the total dose of lidocaine administered is within the accepted safe range.[41] The total amount of injected lidocaine sometimes is a poor predictor of the potential for toxicity since the absorption rates can vary significantly. A significantly better correlation with the potential for toxicity is the peak plasma lidocaine level. The danger for higher-volume, tumescent liposuction outpatient procedures is that lidocaine absorption can peak 10 to 12 hours after infiltration, hours after these patients are typically discharged from the surgical facility.[42,43] Since most of the senior author's liposuction surgeries are circumferential and moderate to high volume, the preference is for general anesthesia. It not only improves patient comfort significantly but also provides a safe airway in the prone and lateral decubitus positions.

The author's preference for wetting solution in these cases is 1 mg of epinephrine 1:1000, a vial of Tranexamic Acid (TXA),[44] (1 gm/10 mL), in a liter of Ringer's lactate at room temperature (21° Fahrenheit). I do not use lidocaine for general anesthesia cases since its effect on postoperative pain is clinically irrelevant.[45] In the occasional small surface area case, where general anesthesia is not utilized, 30 mL of 1% lidocaine is added to each liter of my standard wetting solution. Even though some proponents of local tumescent anesthesia for liposuction will disagree, I strongly believe that the total dose of lidocaine when used in wetting solution should not exceed 35 mg/kg of bodyweight. Peak plasma levels of lidocaine in the 3ug/ml are considered in the toxic range. Since most major circumferential liposuctions require general anesthesia, they do not need lidocaine as part of the wetting solution formula. Smaller liposuction procedures without general anesthesia do not require such high volumes of wetting solution, so there really is no good reason to push the limits of lidocaine toxicity in patients undergoing elective, aesthetic surgery.[46]

Epinephrine is an important component of wetting solutions for liposuction. The vasoconstrictive effects of this drug have significantly decreased blood loss in the aspirate during liposuction cases. Common effects of toxicity include an increase in blood pressure, tachycardia, and arrhythmias. A total dose of 10 mg has been proposed by some authors.[47] The University of Texas Southwestern has reported administering up to 12 mg in some cases without associated complications. I have personally administered up to 14 mg in intermittent fashion, throughout the course of a high-volume extraction case, without signs or symptoms associated with exceeding the toxic dose. It goes without saying that these patients require proper monitoring of their vital signs during the surgery. It is important to note the importance of infiltrating the wetting solution at room temperature. Warm wetting solutions are associated with initial vasodilation with early rapid absorption of the lidocaine component.

If there are concerns about hypothermia, the intravenous fluids can be warmed in conjunction with warmed forced air via a Bair Hugger. The common wetting solution formulas are depicted in (**Table 1**).

Body contouring with VASER-Liposuction employs higher volumes of wetting solution than SAL. This results in higher unquantifiable losses from the infiltration fluid back-leaking through the access incisions due to increased hydrostatic pressure.[48] The loss of infiltration fluid from back-leak can be as high as a third of the volume infiltrated. Approximately another third of the infiltration solution is aspirated during liposuction. Thus, only a third of the initial wetting solution volume stays in the subcutaneous tissues at the conclusion of liposuction and is eventually absorbed and processed through normal physiologic channels.

Anesthesia

Specific positioning and surgical techniques depend on the anatomic areas being treated. It is generally accepted that circumferential body contouring leads to more harmonious aesthetic result than segmental, "spot" liposuction, however those cases are typically associated with higher volume aspirate. The author's experience is that UAL is best performed under general anesthesia since most of our cases involve moderate to high-volume aspirates. While "awake" liposuction procedures have been described and are considered safe,[49–51] they are generally limited to small areas of mild lipodystrophy and yield relatively small volumes of aspirate.

Maintaining homeostasis during moderate-to-high volume liposuction can be challenging. Mild hypothermia is common due to the large quantities of infiltration within the subcutaneous space, the large body surface area exposed and the effects of prolonged general anesthesia. Strategies to mitigate hypothermia include external warming using forced warm air (ie, Bair Hugger) to non-operative areas, infusing warmed IV fluids, and wrapping head/extremities not involved in the surgery (**Fig. 5**).

Table 1
Common wetting solution formulas

Fodor's		**University of Texas Southwestern**	
Ringer's lactate	1L	Ringer's lactate (21*C)	1L
Low volume (<2000 mL)			Low volume (<50,000)
Epinephrine 1:500	1 mL	lidocaine 1%	30 mL
Mod volume (2000–4000 mL)			High volume (>5000 mL)
Epinephrine 1:1000	1 mL	lidocaine 1%	15 mL
High volume (>4000)		epinephrine 1:1000	1 mL
Epinephrine 1:1500	1 mL		
Klein's		**Hunstad's**	
Normal saline	1L	Ringer's lactate (38–40*C)	1L
Lidocaine 1%	50 mL	Lidocaine 1%	50 mL
Epinephrine 1:1000	1 mL	Epinephrine 1:1000	1 mL
Sodium bicarbonate 8.4%	12.5 mL		
Hamburg		**Garcia (Author's Formula)**	
Normal saline	1L	*general anesthesia cases*	
Lidocaine 2%	10 mL	Ringer's lactate (room temp)	1L
Prilocaine 2%	10 mL	Epinephrine 1:1000	1 mL
Sodium bicarbonate 8.4%	6 mL	Tranexamic acid (TXA)	1gm
Epinephrine 1:1000	0.7 mL	*Local anesthesia cases*	
Triamcinolone 10 mg	1 mL	Add Lidocaine 1%	30 mL
		(total dose of lidocaine <35 mg/kg)	

Adapted from Garcia O, Chaustre-Pena PS, Pazmino P. Suction-assisted lipectomy and Brazilian butt lift. In: Thaller S, Panthaki Z, (eds) Tips and Tricks in Plastic Surgery. Springer Nature Publishers. Switzerland, AG. 2022; 151 to 189.

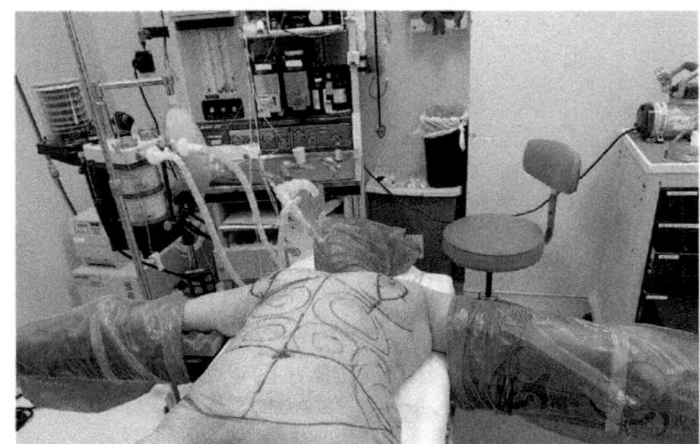

Fig. 5. Wrapping the head and extremities not involved in the surgery is an efficient method of maintaining body temperature.

Patients are usually given preoperative prophylactic antibiotics (such as a cephalosporin), and some even advocate for preoperative steroid dosing to help with edema and post-liposuction fibrosis.[52] Liposuction procedures, particularly high-volume extractions, present distinct challenges for the anesthesiologist. There is the potential for hypothermia, hypovolemia, fluid overload, and toxic effects from lidocaine and epinephrine. Position changes on the operating table can lead to postoperative sequelae of pressure-related injuries. Of particular concern is the fact that peak plasma lidocaine levels can take 10 to 12 hours after infiltration, so toxicity may not manifest itself until hours after the patient has been discharged from the outpatient surgery facility. For these reasons, an experienced anesthesiologist is preferred for the high-volume cases where large amounts of wetting solution are employed. Strict adherence to fluid replacement guidelines, close attention to patient positioning with proper padding of all pressure points, and not exceeding the total recommended doses for both lidocaine and epinephrine will help avoid serious complications.

Preoperative planning and marking

Preoperative markings should be performed on a standing patient, preferably employing waterproof markers of different colors. To avoid iatrogenic contour deformities, surgeons should avoid SAL or UAL in the five anatomic zones of the adhesions: {1} the gluteal crease, {2} the lower the popliteal crease, {4} the mid-medial thigh area and {5} the lateral gluteal depression.[53] These areas should be properly outlined during the preoperative marking.

Surgeons should note and discuss with the patient any pre-existing contour irregularities, hernias, previous treatment areas, and planned fat extraction areas. UAL requires a greater number of slightly longer incisions to better accommodate the skin protectors and avoid placing torque on the ultrasonic probe. Whenever possible, incisions should be hidden in natural creases or areas that are generally covered even when wearing a swimsuit.

Typical VASER settings and instrumentation

The original recommendations for VASER settings came from the original manufacturer of the device. The ultrasound time suggested was approximately 1 min./100 mL of wetting solution employed. Continuous mode was recommended for tight, fibrous, areas and gynecomastia. It was not unusual for surgeons to employ 1-ring probes for tight fibrous areas or a highly aggressive specialized gynecomastia probe for male breast surgery. As surgeons have become more experienced with the device it has become apparent that highly efficient fragmentation can be achieved while delivering much less ultrasound energy to the tissues. This has significantly increased the safety margin for VASER-assisted liposuction. The author makes the following recommendations (**Table 2**) based on over 20 years of experience with the VASER device and over 10,000 VASER procedures.

UAL for gynecomastia

Gynecomastia treatment is one the most common applications for UAL, and even considered by some as the best option for treatment.[54] The cavitation phenomenon with UAL selectively fragments the fatty matrix within the breast tissue. Although UAL is considered more effective than SAL at fragmenting fibrous fat within the breast tissue, a small open resection may still be required to remove the fibrous glandular tissue.[55]

In the senior author's technique, the patient is placed in the supine position and his standard wetting solution is infiltrated at a rapid 500 mL/min to obtain good dispersion. The chest is an area where increased interstitial fluid pressure is advantageous, thus infiltration volumes should be generous. Specialized gynecomastia probes are available however, the author finds the tip too aggressive and unnecessary to achieve adequate fragmentation in these cases. VASER settings for gynecomastia are displayed in (see **Table 2**). Aspiration can then be performed using 3,7 mm and 3 mm Ventx cannulas. In addition to tissue fragmentation, application of ultrasonic energy to the subdermal plane stimulates the dermis, allowing for skin retraction and improved aesthetic outcome for gynecomastia (**Fig. 6**). Patients with significant breast ptosis and large breast skin envelopes, may require mastopexy techniques with skin resection and even free nipple areolar grafts in severe cases.[56]

Table 2
Recommended VASER settings

Procedure	VASER settings	VASER Probe	Ultrasound time
Gynecomastia	80% pulsed	2-ring, 3.7 mm	1 min./100 mL, expected aspirate.
Face/Neck	60% pulsed	5-ring, 2.4 mm	20 s./50 mL, expected aspirate
Abdomen	70% pulsed	5-ring, 3.7 mm	45 s./100 mL, expected aspirate
Upper Back	80% pulsed	5-ring, 3.7 mm	1 min./100 mL, expected aspirate
Posterior Flanks	70% pulsed	5-ring, 3.7 mm	45 s./100 mL expected aspirate
Inner Thighs	60% pulsed	5-ring, 3.7 mm	30 s./100 mL expected aspirate
Outer Thighs	70% pulsed	5-ring, 3.7 mm	45 s./100 mL expected aspirate
Arms	60% pulsed	5-ring, 3.7 mm	30 s./100 mL expected aspirate
Fat Harvest/Graft	60%–70% pulsed	5-ring, 3.7 mm	45 s./100 mL expected aspirate

Delivering ultrasonic energy to a more superficial plane does require prior training experience, and there have been reports of full thickness skin loss when this is performed incorrectly.[57–59] Maximal skin retraction is achieved after 6 to 9 months, thus if redundant skin persists, revisions should not be offered for several months.[60]

UAL of the neck

Neck contouring with UAL is commonly performed since ultrasonic energy is a helpful adjunct for skin contraction.[61] Patient selection is of paramount importance in achieving successful aesthetic results with neck contouring.[62] An accurate assessment of skin elasticity is mandatory, particularly in older patients or those with significant amounts of submental fat. One should never trade fat for loose skin, particularly in a visible area such as the neck. Some patients with extensive submental fat may need to accept a secondary open procedure if prominent platysma bands are exposed following the neck fat extraction. Although complications are rare with this procedure, the informed consent for neck contouring with ultrasonic liposuction should include the possibility of postoperative contour deformities, asymmetry, prolonged edema, exposed platysma bands, thermal injury, pigmentation changes, neck skin paresthesia, and vascular injury.

Most of the fat extracted from the neck is from the submental area. Extensive defatting of the neck may expose underlying, prominent platysma bands and patients may need a secondary open procedure to address these.[63]

Three access incisions are usually needed to avoid torque on the ultrasonic probe: one behind each earlobe and one in the submental crease.

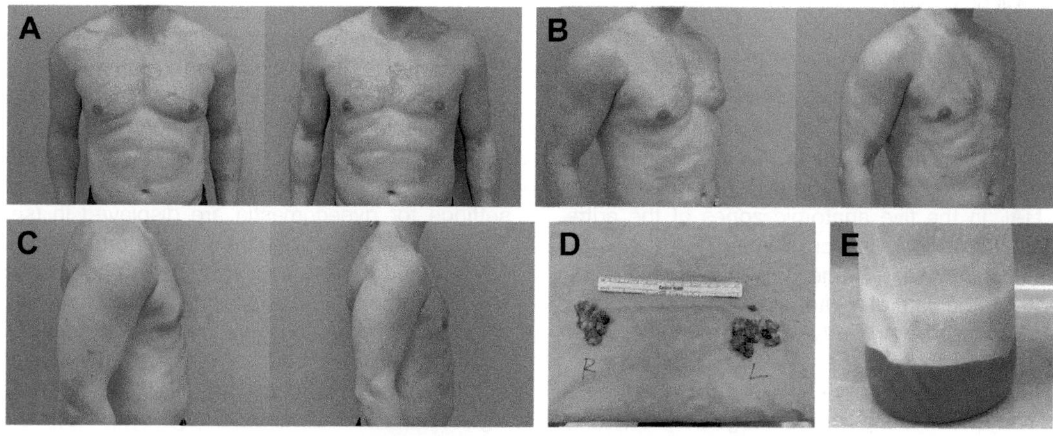

Fig. 6. (*A*) Anterior Views, before and after VASER-assisted resection of gynecomastia, 6 months postoperative. (*B*). Right, anterior oblique views. (*C*). Right, lateral views.(*D*). Gynecomastia glandular specimen. (*E*). Approximately 300 mL VASER supernatant fat aspirate from bilateral breasts.

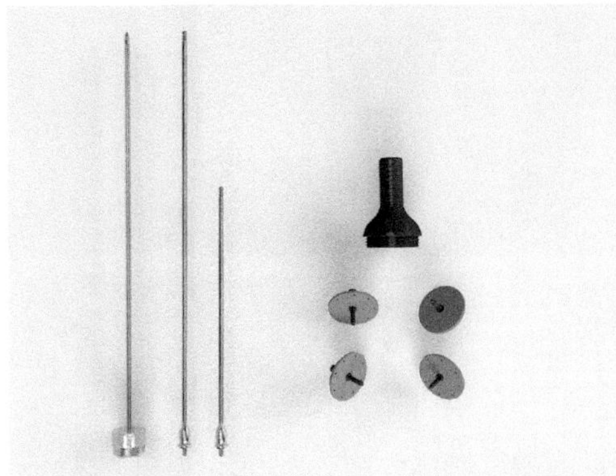

Fig. 7. Shorter and small diameter VASER probes and VENTX cannulas are employed in neck and facial contouring.

Wetting solution should be slowly infused at 150 to 200 mL/min. The probes and cannulas used should also be smaller in diameter and shorter in length (**Fig. 7**). VASER settings for face and neck contouring are displayed in (see **Table 2**). A 2.7 mm and 3 mm Ventx cannulas may be used for aspiration in the face and neck regions (**Fig. 8**).

UAL of the trunk (VASER 360)

The trunk is one of the most common areas for patients seeking body contouring. The term VASER 360 applies to circumferential contouring of the trunk which yields more harmonious aesthetic results than segmental liposuction.

The fat in the back is dense, fibrous, and particularly well suited for UAL. The back skin is also

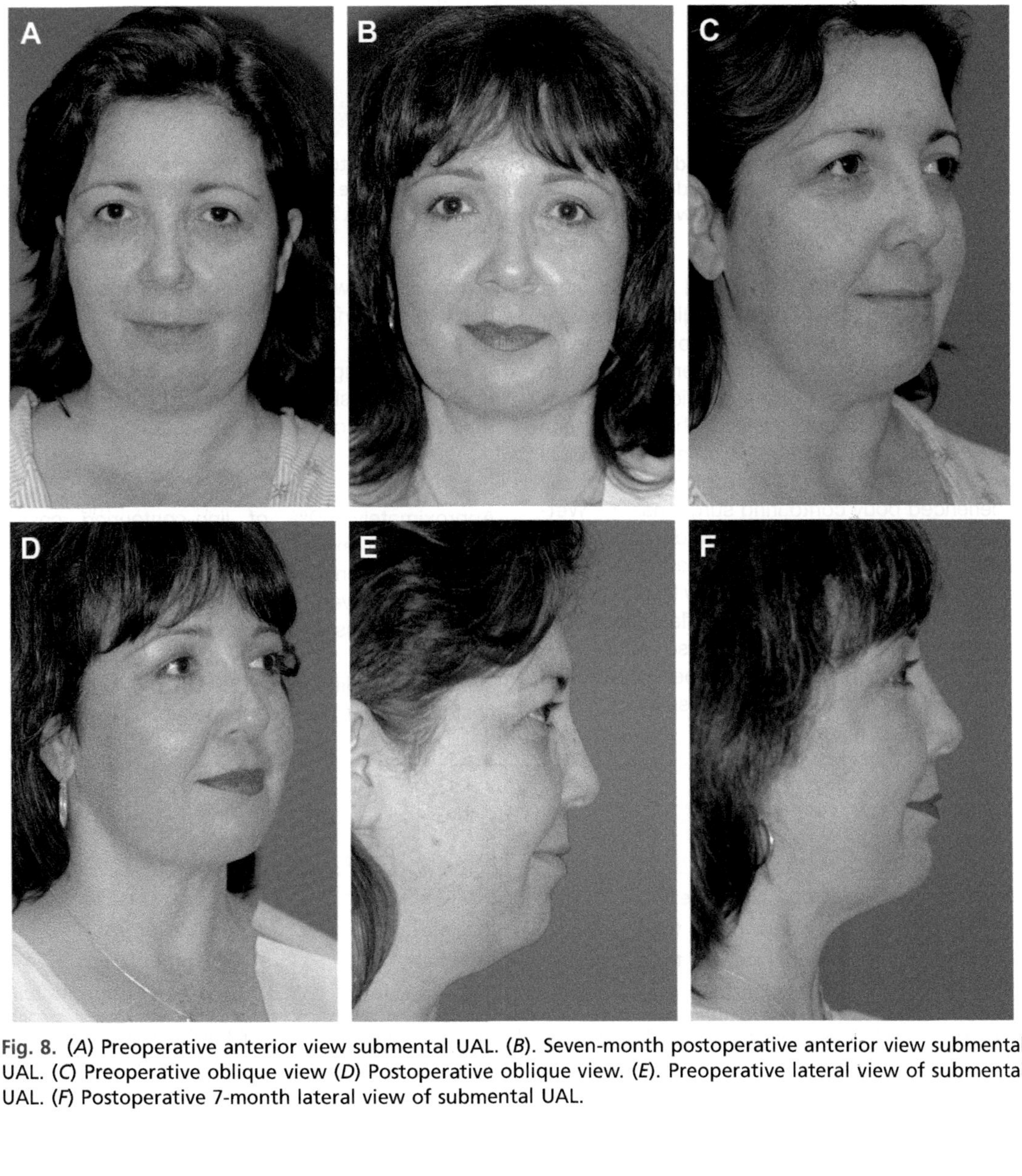

Fig. 8. (*A*) Preoperative anterior view submental UAL. (*B*). Seven-month postoperative anterior view submental UAL. (*C*) Preoperative oblique view (*D*) Postoperative oblique view. (*E*). Preoperative lateral view of submental UAL. (*F*) Postoperative 7-month lateral view of submental UAL.

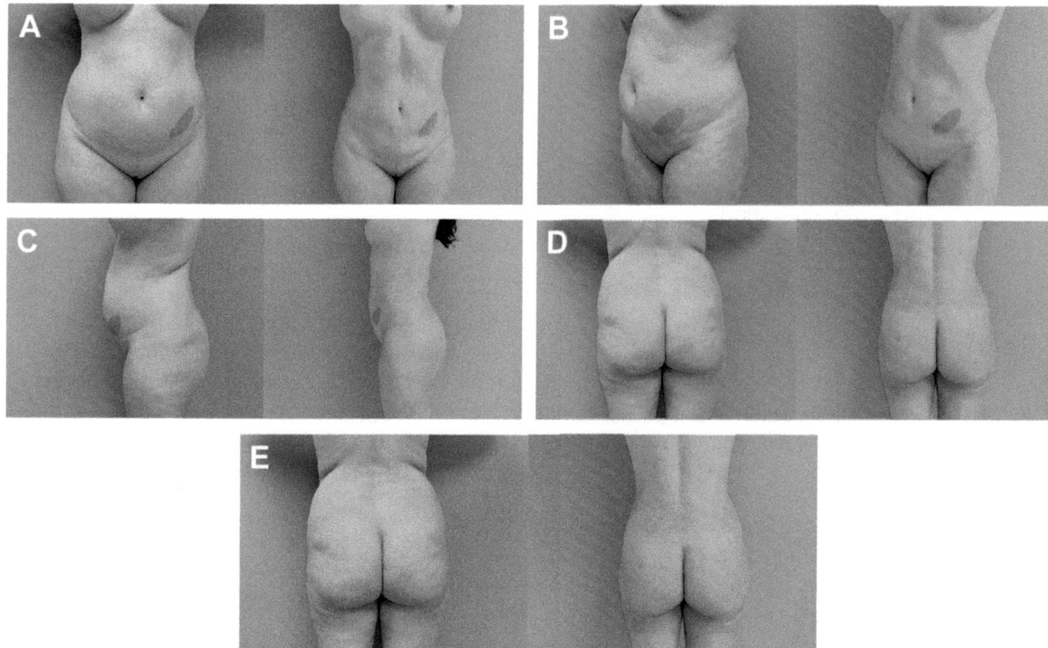

Fig. 9. (*A*) 360 VASER-Lipo, before and after abdomen view, 5 months postoperative. (*B*). Anterior oblique view (note the shadow effects in upper abdomen). (*C*). Lateral views. (*D*). Before and after 360 VASER-Lipo, back and posterior flanks. (*E*). Contouring the waistline and upper lateral thighs has a profound effect on buttock shape.

one of the thickest in body, and thus is more forgiving and capable of camouflaging minor contour irregularities from body contouring procedures. Although the back and posterior flanks can be accessed from the prone position, the author prefers a lateral decubitus approach. This position provides the best access for creating a radical waistline and is currently employed by many experienced body contouring surgeons.[64,65] Wetting solution can be infiltrated rapidly at approximately 500 mL/min. The senior author uses a 3.7 mm 3-ring probe at 80% energy level in pulsed (VASER) mode for the back and flank area. The abdomen wetting solution is also infused at 500 mL/min to achieve proper dispersion. VASER settings for trunk contouring are displayed in (see **Table 2**). Following the ultrasound phase, aspiration can be performed using 3.7 mm and 3.0 mm cannulas.

One advantage of VASER 360 is the improved postoperative skin retraction and enhanced contour of the buttocks (**Fig. 9**).

UAL of the extremities

Approximately 40% of lipo-contouring cases involved the extremities.[66] The extremities are three-dimensional, cylindrical structures that exhibit an uneven distribution of compartmentalized fatty deposits. It is generally agreed that the circumferential liposuction of the extremities, either with traditional SAL or UAL, yields a better aesthetic result than “spot liposuction.”

Table 3
Patient selection criteria for thigh contouring

Type	Skin Assessment	Fat Assessment	Recommendation
1	Good skin tone	Moderate	SAL, UAL, or VAL
2	Moderate skin tone	Moderate	UAL or VAL
3	Moderate skin tone	Minimal	Thighplasty
4	Poor skin tone	Mod. - Large	VAL + Thighplasty

Abbreviaitons: SAL, traditional liposuction; UAL, Ultrasound-Assisted Liposuction; VAL, VASER-Assisted Liposuction.
From Garcia O. Liposuction of the Upper and Lower Extremities. In Ali A, Nahas F, (eds) The Art of Body Contouring: A Comprehensive Approach. 1st Ed. Quality Medical Publishing, St. Louis, MO. 2017; 361 to 395.

Table 4
Patient selection criteria for arm contouring

Type	Skin Assessment	Fat Assessment	Recommendation
1	Good skin tone	Moderate	SAL, UAL, or VAL
2	Moderate skin tone	Moderate	UAL or VAL
3	Moderate skin tone	Minimal	Brachioplasty
4	Poor skin tone	Mod. - Large	UAL, or VAL Brachio

Abbreviaitons: SAL, traditional liposuction; UAL, Ultrasound-Assisted Liposuction; VAL, VASER-Assisted Liposuction.
From Garcia O. Liposuction of the Upper and Lower Extremities. In Ali A, Nahas F, (eds) The Art of Body Contouring: A Comprehensive Approach. 1st Ed. Quality Medical Publishing, St. Louis, MO. 2017; 361 to 395.

Rohrich, Beran, and Kenkle assessed the efficacy of UAL in comparison to SAL according to the anatomic site in their 1998 textbook "Ultrasound-Assisted Liposuction." Those authors rated the efficacy of UAL as good to excellent for the thighs and arms. The calves were rated as fair to good and the ankle area rated as fair to ineffective. Clinical decision-making algorithms for the upper and lower extremities are depicted in (**Tables 3** and **4**)

The surgeon should place special emphasis on access incision planning since scars on the extremities are more difficult to conceal. Wetting solution can be infiltrated rapidly at 500 mL/min. Because the superior medial thigh skin consists of very thin dermis, it is more susceptible to thermal injury from prolonged ultrasound exposure. VASER settings for the lower extremities are depicted in (see **Table 2**). Once fragmented, fat can be easily extracted with 3.7 mm and 3 mm cannulas.

Infusion of the arms should be performed at slower rate, approximately 300 mL/min to the level of tumescence. VASER setting for upper extremities are depicted in (see **Table 2**). The author follows the ultrasound phase with fat aspiration techniques using a 3 mm Ventx cannula. Liposuction of the upper extremities needs to be judicious since the arm skin is not forgiving and over extraction will invariably result in contour deformities and visible skin laxity. Patient selection is of paramount importance in these cases and patients with arm lipodystrophy and skin laxity should consider VASER-assisted brachioplasty to address the excess skin issues (**Fig. 10**).

Lipografting VASER aspirate

Earlier generations of UAL devices delivered high amounts of ultrasound energy to the tissues. The cavitation phenomenon caused implosion of the adipocytes[67] creating a large oil-lipid layer in the aspirate rendering it unsuitable for fat grafting. Fat harvested with VASER-assisted liposuction at the appropriate settings (see **Table 2**), is highly suitable for fat grafting (**Fig. 11**). The senior author has more than 20 years of experience grafting

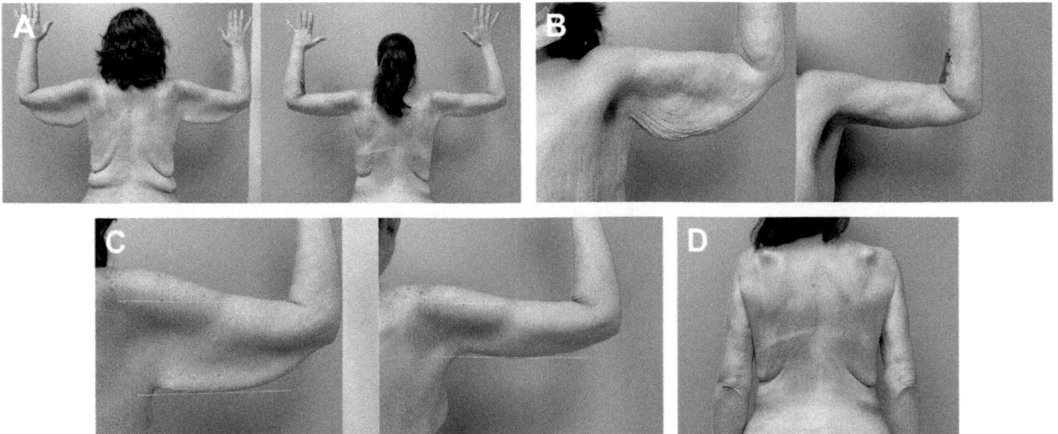

Fig. 10. (A) Before and after posterior view of VASER-assisted, posterior approach, brachioplasty in a massive weight loss patient (225 lbs.), at 9 months postoperative. (*B*). Before and after anterior view. (*C*). Before and after posterior view. The parallel lines provide a perspective of the significant reduction in upper arm surface area. (*D*). Posterior VASER-assisted brachioplasty scars at 9 months.

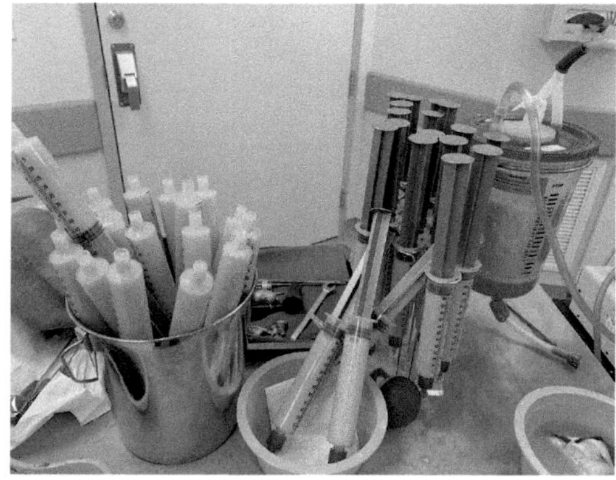

Fig. 11. High-volume VASER-assisted liposuction aspirate is relatively bloodless and highly suitable for lipografting.

VASER harvested fat to a variety of anatomic areas. An example of large volume lipografting in a Brazilian Butt Lift (BBL) patient is depicted in (**Fig. 12**A, B). Note that a significant portion of the aesthetic effect is related to the radical VASER contouring of the waistline and the slight VASER reduction of the upper lateral thighs (**Fig. 12**C, D). A good rule of thumb for BBL surgery is to remove more so you can graft less to achieve the desired aesthetic result. Continuous ultrasound-assisted visualization of the injection cannula is highly recommended and is soon expected to be the standard of care for this operation.[68,69]

Postoperative care

Postoperative care protocols can vary based on areas of treatment, the volume of fat removed and patient factors. Generally, patients are instructed to wear compression garments continuously for 3 to 6 weeks. Patients are then transitioned to intermittent compression garments for approximately 12 hours a day, for another 2 to 6 weeks. Lymphatic massages are helpful in diminishing edema and are started as soon as the patient can tolerate them. Patients are advised

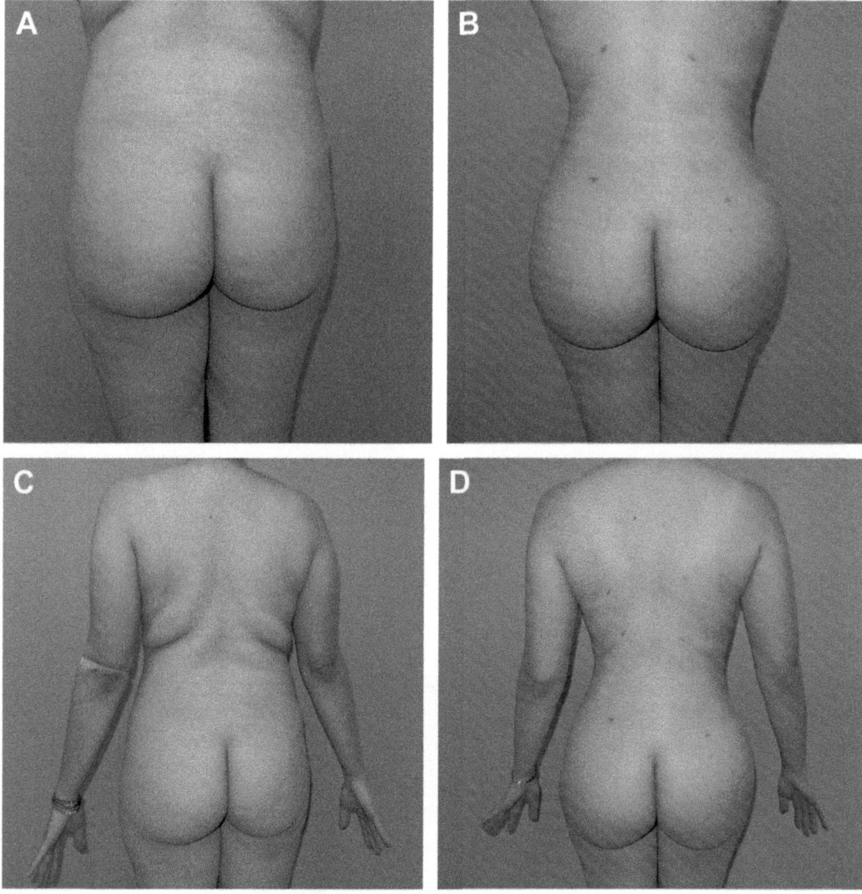

Fig. 12. (A) Preoperative view of buttock.(*B*). Postoperative BBL with VASER harvested lipo-grafting of 450 mL to each buttock, injected strictly into the subcutaneous plane.(*C,D*). Before and after BBL surgery. Note the significant effect of the VASER lipo-harvest on the buttock aesthetics. A significant portion of the aesthetic effect in these cases is related to the extraction not the graft volume. The author's philosophy in these cases is to "remove more, then add less."

to use skin moisturizers liberally over the treated areas, several times a day to avoid the dry skin typically associated with UAL in the early postoperative period. Depending on the volume of lipoaspirate removed, some surgeons include a preoperative and/or post-operative course of dietary supplements such as iron and antioxidant vitamins for several weeks.

Complications and management

Early generation UAL devices had a complication rate of 5%. The most common complications include seroma, prolonged dysesthesia, burns, induration, contour irregularities, hyperpigmentation, cellulitis, and prolonged swelling. Paresthesia or dysesthesia from UAL is usually a transient event and is the result of the ultrasonic energy effects on the phospholipid envelope of sensory nerves.[70] Hyperpigmentation following UAL and SAL may be due to hemosiderin deposits or post-inflammatory hyperpigmentation. Patients with higher Fitzpatrick skin types are at higher risk for post-inflammatory hyperpigmentation and may require laser treatments. Contour irregularities and persistent areas of induration can typically be conservatively managed with compression, injections, and lymphatic massage.[71–73] In some scenarios patients may require minor surgical revisions.

Thermal injury is one of the most feared complications of UAL, and subsequently one of the most extensively discussed.[74,75] Thermal injury can occur at the skin or in the deeper tissue. Skin level thermal injury is usually due to direct contact with the ultrasound probe. This can be avoided with skin protectors and wet drapes to cover any areas of potential contact. Thermal injury to deeper structures can be reduced with technique modifications that avoid end-hits and torque on the probe. Localized points of severe overheating occur when the tip of the ultrasound probe hits the deeper layer of dermis tangentially. Both can be avoided by applying providing direct, linear access for the ultrasound probes. Both the position of the patient on the operating table and the placement of the access incisions in relation to the treatment area determine the extent of lineal access. This is of paramount importance in the avoidance of probe-torque-related complications. Major complications from UAL such as visceral perforation leading to sepsis, necrotizing fasciitis, pulmonary edema from excessive subcutaneous tumescence, and DIC are rare.

SUMMARY

Over the past 40 years, liposuction has evolved from a rudimentary technique into a highly sophisticated method of body contouring. The addition of ultrasound technology to traditional liposuction (SAL), has increased the efficacy of the procedure and expanded the indications for lipo-contouring in multiple anatomic regions.[76] What was once considered large volume SAL, is now accepted as moderate volume for UAL since it is associated with less blood loss and decreased surgeon fatigue.

As UAL devices continue to evolve and improve, tissue fragmentation is maximized while energy delivery to the tissues is minimized. Third-generation UAL, (VASER) is currently considered the gold standard for contouring areas of fibrous fatty tissue, high-definition body sculpting, high-volume cases, as a contouring adjunct to open procedures and for repeat or secondary liposuction. The volume of cases performed and its status as the most common aesthetic surgical procedure are a testament to the high patient satisfaction rate associated with liposuction.

CLINICS CARE POINTS

- Use of skin protectors is recommended at the access incisions during the ultrasound phase of the procedure to avoid thermal injury.
- The gynecomastia VASER probe and the 1-ring VASER probe are extremely aggressive and are not typically used for body contouring. In most VASER liposuction cases, efficient adipose tissue fragmentation can be achieved employing the 3-ring and 5-ring VASER probes.
- Avoid adding Xylocaine to the wetting solution in large volume extractions under general anesthesia. It has no effect on postoperative pain however it places the patient at high risk for Xylocaine toxicity.
- Avoid hypothermia in longer cases with large body surface areas exposed. Strategies to mitigate hypothermia include using warm forced air (Bair Hugger to non-operative areas, warming the IV fluids and wrapping the head and extremities not invoived in the surgery.
- A VASER energy level of 60% to 80% allows efficient adipose tissue fragmentation in most VASER Liposuction surgeries.

DISCLOSURE

The authors have nothing to disclose.

REFERENCES

1. The American Society for Aesthetic Plastic Surgery. Garden Grove, CA: Cosmetic Surgery Data Bank; 2021.
2. Garcia O Jr. Ultrasonic liposuction. In: Shiffman MA, Di Giuseppe A, editors. Body contouring and liposuction E-book: expert consult - online. London, UK: Elsevier Health Sciences; 2012. p. 543–58.
3. Balamuth L. Ultrasonics and dentistry. Sound: Its Uses and Control 1963;2:15.
4. Scuderi N, Devita R, D'Andrea F, et al. Nuove prospettive nella liposuzione la lipoemulsificazone. Giorn Chir Plast Ricostr ed Estetica 1987;2(1):33–9.
5. Zocchi ML. New prospective in liposculpturing: the ultrasonic energy. Zurich, Switzerland: 10th ISAPS Congress; 1989.
6. Zocchi ML. Metodo di trattamento del tessuto adipose con energia ultrasonic. Rome, Italy: Congresso dell Societa Italiana di Medicina Estetica; 1988.
7. Zocchi ML. Clinical aspects of ultrasonic liposculpture. Perspect Plast Surg 1993;7:153–74.
8. Zocchi ML, Vincenzo V. Ultrasonic-assisted lipoplasty. In: Zienowicz RJ, Karacaoglu E, editors. Atlas of whole body contouring: a practical guide. Cham, Switzerland: Springer Nature; 2022. p. 203–36.
9. Fredricks S. Analysis and introduction of A technology: ultrasound-assisted lipoplasty task force. Clin Plast Surg 1999;26(2):187–204. https://doi.org/10.1016/S0094-1298(20)32604-3.
10. Zukowski ML, Ash K. Ultrasound-assisted lipoplasty learning curve. Aesthetic Surg J 1998;18(2):104–10.
11. Cimino WW. Ultrasonic surgery: power quantification and efficiency optimization. Aesthetic Surg J 2001; 21(3):233–40.
12. Chang CC, Commons GW. A comparison of various ultrasound Technologies. Clin Plast Surg 1999;26(2): 261–8.
13. Bond LJ, Cimino WW. Physics of ultrasonic surgery using tissue fragmentation: Part II. Ultrasound Med Biol 1996;22(1):101–17.
14. Jewell ML, Fodor PB, de Souza Pinto EB, et al. Clinical application of VASER-assisted lipoplasty: a pilot clinical study. Aesthetic Surg J 2002;22(2): 131–46.
15. Garcia O, Nathan N. Comparative analysis of blood loss in suction-assisted lipoplasty and third-generation internal ultrasound-assisted lipoplasty. Aesthetic Surg J 2008;28(4):430–5.
16. de Souza Pinto EB, Chiarello de Souza Pinto Abdala P, Montecinos Maciel C, et al. Liposuction and VASER. Clin Plast Surg 2006;33(1):107–15.
17. Bruno G, Amadei F, Abbiati G. Liposculpture with ultrasound: biomedical considerations. Aesth Plast Surg 1998;22(6):401–3.
18. Zocchi M. Ultrasonic liposculpturing. Aesth Plast Surg 1992;16(4):287–98.
19. Schafer ME. Basic science of ultrasound in body contouring. In: Garcia O, editor. Ultrasound assisted liposuction: current concepts and techniques. Switzerland, AG: Springer Nature; 2020. p. 9–21.
20. Panetta NJ, Gupta DM, Kwan MD, et al. Tissue harvest by means of suction-assisted or third-generation ultrasound-assisted lipoaspiration has No effect on osteogenic potential of human adipose-derived stromal cells. Plast Reconstr Surg 2009; 124(1):65.
21. Garcia O, Schafer M. The effects of non-focused external ultrasound on tissue temperature and adipocyte morphology. Aesth Surg J 2013;33:117–27.
22. Schafer ME, Hicok K, Mills D, et al. Acute adipocyte viability after third generation ultrasound-assisted liposuction. Aesth Surg J 2013;33(5):698–704.
23. Jewell JL. Ultrasonic-assisted liposuction: introduction and historic perspectives. In: Garcia O, editor. Ultrasonic-assisted liposuction: current concepts and techniques. New York: Springer; 2019. p. 3–8.
24. Garcia O. Liposuction for body contouring: discussion. In: Cohen MN, Thaller SR, editors. The unfavorable result in plastic surgery: avoidance and treatment. New York: Thieme Medical Publishers; 2018. p. 451–5.
25. Cimino WW. Ultrasound assisted lipoplasty: basic physics, tissue interactions and related results-complications. In: Shiffman MA, Di Giuseppi A, editors. Body contouring: Art, science and clinical practice. Berlin: Springer-Verlag; 2010. p. 389–98.
26. Garcia O. Blood loss in lipoplasty: a comparison of traditional and VASER assisted lipoplasty. In: Shiffman M, Di Giuseppe A, editors. Body contouring: Art, Science and clinical practice. 2nd Edition. Berlin: Springer; 2010. p. 565–73.
27. Garcia O. Contouring of the trunk. In: Garcia O, editor. Ultrasonic-assisted liposuction: current concepts and techniques. New York: Springer; 2019. p. 65–86.
28. Garcia O. VASER-assisted liposuction of gynecomastia. In: Garcia O, editor. Ultrasonic-assisted liposuction: current concepts and techniques. New York: Springer; 2019. p. 87–97.
29. Hoyos A, Millard J. VASER-assisted, high-definition liposculpture. Aesth Surg J 2007;27(6):594–604.
30. Garcia O. Liposuction of the upper and lower extremities. In: Aly A, Nahas F, editors. The Art of body contouring: a comprehensive approach. New York: Thieme Medical Publishers; 2017. p. 361–95.
31. Hurwitz DJ, Beidas O, Wright L. Reshaping the oversized waist through oblique flankplasty with lipoabdominoplasty (OFLA). Plast Reconstr Surg 2019; 143(5):960e–72e.
32. Hurwitz DJ. Ultrasound-assisted liposuction in the massive weight loss patient. In: Garcia O, editor. Ultrasonic-assisted liposuction: current concepts and techniques. New York: Springer; 2019. p. 189–202.

33. Rohrich RJ, Raniere J, Beran SJ, et al. Patient evaluation and indications for ultrasound-assisted lipoplasty. Clin Plast Surg 1999;26(2):269–78.
34. Hughes CE III. Patient selection, planning, and marking in ultrasound-assisted lipoplasty. Clin Plast Surg 1999;26(2):279–82.
35. Glaser DA, Kaminer MS. Body dysmorphic disorder and the liposuction patient. Dermatol Surg. 2005; 31(5):559-560; discussion 561.
36. Perez-Gurri JA. Choosing the correct candidate. In: Garcia O, editor. Ultrasonic-assisted liposuction: current concepts and techniques. New York: Springer; 2019. p. 23–36.
37. Illouz YG. Body contouring by lipolysis; a 5 year experience with over 3,000 cases. Plast Reconstr Surg 1983;72:587–91.
38. Klein JA. The tumescent technique: anesthesia and modified LiposuctionTechnique. Dermatol Clin 1990; 8(3):425–37.
39. de Jong R. Titanic tumescent anesthesia. Dermatol Surg 1998;24:689–92.
40. Shiffman MA. Medications potentially causing lidocaine toxicity. Am J Cosmet Surg 1998;15(3):227–8. https://doi.org/10.1177/074880689801500302.
41. Shiffman MA. Prevention and treatment of liposuction complications. In: Shiffman MA, Di Giuseppe A, editors. Liposuction: principles and practice. Berlin, Germany: Springer; 2006. p. 333–41. https://doi.org/10.1007/3-540-28043-X_5025.
42. Samdal F, Amland PF, Bugge JF. Plasma lidocaine levels during suction-assisted lipectomy using large doses of dilute lidocaine with epinephrine. Plast Reconstr Surg 1994;93(6):1217–23.
43. Fodor PB. Lidocaine toxicity issues in lipoplasty. Aesthetic Surg J 2000;20(1):56–8.
44. Cansancao AL, Condé-Green A, David JA, et al. Use of tranexamic Acid to reduce blood loss in liposuction. Plast Reconstr Surg 2018;141(5):1132–5.
45. Danilla S, Fontbona M, de Velez VD. Analgesic efficacy of lidocaine for suction assisted lipectomy with tumescent technique under general anesthesia: a randomized double masked controlled trial. Plast Reconstr Surg 2003;132(2):327–32.
46. Garcia O. Ultrasonic liposuction. In: Rubin JP, Jewell ML, Richter DF, et al, editors. Body contouring and liposuction. Philadelphia: Saunders; 2013. p. 543–58.
47. Burk RW, Guzman-Stein G, Vasconez LO. Lidocaine and epinephrine levels in tumescent technique. Plast Reconstr Surg 1996;97:1379.
48. Garcia O, Chaustre-Pena PS, Pazmino P. Suction-assisted lipectomy and Brazilian butt lift. In: Thaller S, Panthaki Z, editors. Tips and Tricks in plastic surgery. Switzerland, AG: Springer Nature Publishers; 2022. p. 151–89.
49. Klein JA. The tumescent technique for liposuction surgery. Am J Cosmet Surg 1987;4:263–7.
50. Lillis PJ. Liposuction surgery under local anesthesia: limited blood loss and minimal lidocaine absorption. Dermatol Surg Oncol 1988;80:1145.
51. Klein JA. The tumescent technique for local anesthesia improves safety in large-volume liposuction. Plast Reconstr Surg 1993;92:1085.
52. Kloehn RA. Liposuction with "sonic sculpture": six years' experience with more than 600 patients. Aesthetic Surg J 1996;16(2):123–8.
53. Rohrich RJ, Smith PD, Marcantonio DR, et al. The zones of adherence: role in preventing contour deformities in liposuction. Plast Reconstr Surg 2001; 107:1562.
54. Rohrich RJ, Ha RY, Kenkel JM, et al. Classification and management of gynecomastia: defining the role of ultrasound-assisted liposuction. Plast Reconstr Surg 2003;111:909–23.
55. Novo R, Garcia O. Ultrasound-assisted liposuction for gynecomastia. In: Anh Tran T, Panthaki Z, Hoballah JJ, et al, editors. Operative dictations in plastic surgery. Cham, Switzerland: Springer Medical Publishers; 2017. p. 179–80.
56. Novo R, Reusche R, Garcia O. Subcutaneous mastectomy and free nipple graft for gynecomastia. In: Anh Tran T, Panthaki Z, Hoballah JJ, et al, editors. Operative dictations in plastic surgery. Cham, Switzerland: Springer Medical Publishers; 2017. p. 181–3.
57. Gorney M. Liability in suction-assisted lipoplasty: a different perspective. Clin Plast Surg 1999;26(3): 441–5, ix.
58. Kenkel JM, Robinson JBJ, Beran SJ, et al. The tissue effects of ultrasound-assisted lipoplasty. Plast Reconstr Surg 1998;102(1):213.
59. Zocchi ML, Vindigni V. Invited discussion on: the nipple-areolar complex over time after treatment of gynecomastia with ultrasound-assisted liposuction mastectomy compared to subcutaneous mastectomy alone. Aesth Plast Surg 2021;45(2):438–41.
60. Fischer PD, Narayanan K, Liang MD. The use of high-frequency ultrasound for the dissection of small-diameter blood vessels and nerves. Ann Plast Surg 1992;28(4):326–30.
61. Di Giuseppe A, Commons G. Jowl and neck remodeling with ultrasound-assisted lipoplasty (VASER). In: Shiffman MA, Di Giuseppe A, editors. Cosmetic surgery: Art and techniques. Berlin, Germany: Springer; 2013. p. 539–51.
62. Rohrich RJ, Beran SJ, Kenkel JM. Patient selection and planning. In: Rohrich RJ, Beran SJ, Kenkel JM, editors. Ultrasound-assisted liposuction. St. Louis, MO: Quality Medical Publishing; 1998. p. 87–110.
63. Garcia O. Neck and facial contouring. In: Garcia O, editor. Ultrasound-assisted liposuction: current concepts and techniques. New York, NY: Springer Medical Publishers; 2019. p. 49–64.
64. Garcia O. Aesthetic body contouring of the posterior trunk using third generation pulsed solid probe

internal ultrasound assisted lipoplasty. In: Shiffman, Di Giuseppe A, editors. Body contouring: Art, science and clinical practice. 2nd Edition. Berlin: Springer; 2010. p. 493–504.

65. Mendieta CG. Buttock contouring with liposuction and fat injection. In: Rubin JP, Jewell ML, Richter DF, et al, editors. Body contouring and liposuction. Philadelphia: Saunders; 2013. p. 447–60.
66. Garcia O. Contouring of the extremities. In: Garcia O, editor. Ultrasound-assisted liposuction: current concepts and techniques. New York, NY: Springer Medical Publishers; 2019. p. 99–132.
67. Rohrich RJ, Beran SJ, Kenkle JM. Understanding ultrasound assisted liposuction and safety issues. In: Rohrich RJ, Beran SJ, Kenkle JM, editors. Ultrasound assisted liposuction. St. Louis, MO: Quality Medical Publishing; 1998. p. 21–36.
68. Pazmino P, Garcia O. Brazilian butt lift-associated mortality: the south Florida experience. Aesthet. Surg. J. 2022. https://doi.org/10.1093/asj/asjc224. sjac 224.
69. Garcia O, Pazmino P. Response to commentary on: Brazilian butt lift-associated mortality: the south Florida experience. Aesthet. Surg. J. 2022;sjac325. https://doi.org/10.1093/asj/sjac325.
70. Howard BK, Beran SJ, Kenkel JM, et al. The effects of ultrasonic energy on peripheral nerves: implications for ultrasound-assisted liposuction. Plast Reconstr Surg 1999;103(3):984–9.
71. Perez JA, van Tetering JPB. Ultrasound-assisted lipoplasty: a review of over 350 consecutive cases using a two-stage technique. Aesthetic Plast Surg 2003;27(1):68–76.
72. Graf R. Ultrasound-assisted liposuction: an analysis of 348 cases. Aesthetic Plast Surg 2003;27(2): 146–53.
73. Chacur R, Menezes HS, Chacur NMB da S, et al. Aesthetic correction of lesion by post-liposuction corticoid infiltration using subcision, PMMA filling, and CO2 laser. Case Reports in Plastic Surgery and Hand Surgery 2019;6(1):140–4.
74. Zocchi ML, Vindigni V, Bassetto F. 32 Years of ultrasonic-assisted lipoplasty (U.A.L.): from aesthetic to obesity. Aesth Plast Surg 2020;44(4):1230–40.
75. Wall S. Liposuction for body contouring. In: Cohen MN, Thaller SR, editors. The unfavorable result in plastic surgery: avoidance and treatment. New York: Thieme Medical Publishers; 2018. p. 433–51.
76. Rohrich RJ, Beran SJ, Kenkel JM, et al. Extending the role of liposuction in body contouring with ultrasound-assisted liposuction. Plast Reconstr Surg 1998;101(4):1090.

Lipoplasty in the Overweight Patient

Emmanuel De La Cruz, MD[a,b,*]

KEYWORDS

- Body contouring • Large volume liposuction • VASER liposuction • Ultrasonic-assisted liposuction
- Renuvion • Radiofrequency-assisted liposuction • Liposuction safety
- Synchronous energy-assisted liposuction

KEY POINTS

- Large volume liposuction (LVL), performed by board-certified plastic surgeons using energy-assisted liposuction devices, is safe with improved aesthetic outcomes and minimal complications.
- Utilizing synergistic energy-based devices, VASERLipo and Renuvion, can achieve substantial retraction following LVL.
- Evidence-based protocols, including hypothermia prevention, deep vein thrombosis (DVT) prophylaxis, and perioperative antibiotics, reduces complications.
- For optimal patient safety and high-quality care, LVL should be performed in accredited hospitals or certified ambulatory surgery centers with overnight admission for hemodynamic monitoring for prompt identification and management of complications.
- While the use of advanced devices like VASERLipo and Renuvion has shown promising results, surgeons must exercise caution to avoid seroma, pneumomediastinum/pneumoperitoneum, and subcutaneous emphysema.

INTRODUCTION

The prevalence of obesity has increased for most countries since the 1980s. This global obesity epidemic has contributed directly to the increased incidence of cardiovascular risk factors, such as type 2 diabetes, hypertension, dyslipidemia, and sleep disorders. Despite the ever-changing ideal of feminine and masculine body types, and constantly changing beauty standards imposed throughout the past decade, the increased rates of obesity and the growing pursuit of a slender body contributed to the growing desire for liposuction. Suction-assisted lipectomy remains one of the most common body contouring procedures in the United States.[1] During the last decade, liposuction has undergone significant improvement with regards to technique, technology, safety, and outcomes. This advancement in techniques and energy-based devices has improved the postoperative skin retraction as well as reduced complications, such as blood loss. With the improvement of surgical outcomes and reduction of potential complications, large volume liposuction becomes a viable alternative in body contouring.

HISTORICAL BACKGROUND

The modern technique of liposuction was initially introduced in 1975 by a father and son who were cosmetic surgeons. Arpad and Giorgio Fischer (Rome, Italy) first described the crisscross suctioning of fat of the outer thighs using a blunt hollow cannula attached to a suction source.[2]

Yves-Gerard Illouz[3] and Pierre Fournier (Paris, France) popularized the Fischer technique in 1977 by performing liposuction to the whole body by introducing smaller blunt cannulas of different diameters. In order to reduce bleeding and trauma to the surrounding tissues, Illouz[4] later developed the “wet technique” by injecting saline

[a] American Board of Plastic Surgery; [b] American Board of Surgery
* Corresponding author. 15016 FM 529, Houston, TX 77095.
E-mail address: delacruzplasticsurgery@gmail.com

Clin Plastic Surg 51 (2024) 29–43
https://doi.org/10.1016/j.cps.2023.06.010

solution with hyaluronidase into the localized adipose tissue. Fournier subsequently introduced the use of lidocaine in liposuction as well as the concept of compression techniques during the postoperative period.[5]

The reduction of blood loss associated with suction-assisted lipectomy was further improved when Jeffrey Klein (Southern California, USA),[6,7] a dermatologic surgeon, introduced the Klein tumescent technique, which involved the infusion of a solution consisting of 0.05% lidocaine, 1:1,000,000 epinephrine, and 10 mL sodium bicarbonate per liter of saline into the adipose tissue before the liposuction procedure. A safe upper limit for lidocaine dosage was determined by Klein to be 35 mg/kg with minimal toxicity and was later proven to be safe at 55 mg/kg by Ostad and colleagues.[8,9] The peak plasma level of lidocaine was found to be present around 4 to 8 hours after the infiltration of the tumescent fluid.[9] The large volume of dilute epinephrine also afforded the additional benefit of avoiding tachycardia and hypertension during and after the procedure.[8]

The introduction of ultrasonic liposculpturing by Michele Zocchi[10] (Italy) in 1992 further revolutionized liposuction based on the surgical use of ultrasonic energy.

This liposuction method required a two-stage process involving the emulsification of fat with a solid probe followed by aspiration of fat. Selective lipolysis occurs secondary to cavitation and cellular fragmentation at frequencies in excess of 16 kHz with the vibration of the ultrasonic probe.[11,12] With the benefit of a reduced physical workload on the surgeon, this selective destruction of adipose tissues enhanced the ease of fat extraction as well as facilitated the retraction of skin by the application of ultrasonic heat. This ultrasound-assisted liposuction technique has undergone multiple refinements from a solid probe to a hollowed cannula that allowed simultaneous emulsification and lipoaspiration.[13] Vibration Amplification of Sound Energy at Resonance (VASERLipo; (Solta Medical, Bothell, WA, USA) supplanted the 2 previous generations of ultrasonic liposuction systems that were riddled with seroma and thermal injury complications. The VASER system uses a probe with multiple rings or grooves that redistribute the ultrasonic pulsed energy from the tip to the sides of the probe where the rings are located. This redistribution of ultrasonic energy results in a reduction of applied power and greater fragmentation of adipocytes at a lower-energy setting with either a pulsed or a continuous energy.[14,15]

Further technological advancement in 1998 led to the emergence of power-assisted liposuction that uses a rapidly vibrating cannula reciprocating at 2000 to 4000 cpm with a 2-mm stroke.[16] This rapid oscillating cannula movement allows the breaking up of fibrous fat much more readily, which helps reduce operative time as well as makes liposuction less labor-intensive than the traditional suction-assisted lipectomy.[17]

Several technological advancements contributed further to the improvement of the outcome in liposuction. Whether it is driven by an oscillating tool, ultrasound, laser, or radiofrequency (RF) energy, each of these technologies has its set of benefits as well as its complications.[12,18,19]

LARGE VOLUME LIPOSUCTION

In 1998, the American Society of Plastic Surgery Task Force on Lipoplasty defined large volume liposuction as greater than 5000 cc total aspirate in a single procedure.[11] During this procedure, patients are exposed to a large volume of subcutaneous fluid infiltration, prolonged general anesthesia with hypothermia, and potential higher doses of epinephrine or lidocaine. Profound hemodynamic alterations occur during large volume liposuction. Because of the epinephrine from the infused tumescent fluid, there is an increase in heart rate, cardiac index, mean arterial pressure, and right ventricular stroke work index.[20] A diminished mean arterial pressure and systemic vascular index, however, also occur during large volume liposuction, which may be attributed to the vasodilation effects of general anesthesia.[20]

Intraoperative blood loss in suction-assisted lipoplasty has always been a major concern in the past with blood loss ranging from 20% to 45% in dry lipoplasty when no subcutaneous infiltration was given before liposuction.[21] The introduction of tumescent infiltration in the targeted area of liposuction with dilute lidocaine and epinephrine significantly reduced the blood loss associated with this procedure.[7,8,21] Blood loss diminished from 45% as seen in dry lipoplasty techniques to 1% as seen in tumescent and superwet techniques.[21] With the advent of ultrasound-assisted liposuction using the VASERLipo system (Solta Medical, Bothell, WA, USA), blood loss secondary to liposuction further improved and diminished. A 7.5-fold decrease of blood loss made it more feasible to perform large volume liposuction with the use of the VASERLipo device with 0.61% blood loss of the total aspirate.[22]

The use of the superwet and tumescent techniques in liposuction, as well as the utilization of ultrasonic liposuction devices, has significantly decreased intraoperative blood loss and the potential need for blood transfusion in lipoplasty.

Volume overload resulting in pulmonary edema and acute respiratory distress syndrome, however, can be a potential problem in large volume liposuction because greater volumes of subcutaneous fluid infiltration in addition to the resuscitative fluids are involved in this procedure. Given the lack of randomized controlled clinical studies, controversial debate still surrounds the issues of the optimal fluid strategy in large volume liposuction. Several studies were previously conducted and created guidelines for fluid management in patients who underwent suction-assisted lipectomy using superwet techniques.[23–25] "Intraoperative fluid ratio" as described by Trott and colleagues[23] seemed to be a safe guideline for fluid management in large volume liposuction. Intraoperative fluid ratio was defined as the volume of subcutaneous infiltrated fluid and intravenous fluid divided by the total aspiration volume. Studies have shown that an intraoperative fluid ratio of 1.2 to 1.4 was safe for large volume liposuction.[23–25]

SKIN RETRACTION WITH ENERGY-ASSISTED LIPOSUCTION DEVICES

Lipoaspiration is an excellent tool that can remove excess adipose tissue; however, it cannot remove excess skin, and therefore, techniques are compared based on their ability to contract the skin of the treated area. Approximately 10% of skin retraction occurs after suction-assisted lipectomy.[26,27] There were multiple modalities and technologies used to assist skin retraction in suction-assisted lipectomy, which ranges from the use of ultrasonic energy, LASER, to RF energy. VASER-assisted lipoplasty was shown to cause significant skin retraction of 17% at 6 months in a randomized clinical trial by Nagy and Vanek.[14] This was a 53% improvement in skin retraction relative to suction-assisted lipectomy. LASER-assisted liposuction, however, was reported to have a similar soft tissue contraction of 17.2% as compared with 10.6% skin surface area reduction obtained from suction-assisted lipectomy.[27]

The advent of RF energy-based devices further contributed to the improvement of skin retraction as well as to the contraction of the underlying fibroseptal network underneath the skin.[26,28] A randomized clinical study by Duncan[26] revealed that the subdermal and subcutaneous application of RF energy using BodyTite (InMode Corporation, Toronto, Canada) resulted in a 36.4% skin surface area reduction at 1 year by dermal collagen fiber contraction and neocollagenesis. This RF energy device uses a handpiece that transmits RF energy between 2 electrodes: an external electrode that is in contact with the skin, and an internal electrode that is in contact with the subcutaneous adipose tissue layer and fibroseptal network.[19,29]

The introduction of plasma-converted radiofrequency energy (Renuvion; Apyx Medical, Clearwater, FL, USA) in 2016 as a subdermal coagulation device using RF energy contributed further to the arena of energy-assisted liposuction devices as an alternative to improve soft tissue contraction. This device delivers RF energy at 13.05 MHz to energize a tungsten needle electrode that would ionize helium gas and convert it into cold helium plasma.[30,31] Helium gas is used in this device because of its low electron density, which has a higher thermal conductivity when ionized and uses lower energy than an equipment-operational argon plasma.[30,32] This helium-based plasma RF technology delivers heat to the tissues at temperatures greater than 85°C for 0.040 to 0.080 seconds.[30] This rapid heating in the form of cold helium plasma results in rapid cooling after the application of the RF energy to the surrounding tissues. Thus, soft tissue contraction from the heat generated from the Renuvion device is achieved without overheating the full thickness of the dermis. Because the RF plasma energy is conducted to lower impedance targets, such as the fibroseptal networks that encase the fat globules, the redirection of the flow of energy allows soft tissue contraction without excessive heating.[33] This helium-based plasma RF technology not only had shown to improve skin laxity but also affords a treatment time efficiency advantage because it delivers heat within 0.044 seconds.[18,30]

With all these technological innovations, the ideal liposuction technology would be the ability to remove fat easily with minimal morbidity, and concomitantly tighten skin without the need for excisional surgery. Synchronous energy-assisted lipectomy (SEAL) has recently emerged by combining multiple technologies to improve surgical efficiency as well as improve the aesthetic outcome of lipoplasty. Studies have shown that skin and soft tissue retraction that results from the subdermal application of energy-based liposuction devices is also secondary to contraction of the collagen fibers of the fibroseptal network.[18,31,34]

CURRENT STUDY

A retrospective chart review study was conducted on patients who underwent large volume liposuction (>5 L Liposuction aspirate) using either the ultrasonic-assisted lipectomy (VASER only) or the SEAL technique from a single surgeon's institution from January 2018 to February 2023. This SEAL technique included 4 stages consisting of tumescent infiltration; emulsification of fat using the VASER probe; suction-assisted lipectomy using a power-assisted liposuction device (MicroAire Surgical Instruments, Charlottesville, VA, USA); and subdermal application of plasma-converted RF energy (Renuvion). Inclusion criteria included male and female subjects greater than 21 years of age who underwent large volume liposuction. The exclusion criteria include any previous abdominal or chest surgery, history of ventral hernia, congestive heart failure, myocardial infarction, deep vein thrombosis (DVT), or any combined procedures, such as abdominoplasty or breast augmentation. All patients were also evaluated for the presence of an umbilical hernia. When an umbilical hernia was present, a concomitant umbilical hernia repair was planned before the lipoplasty procedure.

Informed consent was obtained on every patient before each procedure to be included in a potential clinical research study and informed of the potential risks of the surgical devices used. All patients provided informed consent for the procedure to be performed, as well as authorization for the usage of photographs for research purposes. Deidentified information was collected on the following patient demographics: sex, age, race, body mass index (BMI), and comorbidities. The following surgical variables were included: tumescent infiltration volume, liposuction aspirate volume, concomitant procedures, and intraoperative complications.

EVALUATION

All patients were clinically screened for cardiovascular and blood pressure disorders by obtaining a cardiology clearance from a board-certified cardiologist. It is imperative to evaluate cardiac function of patients undergoing this procedure to determine that their compliant right ventricles can accommodate large fluid shifts during surgery.[35]

Attempts to reduce hypothermia during the procedure were obtained by prewarming the patient with forced warm air using the Bair Hugger before surgery; raising the temperature of the operating room to at least 74°F with a relative humidity of 30% to 60%; using warmed forced air intraoperatively; warmed intravenous and tumescent fluids using a fluid warmer at ≤104°F (40°C); and warmed blankets.[36]

Caprini score was calculated by the surgeon in all patients. An intermittent sequential compression device was used before induction of general anesthesia for DVT prophylaxis in all patients. Heparin 5000 units was given subcutaneously at the end of the procedure, and the patients were then prescribed an oral anticoagulant (rivaroxaban) for 10 to 14 days for chemothromboembolic prophylaxis.

Perioperative intravenous antibiotics were given within 30 minutes of the procedure. A Foley urinary catheter was placed, and urine output was monitored throughout the case in all patients. No invasive hemodynamic monitoring was performed.

Intravenous fluids were maintained based on vital signs and urine output of the patient during the entire procedure and postoperatively. All patients were admitted overnight at an accredited hospital or accredited outpatient ambulatory surgery center. Fluid boluses were given if needed under the discretion of the anesthesiologist and surgeon, but maintenance intravenous fluids were administered postoperatively during the 23-hour observation period.

OPERATIVE TECHNIQUE

The patients were marked in the standing position in the preoperative recovery room area and were reevaluated for the presence of umbilical hernia and other hernias. They were then prepared in the standing position using 2% Chlorhexidine gluconate in 70% Isopropyl alcohol (ChloraPrep).

After general anesthesia was induced, surgery was then initiated by performing a simple umbilical hernia repair with a 2-0 nonabsorbable suture if an umbilical hernia was present. It is crucial to repair any umbilical hernia before suction-assisted lipectomy in order to avoid any iatrogenic bowel or intraabdominal organ injuries. Umbilical hernia repair may also mitigate the risk of pneumoperitoneum secondary to the diffusion of helium gas during the Renuvion application phase of the procedure.

Liposuction was then performed by either VASER-assisted liposuction or using a four-stage SEAL technique consisting of tumescent infiltration; emulsification of fat using the VASER probe (Solta Medical); suction-assisted lipectomy using a power-assisted liposuction device (MicroAire); and subdermal application of plasma-converted RF energy (Renuvion).

The superwet technique for infiltration and liposuction was used with 1:1 volume of infiltrate/volume of aspirate. The infiltration solution consisted of 20 mL of 1% lidocaine, 1:1000 (1 mg) of epinephrine, and 8.45% sodium bicarbonate in 1 L of lactated Ringer solution. The author continued to use lidocaine in the wetting solution even though some investigators suggested that lidocaine can be completely eliminated from the infiltration fluid if liposuction is performed under general anesthesia.[37] The reasoning to continue its usage in wetting solutions is that lidocaine affords better postoperative pain control and reduced systemic anesthesia requirements.[38] Although the safe dosage of lidocaine for tumescent liposuction had been shown to be safe at 55 mg/kg,[9] the author selected the maximum lidocaine dosage in his institution to be less than 35 mg/kg in all patients.

Skin protection using the VASERLipo designed skin ports as well as wet towels adjacent to the port locations was used. The emulsification process was performed using a 5-ring VASER probe at 50% amplitude using the VASER-mode (pulsed energy) at a maximum of 1 minute of treatment time per 100 mL of infused wetting solution. The 5-ring VASER probe was used to achieve more fragmentation of the surrounding tissues/fat and to deliver a higher ultrasonic energy parallel to the probe.

Extraction of the fat was performed using a 3.7-mm Vent-X cannula and a power-assisted liposuction device (MicroAire). Standard manual suction-assisted lipectomy using a 3.0-mm and 3.7-mm Vent-X cannula was performed for the lipoplasty of the abdomen and thighs to minimize contour irregularities. Power-assisted liposuction using a 4.0-mm "candy cane" pattern cannula was performed on the flanks and back. The endpoint of liposuction was when the liposuction aspirate changed from a pure yellow color to a bloody appearance.

The Renuvion device was used at 80% power and 2.0 L of helium flow. The RF-helium plasma was applied subdermally with up to 5 subcutaneous passes applied at the same point of location at different levels. Aspiration of the residual helium gas was performed using a 3.7-mm Vent-X cannula. The small stab incisions were left open to allow egress of the remaining tumescent fluid infused.

POSTOPERATIVE ASSESSMENT

All patients were placed in a foam corset garment and a highly compressive garment immediately after surgery. Highly compressive garments are essential to minimize fluid sequestration into the tissues and thus minimize fluid shifts that may result in intravascular fluid depletion postoperatively. Patients were instructed to wear the foam corset garment for 2 months, and the highly compressive garment for 6 months. The foam corset garment was designed to minimize the risk of seroma formation and compression garment ulcers. Furthermore, all patients received lymphatic massage therapy the following day after surgery for 10 consecutive days. All patients were followed up in clinic the following day after surgery, and 1 week, 4 weeks, 8 weeks, and 6 months after the procedure.

Table 1
Patient demographics and operative data

Sex	
Female	63 (71.59%)
Male	25 (28.41%)
Ethnic background	
African American	43 (48.87%)
Asian	1 (1.14%)
Caucasian	21 (23.86%)
Hispanic	22 (25%)
Middle Eastern	1 (1.14%)
Liposuction of trunk	
No	4 (4.55%)
Yes	84 (95.5%)
Liposuction of bilateral arms	
No	14 (15.91%)
Yes	74 (84.09%)
Liposuction of bilateral thighs	
No	25 (28.41%)
Yes	63 (71.59%)
Fat transfer area	
Butt	44 (50%)
Correction of gynecomastia	
No	80 (90.91%)
Yes	8 (9.09%)
Concomitant procedure	
Bilateral medial thigh lift	4 (4.55%)
Excision of right torso lipoma	1 (1.14%)
No	77 (87.5%)
Umbilical hernia repair	6 (6.82%)
Renuvion	
No	63 (71.59%)
Yes	25 (28.41%)
Drains	
No	63 (71.59%)
Yes	25 (28.41%)
23 Hour Observation	
Yes	88 (100%)
History of previous laparotomy or midline incision scar	
No	88 (100%)
Hospitalization after discharge	
No	88 (100%)

STATISTICS

The data were analyzed by an independent academic biostatistician and clinical researcher who had full access to all study data. The results of this analysis were the results reported in this article. Data were verified, coded, and analyzed using IBM-SPSS 27.0. Descriptive statistics: Means, standard deviations, frequency, and percentages, were calculated. Normality of continuous variables was tested using Kolmogorov-Smirnov test/Shapiro-Wilk test as appropriate. Paired *t* test analysis was carried out to compare the means of continuous outcomes. A significant *P* value was considered when it is less than .05.

RESULTS

Eighty-eight patients with BMI greater than 30 kg/m^2, aged 21 to 64 years (mean age, 40.8; median age, 41), who underwent large volume liposuction (>5 L liposuction aspirate) with either the VASER-assisted liposuction alone versus the Synchronous Energy-assisted lipoplasty (VASERLipo and Renuvion) were included in this retrospective chart review (**Table 1**). The average BMI of the patients included in this chart review was 35.4 kg/m^2 with a mean weight of 99.06 kg (218.4 lbs). The average Caprini score for venous thromboembolism was 3.68, and all patients were given thromboembolism prophylaxis with heparin 5000 units

Table 2
Patient demographics, operative characteristics, and metabolic parameters

	N	Range	Minimum	Maximum	Mean	SE	SD	Median
Age, y	88	43.00	21.00	64.00	40.8068	1.05118	9.86094	41
BMI	88	20.00	30.00	50.00	35.4069	0.45493	4.26762	34.39
Weight	88	145.00	155.00	300.00	218.4659	3.74661	35.14631	209.5
Height	88	50.80	149.86	200.66	167.6977	1.31865	12.37005	163.83
Tumescent fluid infused	88	8.50	5.00	13.50	10.1681	0.17435	1.61687	10.29
Liposuction aspirate volume (L)	88	8.10	5.00	13.10	7.2697	0.19871	1.84279	6/85
Duration of surgery (min)	88	410.00	115.00	525.00	337.8295	6.51462	61.11253	330
Initial systolic BP	88	90.00	94.00	184.00	129.7907	1.94142	18.00400	128.5
Initial diastolic BP	88	82.00	31.00	113.00	83.0233	1.37855	12.78416	83
Systolic BP (1st week)	82	84.00	80.00	164.00	121.5854	1.58916	14.39046	120
Diastolic BP (1st week)	82	46.00	60.00	106.00	80.3537	1.05871	9.58699	78
Systolic BP (1st month)	77	76.00	81.00	157.00	124.5195	1.62428	14.25299	122
Diastolic BP (1st month)	77	47.00	54.00	101.00	81.5065	1.04014	9.12721	79
Hb (preoperative)	69	7.90	10.20	18.10	13.4870	0.18731	1.55591	13.3
Hb (postoperative)	13	7	8	15	11.82	0.591	2.129	12.2
Hct (preoperative)	69	55.90	31.50	87.40	41.6838	0.84386	6.95865	40.7
Hct (postoperative)	13	19	28	46	36.65	1.429	5.153	36.8
Glucose (preoperative)	66	90.00	74.00	164.00	95.9682	2.02112	16.41966	93.45
Glucose (postoperative)	8	55	75	130	101.88	6.996	19.788	99.5
HbA_{1c} (preoperative)	32	3.70	4.90	8.60	5.7500	0.14438	0.81676	5.6
HbA_{1c} (postoperative)	2	0	6	6	5.60	0.000	0.000	5.6
BUN (preoperative)	62	19.00	7.00	26.00	13.4726	0.54167	4.26508	12
BUN (postoperative)	8	13	9	22	13.63	1.647	4.658	12.5
Crt (preoperative)	63	1.57	0.30	1.87	0.8333	0.03013	0.23916	0.8
Crt (postoperative)	8	0	1	1	0.80	0.043	0.121	0.775
Caprini score	88	3.00	3.00	6.00	3.6818	0.07326	0.68725	4

Abbreviations: BP, blood pressure; Crt, Creatinine; Hb, Hemoglobin; Hct, Hematocrit; SD, standard deviation; SE, standard error of mean.

subcutaneously perioperatively and an oral anticoagulant postoperatively.

The average volume of tumescent fluid infiltrated per patient was 10.16 L, and the average volume of liposuction aspirate was 7.27 L (**Table 2**). The mean duration of surgery was 337 minutes (median, 330 minutes). Sixty-eight patients (77.27%) had the SEAL, and 6 patients (6.82%) had a simple umbilical hernia repair performed concomitantly before lipoplasty. Only 25 (28.41%) patients had a drain placed intraoperatively at the end of the procedure. All patients were admitted overnight at either a certified hospital or an accredited ambulatory surgery center.

There were no thromboembolic complications and no cardiac events, such as myocardial infarction or pulmonary edema, in any of the patients. No patient required any blood transfusions. There were no pneumoperitoneum or mediastinal emphysema on any of the patients who underwent either the VASER liposuction alone or synchronous energy-assisted lipoplasty with VASERLipo and Renuvion. However, there were 2 patients who developed a seroma postoperatively requiring aspiration (n = 2; 2.27%), and both patients had Renuvion during their procedure (**Table 3**). One patient developed blister formation and subcutaneous emphysema (1.47% of Renuvion patients) on the left forearm the day after surgery secondary to migration of helium gas from the left arm where the Renuvion device was applied (**Fig. 1**). Moreover, there were 3 patients who developed mild cellulitis that resolved with oral antibiotics (n = 3; 3.34%).

Analysis of systolic/diastolic blood pressure, hemoglobin, hematocrit, glucose, blood urea nitrogen (BUN), and creatinine was also performed. Using a paired *t* test for statistical analysis, postoperative outcomes were compared with baseline (**Table 4**). The analysis shows that, after liposuction, systolic blood pressure measurements were significantly lower after 1 week ($P<.001$) and after 1 month ($P = .015$). However, diastolic BP measurements were not significantly reduced ($P = .063$ after 1 week and $P = .421$ after 1 month). Hemoglobin and hematocrit levels were significantly reduced ($P = .001$ and $P = .006$, respectively) with an average decrease of hemoglobin of 1.23 g/dL and hematocrit of 3.02% after large volume liposuction. Regarding glucose, BUN, and creatinine levels, the analysis revealed a nonsignificant difference between baseline and postintervention values ($P = .621$, $P = .595$, and $P = .09$, respectively).

DISCUSSION

Because of concerns regarding patient safety, the volume of fat to be aspirated in one session of suction-assisted lipectomy is limited. The volume of fat to be aspirated is limited owing to 2 factors: (1) the volume of fat that can be extracted without causing significant blood loss, and (2) the amount

Table 3
Postoperative complications

Complication	n (%)
Thromboembolism	0 (0.00%)
Pulmonary edema	0 (0.00%)
Pressure garment sore	1 (1.13%)
Seroma	2 (2.27%)
Brachial plexus neuropraxia secondary to prone positioning	2 (2.27%)
Infection (cellulitis)	3 (3.34%)
Burn injury	0 (0.00%)
Bullae formation & subcutaneous emphysema	1 (1.13%)
Wound dehiscence (thigh lift)	1 (1.13%)
Pneumomediastinum	0 (0.00%)
Return to operating room	0 (0.00%)
Any return to hospital	0 (0.00%)
Mortality	0 (0.00%)

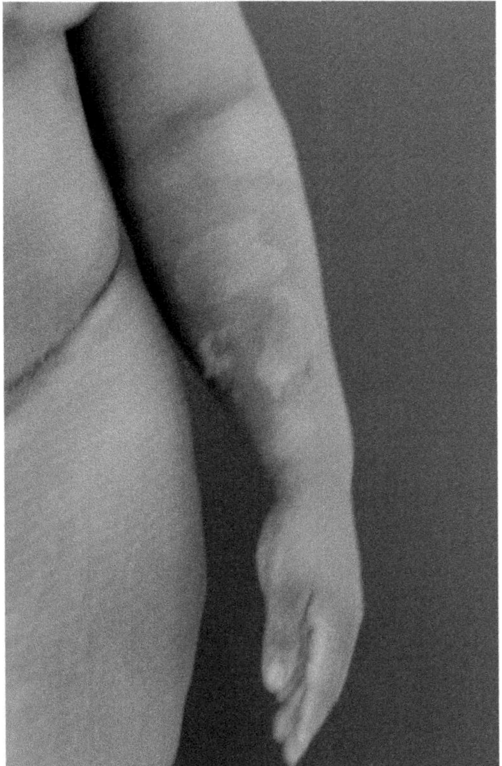

Fig. 1. Subcutaneous emphysema and blister formation of the forearm secondary to helium gas migration from the arm 2 days after Renuvion subdermal coagulation.

Table 4
Postoperative outcomes compared with baseline

	Mean Difference	SD Difference	SE Difference	Lower 95% CI	Upper 95% CI	t	*df*	*P* Value[a]
Systolic BP after 1 wk	−8.82500	20.03843	2.24036	−13.28433	−4.36567	−3.939	79	.000
Systolic BP after 1 mo	−5.33766	18.85444	2.14866	−9.61709	−1.05823	−2.484	76	.015
Diastolic BP after 1 wk	−3.16250	14.97377	1.67412	−6.49475	0.16975	−1.889	79	.063
Diastolic BP after 1 mo	−1.40260	15.21016	1.73336	−4.85488	2.04969	−0.809	76	.421
Hb	−1.23847	1.06578	0.29560	−1.88251	−0.59441	−4.190	12	.001
Hct	−3.02308	3.28815	0.91197	−5.01009	−1.03607	−3.315	12	.006
Glucose	−4.20000	17.55563	7.85111	−25.99819	17.59819	−0.535	12	.621
BUN	1.80000	6.97854	3.12090	−6.86500	10.46500	0.577	4	.595
Crt	0.07600	0.07635	0.03415	−0.01881	0.17081	2.226	4	.090

[a] Results were calculated using the paired *t* test.

of infiltration and intravenous fluid that can be infused during liposuction without causing fluid overload.

Blood loss had been a major factor limiting surgeons from performing large volume liposuction. The advent of tumescent and superwet techniques a few decades ago led to the increase in the amount of fat to be removed from suction-assisted lipectomy. Despite the fact that the Klein formula described in 1987 contributed to a significant reduction of blood loss from 45% to 1% of the liposuction aspirate, there is still apprehension with regards to performing large volume liposuction of more than 5 L of fat.[7,8]

Minimizing blood loss during surgery had always been the objective of many surgeons in the past few decades. In a meta-analysis involving 3583 patients who had large volume liposuction, the most common complication was blood loss requiring blood transfusion with an incidence of 3.35%.[39] In pursuit of mitigating perioperative hemorrhage, plastic surgeons have started to incorporate the usage of tranexamic acid in suction-assisted lipectomy.[40–42] Hoyos and colleagues[41] had shown in a double-blind randomized clinical trial that the use of intravenous tranexamic acid was associated with a decrease in postoperative bleeding from liposculpture procedures. In the author's retrospective study, they found that the mean decrease of hemoglobin and hematocrit using the superwet technique and ultrasonic-assisted liposuction (with or without the use of Renuvion) in large volume liposuction (>5 L lipoaspirate) was 1.23 g/dL and 3.02%, respectively.[41] Although they did not use tranexamic acid in their patients, the use of tranexamic acid is very promising in large volume liposuction and may lead to a further increase in the amount of fat that can be aspirated.

The volume of tumescent or infiltration fluid, however, may still be a limiting factor to the amount of fat that can be aspirated without causing significant hemodynamic shifts and fluid overload. Fluid overload occurs when there is more than 20% gain of total body fluid.[43] In healthy individuals who do not have a history of renal or cardiopulmonary disorders, the amount of excessive fluid administration that may lead to pulmonary edema occurs when the Net Fluid Retention (NFR) Index exceeds 67 mL/kg/d or an NFR of 7 L over the initial 27 postoperative hours.[44] Thus, the NFR volume in a patient undergoing liposuction would be the total amount of fluids received minus the liposuction aspirate and urine output [Net Fluid Retention Volume = (IVF + Infiltration Fluid) – (Total Liposuction Aspirate Volume + Urine Output)]. Total liposuction aspirate volume as opposed to total

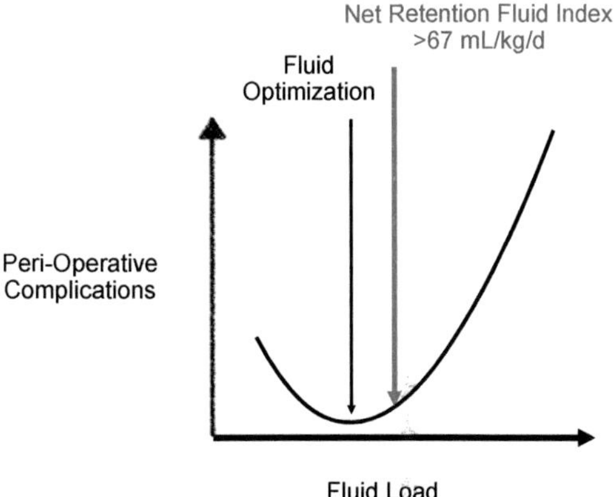

Fig. 2. Correlation between fluid load and perioperative complications in large volume liposuction with a parabolic distribution curve [$f(X) = a(X - 1)^2 + 3$)]. Pulmonary edema occurs when net retention fluid exceeds 67 mL/kg/d. NFR Volume = [(IV Fluid + Infiltration fluid) – (Total Liposuction Aspirate Volume + Urine Output)].

aspirated wetting solution as suggested by Commons and colleagues[45] in 1999 is used in the calculation because most lipoaspirate is pure fat. This modified calculation correlates more with the safe upper limit of an NFR index of 67 mL/kg/d. The total volume of intravenous and infiltration fluids given during suction-assisted lipectomy, and the occurrence of major postoperative complications are correlated in a parabolic distribution curve [$f(X) = a(X - 1)^2 + 3$)] (**Fig. 2**).[46,47] This parabolic distribution curve is the reciprocal of the Frank-Starling curve. Although the mathematical formula is not precise because the time factor is not considered in the equation, knowledge of the potential NFR Volume during the lipoplasty perioperative period may be helpful in managing and mitigating the risks and postoperative complications associated with fluid overload.

Further technological advancements in liposuction, such as the ultrasonic-assisted liposuction using the VASERLipo and power-assisted liposuction device, made large volume liposuction a viable alternative for body contouring in the overweight patient. The emulsification of fat using ultrasonic energy further reduced bleeding in addition to the blood loss reduction from the Klein formula. The power-assisted liposuction device, however, contributed to the ease of fat extraction in the massively obese patient.

Major strides have been made with regards to the innovation of the ideal liposuction device. The optimal liposuction technology should exhibit efficient fat removal; minimal bleeding and contour irregularities; and simultaneous enhancement of

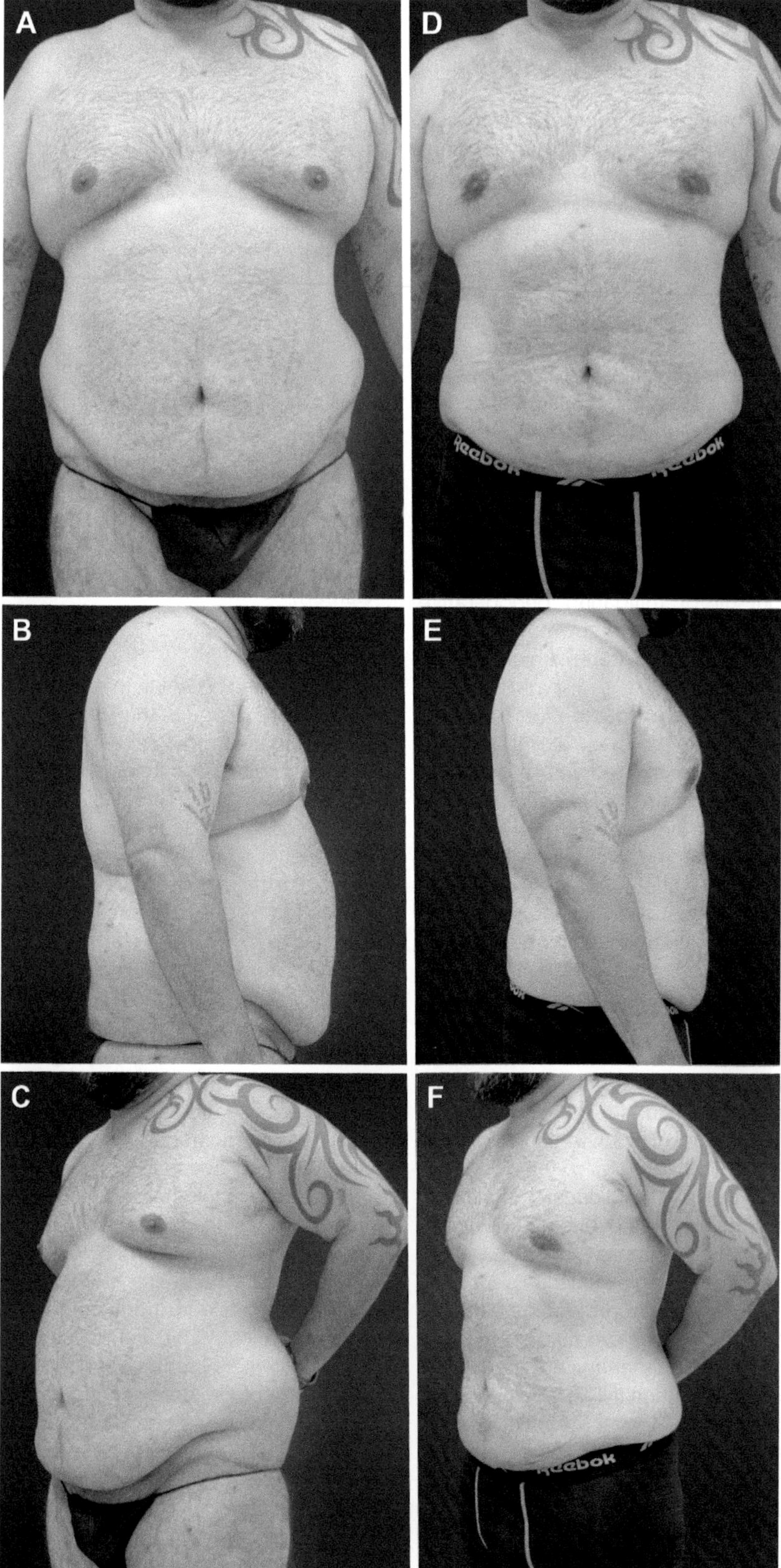

Fig. 3. A 41-year-old man who underwent synchronous energy-assisted lipoplasty of the abdomen, flanks, and back with Renuvion. He also underwent gynecomastia surgery. A total of 6500 mL of fat was removed. The patient lost 18.14 kg 3 months after surgery. (*A–C*) Preoperative views of the front, side, and oblique, respectively. (*D–F*) Postoperative views of the front, side, and oblique at 3 months.

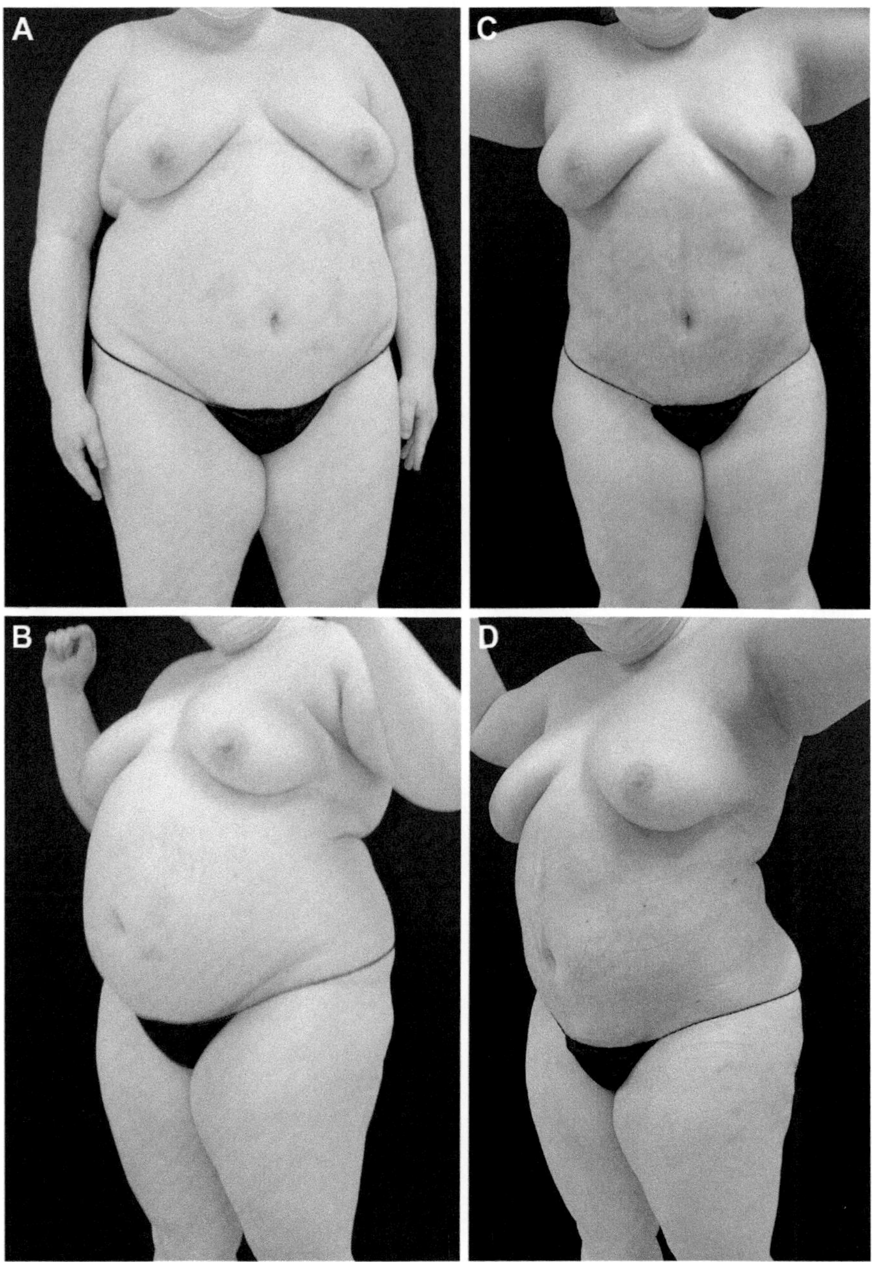

Fig. 4. A 21-year-old woman who underwent large volume liposuction of the trunk and thighs with VASERLipo and Renuvion. A total of 8 L aspirate was removed. (*A, B*) Preoperative views of front and oblique, respectively. (*C, D*) Postoperative views at 2 weeks.

skin and soft tissue retraction. Regrettably, the current market lacks a device that fulfills all these criteria. However, the recent trend in SEAL has introduced promising advancements. By combining multiple cutting-edge technologies, such as VASERLipo, Renuvion, and MicroAire, surgical outcomes have significantly improved in terms of skin and soft tissue retraction while minimizing complications. Although there is no current study evaluating the amount of skin retraction using the combined-energy devices, clinically there is a significant improvement with regards to skin retraction and the quality of skin postoperatively (**Figs. 3–5**.) Skin and soft tissue contraction varies individually and may be influenced by age, ethnic background, Fitzpatrick scores, and/or history of bariatric surgery. Despite the theoretical advantages of synchronous energy-assisted lipoplasty, new potential

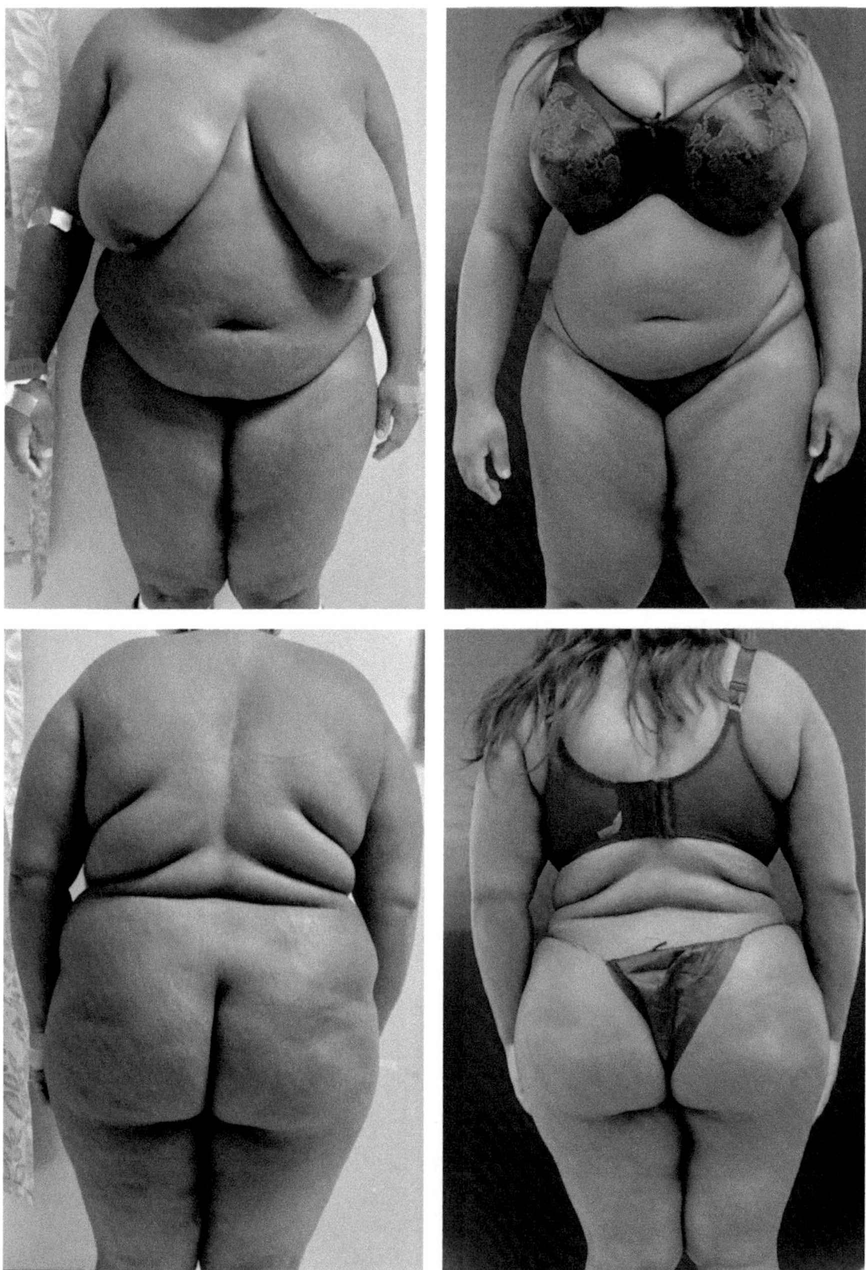

Fig. 5. A 29-year-old woman with a BMI of 44.3 who underwent large volume liposuction of the trunk and thighs with VASERLipo and Renuvion with fat transfer to bilateral buttocks. A total of 11.95 L infiltration fluid was infused, and 11.2 L of liposuction aspirate was obtained. Approximately 700 mL of fat was transferred subcutaneously on each side of the buttocks.

complications may arise from these novel devices, such as Renuvion. Excessive residual helium gas with the usage of Renuvion may potentially result in subcutaneous emphysema, pneumomediastinum, and possibly pneumoperitoneum if the residual helium gas is not aspirated after the procedure.[48] Although the author had no pneumoperitoneum or pneumomediastinum in the retrospective study, they had one patient who developed subcutaneous emphysema and a bullae distal to the treated area of Renuvion (see **Fig. 1**). The use of Renuvion is also associated with an increased seroma rate. Although the seroma rate was minimal (n = 2; 2.27%), all patients who developed seroma requiring aspiration in the study underwent Renuvion subdermal coagulation.

When combining multiple energy devices, it is essential to reduce the power and amplitude of the VASER device to 50% using the VASER mode in order to reduce the risks of potential burn injury and reduce the seroma formation.[45] Aspiration of the residual helium gas at the end of the procedure, and reduction of the flow rate of the Renuvion device can also dampen the excessive residual helium gas. It is also imperative to evaluate and repair any incidental or occult umbilical hernia to reduce any iatrogenic bowel injury for every liposuction procedure. The repair of an occult umbilical hernia may also mitigate the risk of pneumoperitoneum that may result from the Renuvion device.

SUMMARY

Large volume liposuction using multiple energy-assisted liposuction devices is safe with improved aesthetic outcome and with minimal complications. By using techniques to minimize blood loss, such as the superwet technique and ultrasonic-assisted liposuction, and being cognizant of the maximal volume of infiltration fluid that can be safely infused, large volume liposuction can be safely performed by board-certified plastic surgeons. Evidenced-based surgical protocols for hypothermia prevention, DVT prophylaxis, and perioperative antibiotic prophylaxis should be followed to mitigate the risk of postoperative complications. Large volume liposuction should be performed, and patients should be admitted overnight in an accredited hospital or certified ambulatory surgery center for proper hemodynamic monitoring immediately after surgery. While improving skin and soft tissue contraction, the synergy of multiple devices, such as VASERLipo and Renuvion, is associated with a higher seroma rate formation (2.27%) and risk of subcutaneous emphysema (1.47%). One should exercise caution when using these new medical devices to prevent any untoward events.

CLINICS CARE POINTS

- While adhering to safe infiltration fluid volume limits, superwet technique and ultrasonic-assisted liposuction minimizes blood loss.
- Technological advancements, such as ultrasonic-assisted liposuction and power-assisted liposuction, make large volume liposuction (LVL) a viable option for overweight patients, but should be carefully managed to minimize risks.
- Adherence to evidence-based protocols, including hypothermia prevention, deep vein thrombosis (DVT) prophylaxis, and peri-operative antibiotic prophylaxis, reducesthe incidence of complications.
- Use accredited hospitals or certified ambulatory surgery centers for LVL to ensure the highest standards of care and patient safety.
- Monitoring of fluid administration with overnight stay is crucial to prevent overload in LVL, which can lead to hemodynamic shifts and complications.
- Synchronous energy-assisted liposuction, combining multiple cutting-edge technologies, improves outcomes and skin retraction, but long-term studies are needed.
- Surgeons should be aware of complications associated with novel devices, such as Renuvion, including subcutaneous emphysema and increased seroma rate, and take appropriate precautions.

DISCLOSURE

The author has no commercial or financial disclosures.

ACKNOWLEDGMENTS

We would like to show our gratitude to Gina Stepaniants BS who assisted in our medical research. We are also immensely grateful to Ahmed Masoud MD (Director of Clinical Research, Marchand Institute for Minimally Invasive Surgery, AZ, USA) for his expertise in biostatistics.

REFERENCES

1. American Society of Plastic Surgeons. Report of the 2020 plastic surgery statistics. Arlington Heights, Ill: ASPS; 2021.
2. Fischer A, Fischer G. First surgical treatment for molding body's cellulite with three 5 mm incisions. Bull. Int. Acad. Cosmet. Surg. 1976;3:35.
3. Illouz Y. Body contouring by lipolysis: a 5 year experience with over 3000 cases. Plast Reconstr Surg 1983;72:511.
4. Illouz YG. History and current concepts of lipoplasty. Clin Plast Surg 1996;23:721–30.
5. Fournier PF, Otteni FM, Fournier PF. Lipodissection in body sculpturing: the dry procedure. Plast Reconstr Surg 1983;72(5):598–609.

6. Klein JA. The tumescent technique for liposuction surgery. Am J Cosmet Surg 1987;4:263–7.
7. Klein JA. Tumescent technique for local anesthesia improves safety in large volume liposuction. Plast Reconstr Surg 1993;92:1085–98.
8. Klein JA. Tumescent technique for regional anesthesia permits lidocaine doses of 35 mg/kg for liposuction. J Dermatol Surg Oncol 1990;16(3):248–63.
9. Ostad A, Kageyama N, Moy RL. Tumescent anesthesia with lidocaine dose of 55 mg/kg is safe for liposuction. Dermatol Surg 1997;22:921–7.
10. Zocchi M. Ultrasonic liposculpturing. Aesthetic Plast Surg 1992;16(4):287–98.
11. Rohrich RJ, Beran SJ, Kenkel JM, et al. Extending the role of liposuction in body contouring with ultrasound-assisted liposuction. Plast Reconstr Surg 1998;101(4):1090–102 [discussion: 1117-9].
12. Shridharani SM, Broyles JM, Matarasso A. Liposuction devices: technology update. Med Devices (Auckl) 2014;7:241–51.
13. Zocchi ML. Ultrasonic assisted lipoplasty. Technical refinements and clinical evaluations. Clin Plast Surg 1996;23:575–98.
14. Nagy MW, Vanek PF Jr. A Multicenter, prospective, randomized, single-blind, controlled clinical trial comparing VASER-assisted lipoplasty and suction-assisted lipoplasty. Plast Reconstr Surg 2012; 129(4):681e–9e.
15. Jewell ML, Fodor PB, de Souza Pinto EB, et al. Clinical application of VASER – assisted lipoplasty: a pilot clinical study. Aesthet Surg J 2002;22:131–46.
16. Fodor PB, Vogt PA. Power-assisted lipoplasty (PAL): a clinical pilot study comparing PAL to traditional lipoplasty (TL). Aesthetic Plast Surg 1999;23(6):379–85.
17. Fodor PB. Power-assisted lipoplasty versus traditional suction-assisted lipoplasty: comparative evaluation and analysis of output. Aesthetic Plast Surg 2005;29(2):127.
18. DiBernardo BE, Reyes J. Evaluation of skin tightening after laser- assisted liposuction. Aesthet Surg J 2009;29:400–7.
19. Theodorou SJ, Paresi RJ, Chia CT. Radiofrequency-assistedliposuction device for body contouring: 97 patients under local anesthesia. Aesthetic Plast Surg 2012;36:767–79.
20. Kenkel JM, Lipschitz AH, Luby M, et al. Hemodynamic physiology and thermoregulation in liposuction. Plast Reconstr Surg 2004;114:503–13.
21. Rohrich RJ, Beran SJ, Fodor PB. The role of subcutaneous infiltration in suction-assisted lipoplasty: a review. Plast Reconstr Surg 1997;99:514–9.
22. Garcia O Jr, Nathan N. Comparative analysis of blood loss in suction-assisted lipoplasty and third-generation internal ultrasound-assisted lipoplasty. Aesthet Surg J 2008;28:430–5.
23. Trott SA, Beran SJ, Rohrich RJ, et al. Safety considerations and fluid resuscitation in liposuction: an analysis of 53 consecutive patients. Plast Reconstr Surg 1998;102:2220–9.
24. Rohrich RJ, Leedy JE, Swamy R, et al. Fluid resuscitation in liposuction: a retrospective review of 89 consecutive patients. Plast Reconstr Surg 2006; 117:431–5.
25. Jain AK, Khan AM. Stroke volume variation as a guide for fluid resuscitation in patients undergoing large-volume liposuction. Plast Reconstr Surg 2012;130(3):462e–9e.
26. Duncan DI. Nonexcisional tissue tightening: creating skin surface area reduction during abdominal liposuction by adding radiofrequency heating. Aesthet Surg J 2013;33:1154–66.
27. DiBernardo BE. Randomized, blinded split abdomen study evaluating skin shrinkage and skin tightening in laser-assisted liposuction versus liposuction control. Aesthetic Surg J 2010;30(4):593–602.
28. Kenkel J. Response to evaluation of skin tightening after laser-assisted liposuction. Aesthet Surg J 2009;29(5):407–8.
29. Spero J Theodorou MD, Daniel Del Vecchio MD, Christopher T Chia MD. Soft tissue contraction in body contouring with radiofrequency-assisted liposuction: a treatment gap solution. Aesthetic Surg J 2018;38(suppl_2):S74–83.
30. Gentile RD. Renuvion/J-plasma for subdermal skin tightening facial contouring and skin rejuvenation of the face and neck. Facial Plast Surg Clin North Am 2019;27(3):273–90.
31. Irvine Duncan D. Helium plasma-driven radiofrequency in body contouring. The art of body contouring. Int Ophthalmol 2019. https://doi.org/10.5772/intechopen.84207.
32. Jonkers J, Sande M, Sola A, et al. On the differences between ionizing helium and argon plasmas at atmospheric pressure. Plasma Sources Sci Technol 2002;12:30.
33. Paul M, Mulholland RS. A new approach for adipose tissue treatment and body contouring using radiofrequency-assisted liposuction. Aesthetic Plast Surg 2009;33:687–94.
34. Ruff PG 4th. Thermal effects of percutaneous application of plasma/radiofrequency energy on porcine dermis and fibroseptal network. J Cosmet Dermatol 2021;20(7):2125–31.
35. Holte K, Sharrock NE, Kehlet K. Pathophysiology and clinical implications of preoperative fluid excess. Br J Anaesth 2002;89:622–32.
36. Young VL, Watson ME. Prevention of perioperative hypothermia in plastic surgery. Aesthetic Surg J 2006;26:551–71.
37. Perry AW, Petti C, Rankin M. Lidocaine is not necessary in liposuction. Plast Reconstr Surg 1999;104: 1900–2 [discussion: 1903–1906].
38. Matarasso A. Lidocaine in ultrasound-assisted lipoplasty. Clin Plast Surg 1999;26:431–9, viii.

39. Kanapathy M, Pacifico M, Yassin AM, et al. Safety of large-volume liposuction in aesthetic surgery: a systematic review and meta-analysis. Aesthet Surg J 2021;41(9):1040–53.
40. Cansancao AL, Condé-Green A, David JA, Cansancao B, Vidigal RA. Use of tranexamic acid to reduce blood loss in liposuction. Plast Reconstr Surg 2018;141(5):1132–5.
41. Hoyos AE, Duran H, Cardenas-Camarena L, et al. Use of tranexamic acid in liposculpture: a double-blind, multicenter, randomized clinical trial. Plast Reconstr Surg 2022;150(3):569–77.
42. Abboud NM, Kapila AK, Abboud S, et al. The Combined effect of intravenous and topical tranexamic acid in liposuction: a randomized double-blinded controlled trial. Aesthet Surg J Open Forum 2021; 3(1):ojab002.
43. Lowell JA, Schifferdecker C, Driscoll DF, et al. Postoperative fluid overload: not a benign problem. Crit Care Med 1990;18:728–33.
44. Arieff AI. Fatal postoperative pulmonary edema: pathogenesis and literature review. Chest 1999 May;115(5):1371–7.
45. Commons GW, Halperin B, Chang CC. Large-volume liposuction: a review of 631 consecutive cases over 12 years. Plast Reconstr Surg 2001;108(6):1753–63.
46. Licker M, Hagerman A, Bedat B, et al. Restricted, optimized or liberal fluid strategy in thoracic surgery: a narrative review. Saudi J Anaesth 2021;15:324–34.
47. Bellamy MC. Wet, dry or something else? Br J Anaesth 2006;97:755–7.
48. Alqahtani M, Mahabbat N, Fayi K. Rare complication of coupled VASER liposuction and Renuvion technologies: a case report. Case Reports Plast Surg Hand Surg 2023;10(1):2181175.

Lipoabdominoplasty with Anatomical Definition

Update

Osvaldo Saldanha, PhD[a,*], Osvaldo Saldanha Filho, MD[a], Cristianna Bonetto Saldanha, MD[a], Karin Luiza Mokarzel, MD[b], Aline Curado Machado Borges, MD[c], Eduar Arnaldo Murcia Bonilla, MD[d]

KEYWORDS

- Lipoabdominoplasty • Body contouring • Scarpa fascia • Abdominoplasty • Umbilical surgery • Safety score

KEY POINTS

- The anatomical definition achieved with liposuction optimizes esthetic results.
- This technique reduces morbidity by preservation of perforating blood vessels and suspension of Scarpa's fascia. Standardizing this technique makes the procedure safe and reproducible.
- Results provide a harmonic body contour, highlighting the muscular anatomy and making the surgery imperceptible, achieving the appearance of an athletic abdomen and back.

INTRODUCTION

There is a continuous search for better technical alternatives for the treatment of abdominal contour deformities in the practice of plastic surgeons. Such deformities, whether cosmetic or functional, may be characterized by flaccidity, lipodystrophy, and diastasis of the rectus abdominis.

Lipoabdominoplasty (LAP)[1] changed the concepts of abdominal plastic surgery, proposing a narrow tunnel in the superior abdominal flap and changing the taboo of associating liposuction. Because it efficiently treats deformities of the abdomen and back, it has become the first choice for plastic surgeons today. Preservation of the abdominal perforators of the deep inferior epigastric artery (responsible for 80% of the blood supply to the abdominal wall) reduces the postoperative risks of flap ischemia.[1–3]

This current began with Illouz,[4] in 1992. Twelve years after developing liposuction (1980), he published "*Abdominoplasty mesh undermining*," without release of the abdominal flap and performing liposuction in selected cases.

Subsequently, in 2001, Saldanha and colleagues[1] published "*Lipoabdominoplasty without undermining*," and in 2003 with "Lipoabdominoplasty"[2]—standing out among several other publications on the subject. Such a technique is reproducible and esthetically satisfactory for most patients; however, in some cases, it may result in an excessively flat lower abdomen.

Using the same principles as Illouz, Villegas[5] developed the Tulua technique, performing abdominal liposuction in a comfortable way, with "transverse" infraumbilical plication and neomphaloplasty, with interesting and reproducible results.

The first article on the importance of highlighting the muscles of the abdomen and thorax—*Abdominal etching: differential liposuction to detail abdominal musculature*—was written by Mentz and colleagues[6] in 1993 and caught the attention of the scientific community due to its anatomical detail. In this way, the abdominal anatomical definition began a new era of abdominal contouring.

After numerous publications demonstrated the effectiveness of lipodefinition of the abdominal

[a] Av. Ana Costa, 146 cj 1201, Santos, São Paulo 11060-000, Brazil; [b] Rua D. Egydio Martins 160, cj 54, Santos, São Paulo 11030-160, Brazil; [c] Rua José Caballero 60, cj 1903, Santos, São Paulo 11055300, Brazil; [d] Avenida Ana Costa 516, cj 12, Santos, São Paulo 11060002, Brazil
* Corresponding author.
E-mail address: clinicasaldanha@hotmail.com

Clin Plastic Surg 51 (2024) 45–57
https://doi.org/10.1016/j.cps.2023.06.011

contour, Saldanha and colleagues[7,8] consolidated the new standardization of LADE—LAP with anatomical definition that incorporated the principles of highlighting the definition of the abdominal musculature, achieving more natural results with fewer reminders of surgical intervention.

THE PRINCIPLES OF THE LIPOABDOMINOPLASTY

The fundamental principle of this technique remains the preservation of the perforating vessels of the abdominal wall between the inner edges of the 2 abdominal muscles through selective surgical undermining. This one must be meticulous, rigorous, and selective, owing to the greater intensity of liposuction required to achieve anatomical definition (**Fig. 1**).

Some areas will have deep liposuction, others will have both superficial and deep, depending on the areas to be defined.

The preservation of Scarpa's fascia brings important benefits that have already been well defined in previous publications, mainly being the following: reduction of bleeding, homogeneous support for the superior flap, containment of the lateral extension of the scar, better adherence between the flaps, rejuvenation of the pubis and deep planes, and, above all, the improvement of lymphatic drainage.

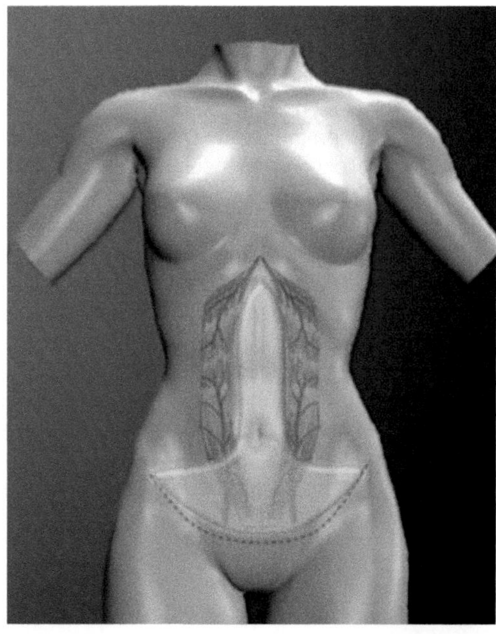

Fig. 1. Schematic of lipoabdominoplasty: preservation of perforating vessels of the rectus muscle and avascular tunnel in the midline. The dotted line indicates the incision.

SURGICAL TECHNIQUE

Patient Selection and Surgical Safety

Ideal patients for the procedure have a body mass index (BMI) less than 30, presenting with lipodystrophy with flaccid abdominal skin. Special attention is given to patients who have undergone previous abdominal surgery, including abdominal liposuction. Abdominal scars and hernias are examined and noted. These patients may be more susceptible to traditional LAP without definition.

Long-lasting surgery and the association of other procedures at the same surgical time are 2 important predictors of complications.[9] It is worth mentioning that the advent of modern concepts and technologies used during the procedure have also been responsible for the increase in surgical time.

The adoption of safety measures to reduce trans and postoperative morbidity is of the utmost importance. To this end, we can use the Safety Score, a valuable tool developed and published in the study "Predictive factor of complications in plastic Surgery—Suggestions for Safety Scores"[9] (**Tables 1** and **2**).

About the Definition

It is important to understand that not all patients are candidates for lipodefinition procedures. The results depend on the patient's requirements, previous anatomy, BMI, skin quality, and abdominal wall musculature. A small, medium or high abdominal definition can be achieved, always paying attention to the intensity of the liposuction and the degree of vascular impairment that may occur. In general, BMI greater than 27 and poor skin quality attenuate significant definition.

Marking of abdominal flap and liposuction areas

We use the principles of lipodefinition marking developed by Ricardo Ventura. We begin by marking the medial and lateral borders of the rectus abdominis muscle, with the patient standing, contracting the abdominal muscles, delimiting the diastasis, and obtaining the necessary orientation for selective liposuction in this area. We can use indirect lighting to identify the patient's preexisting anatomy, which may be "camouflaged" by current flaccidity and lipodystrophy.

For superficial liposuction, we draw 3 lines: the central line of the abdomen (alba line) and the lines that join the lateral edges of the rectum and the oblique muscles (semilunar lines), which correspond to negative areas. The costal margin is also marked (**Fig. 2**).

Table 1 Predictive score of safety parameters in plastic surgery	
1. Surgery Duration	*Scoring*
<4 h	1
4–6 h	2
>6 h	4
2. Surgical Time/*Association*	*Scoring*
Small surgery	1
Medium Surgery/large Surgery or 2 surgical associations	2
Three or more surgical associations	4
3. Body mass index	*Scoring*
18–29.0 kg/m^2	1
30–35 kg/m^2	2
>35 kg/m^2	4
4. Body Area	*Scoring*
Until 20%	1
From 20% to 30%	2
From 30% to 40%	4
5. ASA	*Scoring*
ASA I	1
ASA II	2
ASA III or Greater	4
6. Thromboembolic Factors	*Scoring*
No factor	1
One factor	2
Two or more factors	4

The horizontal suprapubic line is 12 to 14 cm, depending on the width of the patient's pubis, 5 to 7 cm from the vulvar commissure. Two oblique lines of 7 to 8 cm each are drawn in the direction of the iliac crest, with an inclination of approximately 40° to 45°, inside the bikini line, completing the lower incision line (see **Fig. 2**).

These measurements may vary depending on the patient's BMI and the degree of sagging skin. Subsequently, the supraumbilical limit of the abdominal flap to be resected is marked, joining it to the lateral limit of the lower line.

Table 2 Total safety parameter scoring for evaluation of plastic surgery risks	
Final Scoring	Scoring
Ideal parameter	6–12
Acceptable parameter	13–14
Inadequate parameter or exception	>14

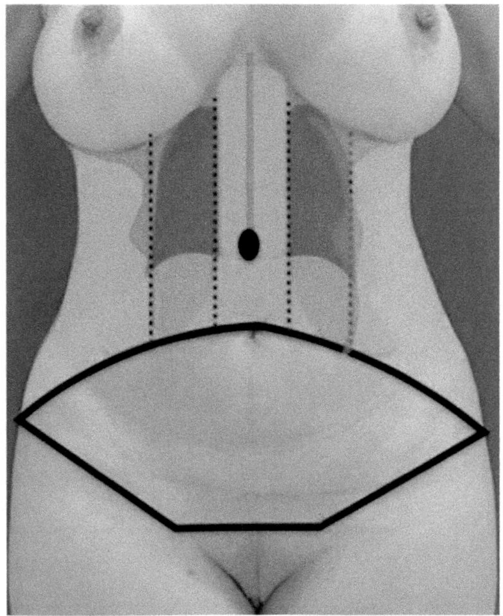

Fig. 2. Light green zone: superficial and deep traditional liposuction; dark green zone: superficial and deep definition liposuction; yellow zone: limited liposuction at the ends of the abdominal flap; red zone: careful liposuction in the area where the perforating vessels are located.

The location of the new umbilicus is marked approximately 4 finger widths above the original umbilicus. The lower area (yellow zone) is a reference line to avoid too aggressive liposuction because it is the distal zone of the flap and it will be the infraumbilical region of the abdominal flap (see **Fig. 2**).

Finally, the demarcation of the pubic region, flanks, iliac crest, or dorsal region is performed if necessary (light green areas) (**Figs. 2** and **3**).

Infiltration

The wet technique is used, infiltrating the entire abdominal region with a saline solution with adrenaline (1:500,000), between 1 and 2 L in the abdominal region, prioritizing the areas where the most intense liposuction will be performed. The addition of an infiltration set and cannulas can significantly shorten the infiltration time.

Liposuction

For greater safety in performing liposuction, the patient is placed in a hyperextended position on the surgical table (Pillét's position), both in ventral and dorsal positions. The surgery begins with the lipodefinition of the back, flanks, and buttocks, seeking the definition and limits of each of these regions (**Fig. 4**A, B).

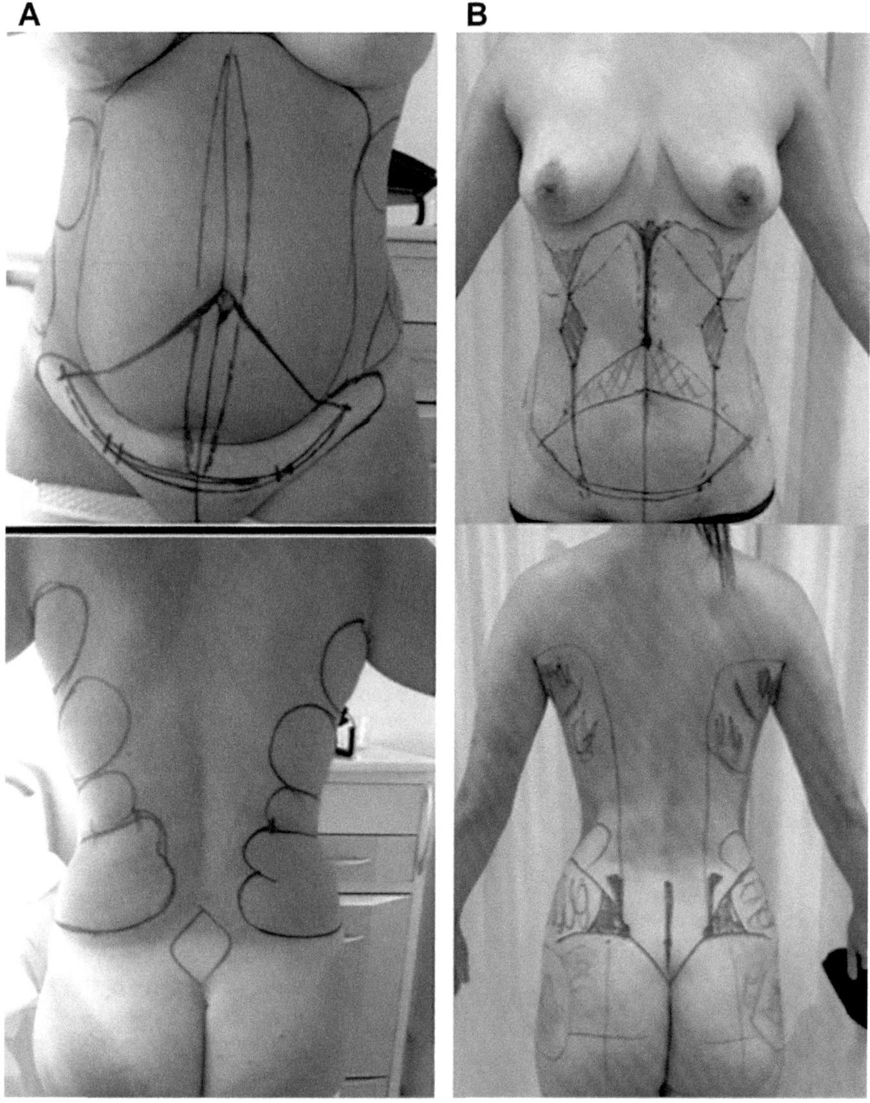

Fig. 3. (*A*) LAP markings where only localized fat and the area to be resected in the abdomen were identified. (*B*) LADE marking, detailing the anatomical limits, with fat and muscle definition of the abdominal and dorsal regions.

Sequentially, the abdomen is aspirated, beginning with the central region (alba line), continuing with the regions of the semilunar lines, with conventional 3 and 4 mm cannulas, extracting fat from the deep and superficial layers. In these (negative) areas, liposuction is more intense, with the aim of achieving a more natural and harmonious result in the contour of the abdominal wall, without traumatizing the subdermal plexus. We emphasize the liposuction of the alba line, which must be limited between the black point (point A—possible location of the new navel) and the xiphoid process. The region below the black dot corresponds to the yellow zone that will replace the skin of the lower abdomen and should not have a central depression area (see **Fig. 2**).

Liposuction in the light green areas (flanks and eventual posterior areas) is performed in the deep and superficial layers, evenly, leaving a fat thickness of about 2 cm until a more natural and harmonious contour of the abdominal wall is achieved. This new concept of selective liposuction aims to define the natural curves of the abdomen, accentuating the muscle insertion areas.[3]

Next, a deep and controlled liposuction of the red zone is performed, with a 3 mm cannula, avoiding trauma to the perforating vessels of the rectus abdominis. In the same way, a deep

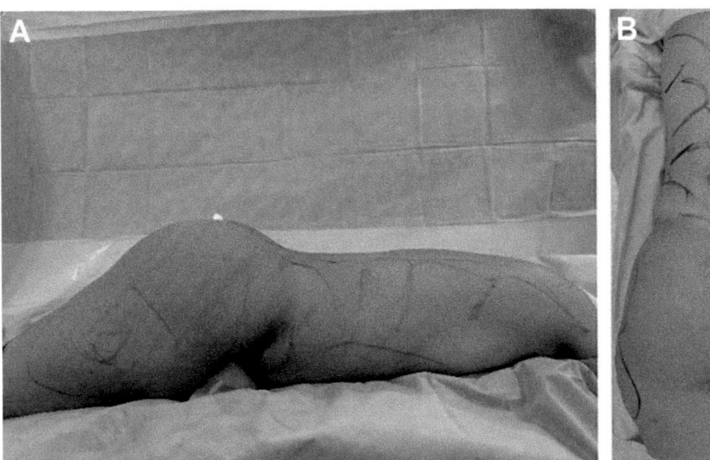

Fig. 4. (*A*) Pillét's position: Hyperextended patient-cushion placed in the pubic region, with the upper limit on the iliac crest, a slight inclination was performed in the Trendelenburg position with a slope in the region of the legs, to facilitate the performance of liposuction. (*B*) Patient in the prone position, in Pillét position, to start liposuction of the back, flanks, and buttocks.

liposuction is performed in the yellow zone. After resection of the lower abdomen, the deep fat in this yellow region is excised, trying to balance the thickness of the flap with the pubis (**Fig. 5**A, B).

The pinch test should be 1:3 in the ratio of negative to positive areas.

Preservation of Scarpa's fascia

Preserving Scarpa's fascia is the next surgical step that we perform. After skin incision in the suprapubic region, Scarpa's fascia is visualized and release is performed in the suprafascial plane up to the level of the anterior superior iliac crest. Although it is not a mandatory procedure, we recommend its conservation for the benefit of reducing the lateral extension of the scar, reducing the risk of seroma and bleeding, in addition achieving pubic suspension, without creating a lower abdominal bulge.[10–18] From there, we proceed to the aponeurotic dissection plane until reaching the umbilicus (**Fig. 6**A–D).

Creation of the Supraumbilical Tunnel

After isolating the umbilicus, the central supraumbilical tunnel is undermined between the inner edges of the rectus abdominis muscles to the xiphoid process, preserving most of the abdominal perforating vessels. The width of the tunnel varies depending on the size of the diastasis. To facilitate muscle plication and a better visualization of the anatomical

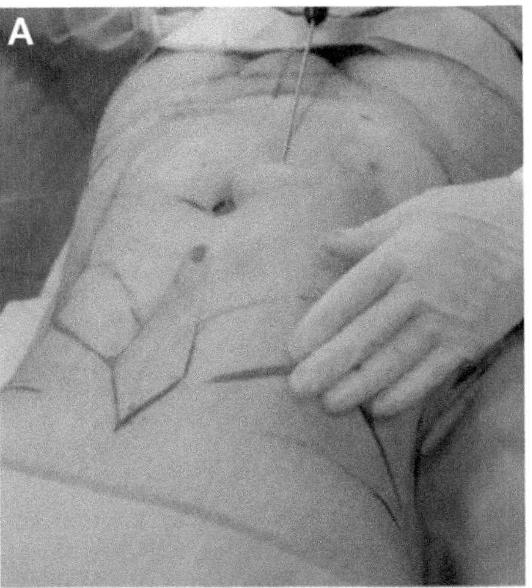

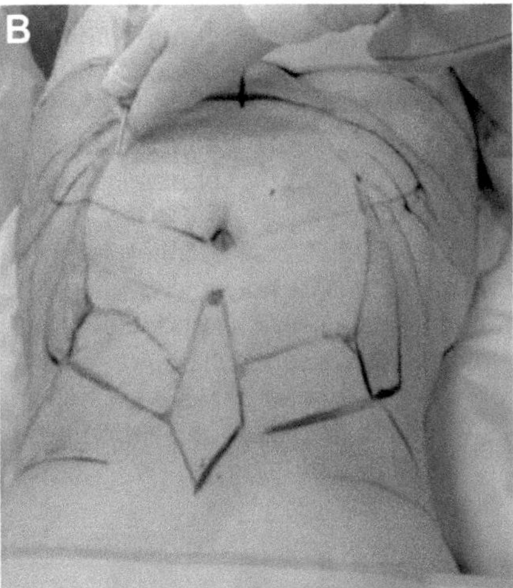

Fig. 5. (*A*) Liposuction of linea alba. (*B*) Liposuction of semilunaris.

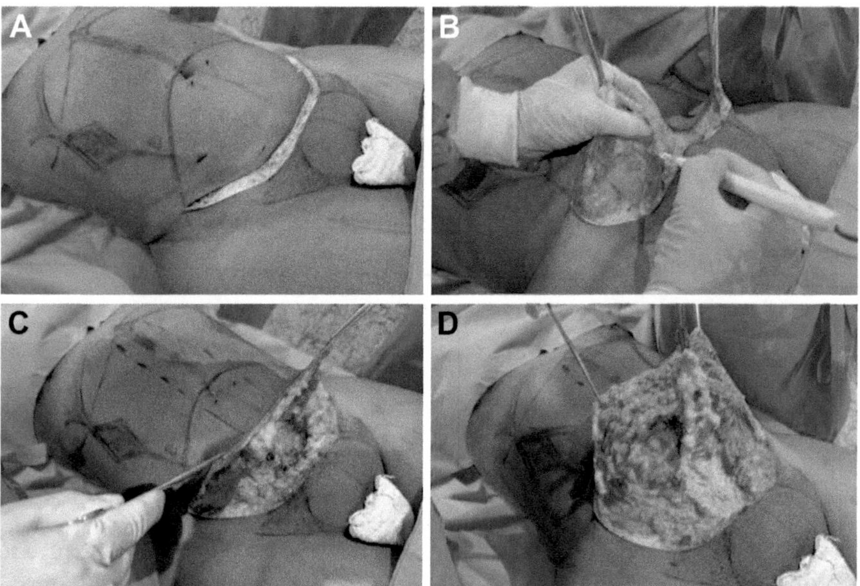

Fig. 6. (*A*) Superficial skin incision, avoiding damage to Scarpa's fascia. (*B*) Release of the suprafacial plane up to the level of the iliac crest. (*C*) Central portion of the fascia marked according to the diastasis. (*D*) Central portion of Scarpa's fascia excised together with fatty tissue for subsequent plication of the entire rectus abdominis, from the xiphoid process to the pubis.

structures, the Saldanha retractor is used. This is the most important part of the LADE, as the preservation of the vascularization of the abdominal wall is the fundamental principle of the technique and its low rate of complications[19,20] (**Fig. 7**).

Plication

In the infraumbilical area, the central portion of Scarpa's fascia over the diastasis is removed along with the fatty tissue, to expose the aponeurosis of the inner edges of the rectus abdominis for a complete plication from the xiphoid process to the pubis. At this stage, the edges of the rectus abdominis are joined by a running suture with Stratafix 0. Scarpa's fascia is then closed, brought back to the midline, and attached to the rectus abdominis aponeurosis, creating a pubic suspension and a shortening of the abdominal scar (**Figs. 8**A, B and **9**A, B).

The low abdominal transverse plication is made in specific cases, with BMI between 30 and 32, and patients that have a previous abdominal surgery with supraumbilical scars, which may represent a risk of necrosis. In that cases, we perform the TULANHA technique (Tulua and Saldanha's technique).

Removal of Excess Infraumbilical Skin

Excess skin from the lower abdomen should be removed after the surgeon has ensured that the flap easily reaches the symphysis pubis. Liposuction facilitates flap mobilization. Blunt cannulas are used to create additional blunt dissection and greater flap release, avoiding excessive tension on the suture line.

Complementary liposuction could be done after resecting the infraumbilical skin in some cases to optimize details and looking the balance of thickness between the flap and the pubis, always maintaining the safety and viability of the flap.

With the patient seated at 25° to 30°, excess skin from the abdominal flap is marked and excised. Also, at this stage, excess subfascial fat in the

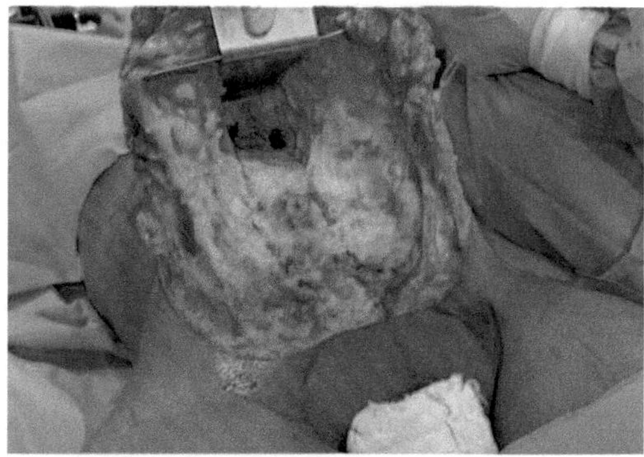

Fig. 7. Tunnel between the internal edges of the rectus abdominis muscles, going to the xiphoid process, according to the width of the diastasis; preserving most of the abdominal perforators.

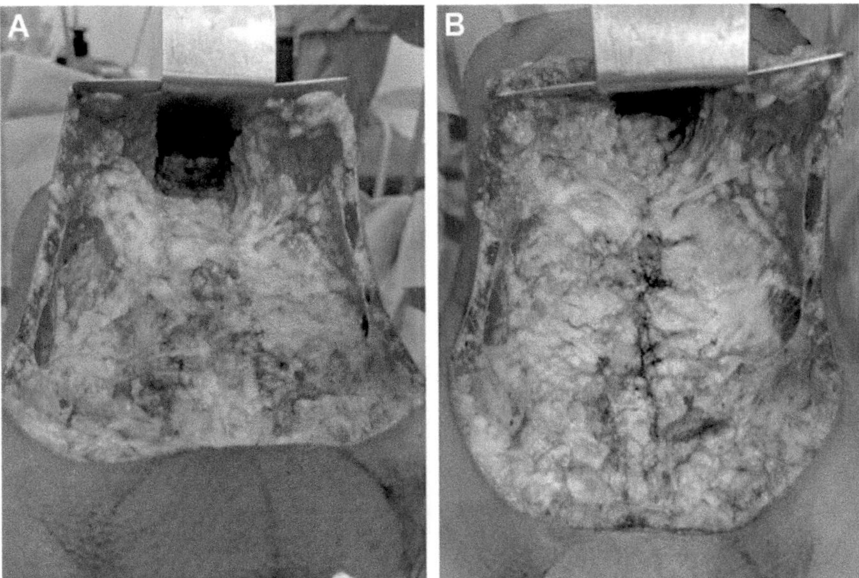

Fig. 8. (*A, B*) Approximation of the internal edges of the rectus abdominis by continuous suture with Stratafix® 0 thread.

lower third of the flap (yellow area) is resected (**Fig. 10**A, B).

Omphaloplasty

We used the "star-shaped omphaloplasty" technique. It is performed through a cross-shaped incision on the abdominal wall and a rectangular incision on the umbilical pedicle (**Fig. 11**).

The cardinal points of the umbilical pedicle are sutured, with subdermal points with Monocryl® 4-0, adjusting to the skin of the cruciform incision of the abdominal skin, repositioning the umbilical pedicle to the abdominal wall. Subsequently, the ends of the flaps are resected, and we finish with 4 complementary subdermal stitches (see **Fig. 10**).

The scar results in a continuous w-plasty, which presents less possibility of retraction. The pedicle

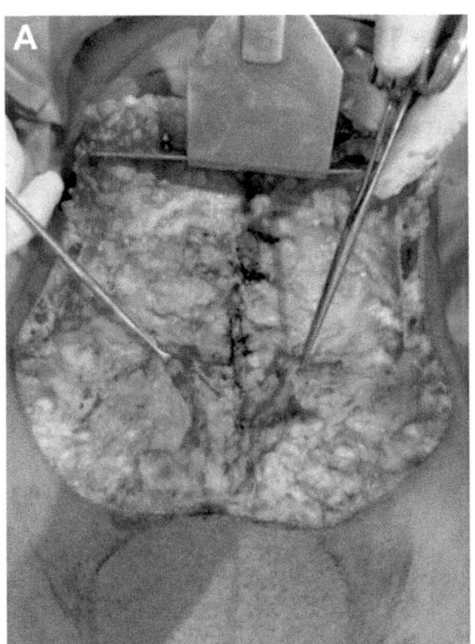

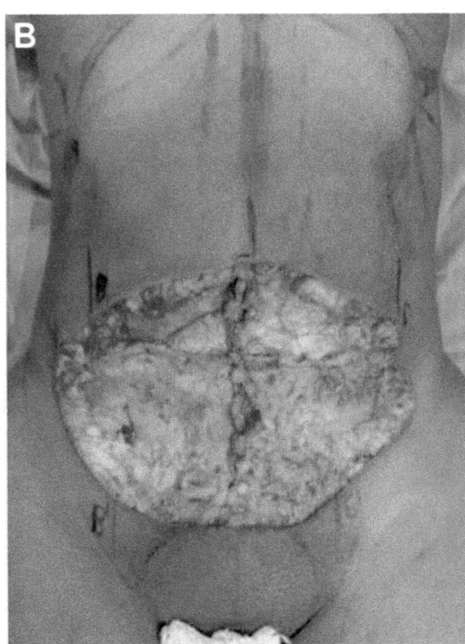

Fig. 9. (*A, B*) Closure of Scarpa's fascia with 4-0 nylon with continuous suture, fixing it to the aponeurosis of the rectus abdominis and bringing the edges together, without tension.

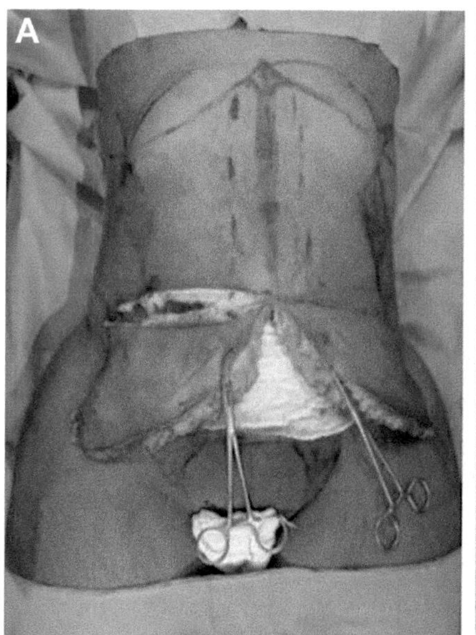

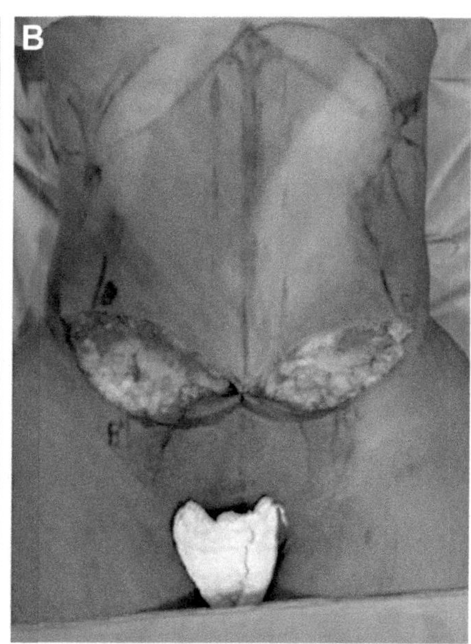

Fig. 10. (*A*) With the patient seated at 25° to 30°, confirm the arrival of the flap at the public symphysis to mark and resect. (*B*) Subsequently, when closing by layers, join points B with B′ and C with C′, avoiding folds and excess skin at the ends of the suture.

is fixed in a deep position in the plication line, which provides navels with excellent esthetic results, also masking the surgical intervention (see **Fig. 10**).

Suture, Drainage, Dressings, and Postoperative Care

The suture is performed in 2 planes with Monocryl® 3-0, one in the deep layer (connective tissue) and another subdermal with Monocryl® 4-0.

It is important to make a symmetric suture of the linea semilunaris, which should be directed to the pubic tubercle on each side (see **Fig. 10**B). We use a continuous aspiration drain that is removed when the drainage debit is less than 50 mL in 24 hours. This usually occurs on the first postoperative day, when the patient is discharged. The dressing is made with Micropore® directly over the suture line. External stitches are not used (**Fig. 12**).

We use intermittent pneumatic compression on the legs, between 30 and 40 mm Hg, during the procedure and in the immediate postoperative period. We continue to use it until the patient is capable of active mobilization. We recommend the use of medium compression stockings at home for a period of five days.

Silicone tapes (for compression of the negative areas of the sacral region and abdomen), straps (depending on the liposuction areas) are used for

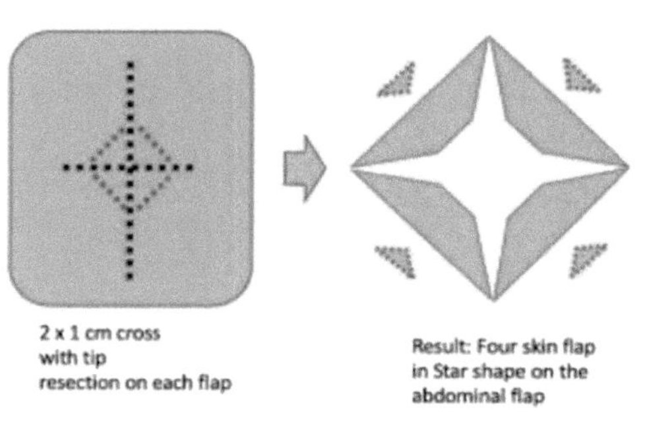

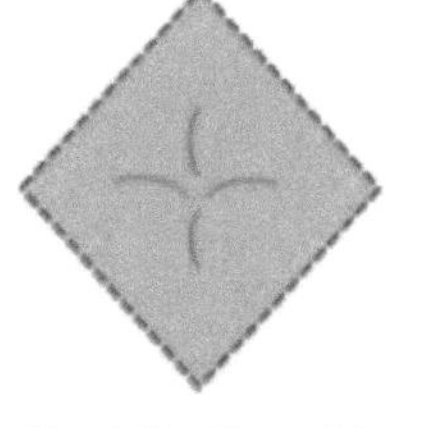

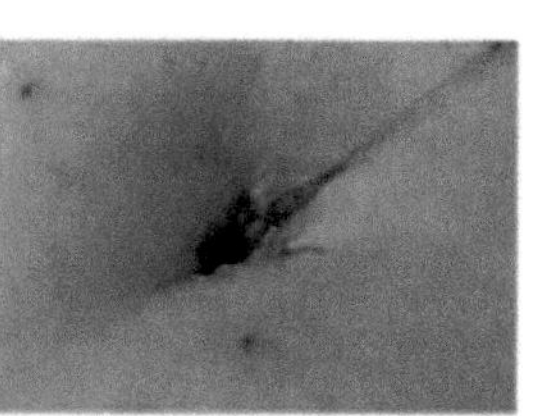

Fig. 11. Star omphaloplasty technique.

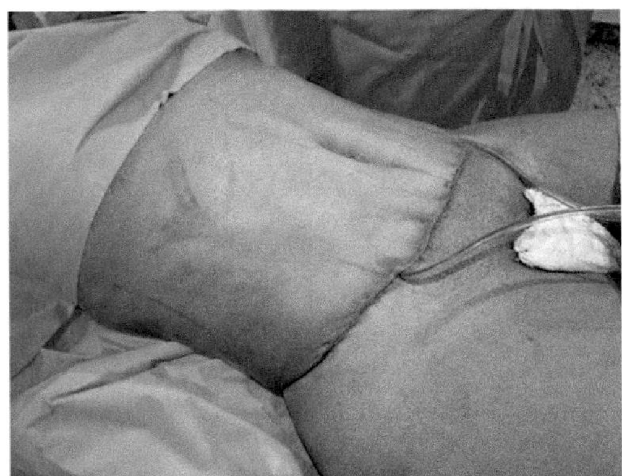

Fig. 12. Closing suture performed in 2 layers and continuous suction drain placement.

a period of 12 to 15 days. Care must be taken that there is no excessive compression on the abdominal flap (Fig. 13).

We routinely prescribe low-molecular-weight heparin (40 mg)—6 hours after the end of the procedure and the next day before walking. We also prescribe it for 7 days after hospital discharge. If there are risk factors for thromboembolic events present in the preoperative evaluation, an evaluation by the vascular surgeon is requested to guide a specific individualized protocol.

Antibiotic prophylaxis is prescribed intraoperatively and is maintained on an outpatient basis with first-generation cephalosporins for 7 days. Guaranteed analgesia with dipyrone 1 g every 6 hours and paracetamol + codeine (500/30 mg) every 8 hours, only if necessary.

As additional measures, we suggest performing lymphatic drainage, which should start on the fifth postoperative day. It should ideally be scheduled 2 to 3 times a week, totaling 10 to 15 sessions, as needed.

RESULTS

LADE is a step ahead of the traditional LAP technique. In the opinion of the author and as perceived by the patients, the esthetic results obtained are superior to the traditional technique. The contour is improved in a natural and harmonious way, because the anatomical limits are followed individually. Such results are possible while maintaining the security of traditional LAP (Figs. 14A, B; 15A, B; 16A, B; 17A, B).

Complication rates are low: seromas in 0.5%, small skin epitheliolysis in 0.2%, dehiscence in 0.5%, and necrosis in 0.1% of cases. We had no cases of major complications with systemic repercussions such as deep vein thrombosis. Complaints of irregularities or the need for secondary revision liposuction are rare, as we prioritize natural definition.

DISCUSSION

Liposuction techniques have significantly changed and evolved over time. We acquired a highly refined approach, with the aim of obtaining better esthetic

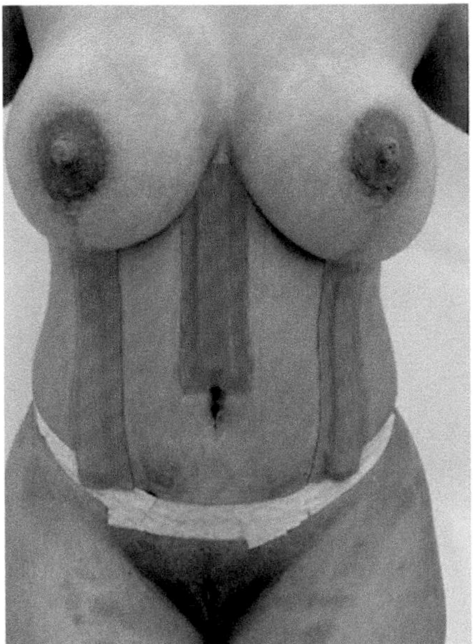

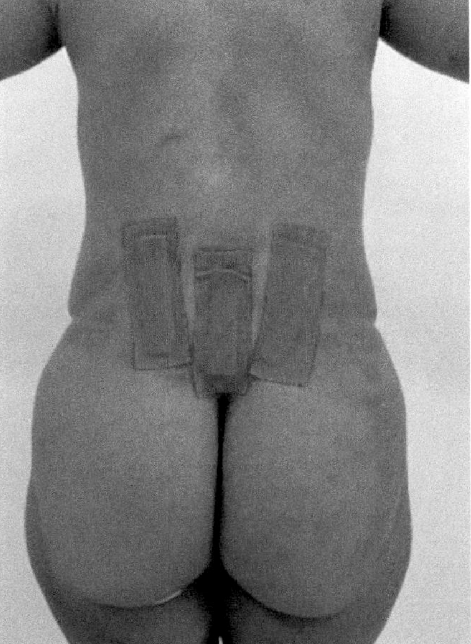

Fig. 13. Silicone surgical gutters placed on the second postoperative day, used for a period of 12 to 15 days, maintained during the drainage sessions.

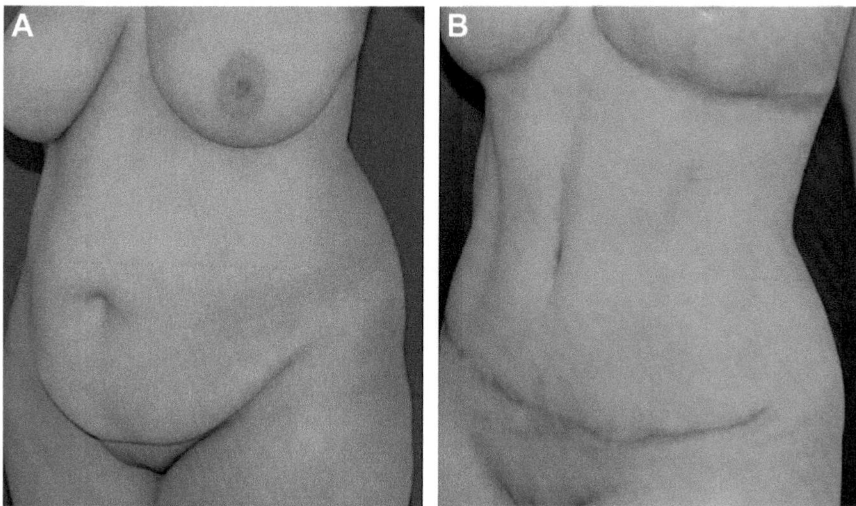

Fig. 14. (*A*) Preoperative photograph of a patient who underwent the LADE technique. (*B*) Postoperative photo 3 months after LADE.

results, defining the natural curves of the abdomen and highlighting muscle projections and insertions. The main objective is the incorporation of the anatomical variability of the patients in the marking, obtaining an individualized definition.

We must be rigorous in maintaining surgical safety, considering that there was a time when the combination of liposuction and abdominoplasty presented so many complications that their combination was almost prohibited.[2–4,8,9,21–25]

With the consolidation of the techniques described by Saldanha and colleagues[1]—widely studied until today—the standardization of LADE, its concepts and applicability is acknowledged worldwide—breaking the taboo on the high risk of this association. To perform it safely, the vascular territories of the abdominal wall must be known.[18,26–28]

Thanks to the studies carried out by Graf and Munhoz (2006), it was possible to observe the importance of maintaining the perforating vessels.[21,22] The greater the number of perforators in the flap, the greater the safety for the patient and the lower the risk in performing a more intense liposuction.[25–33]

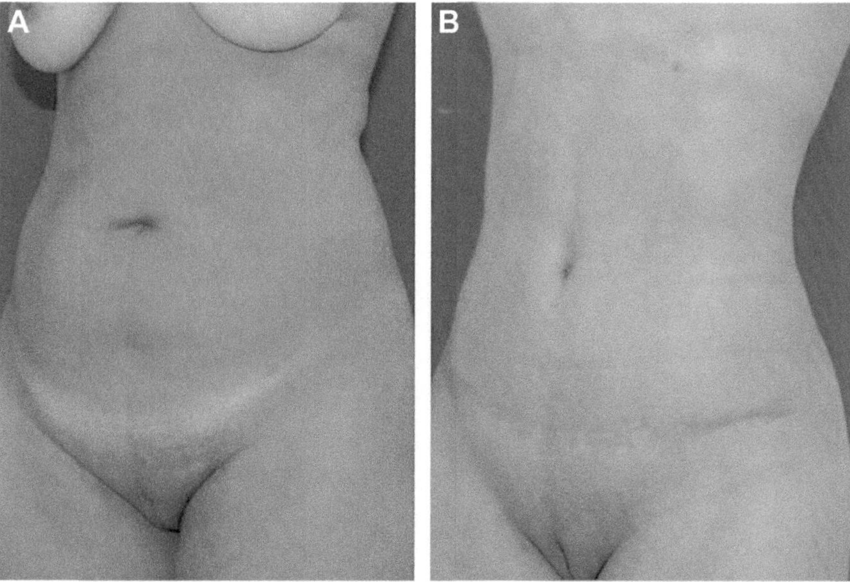

Fig. 15. (*A*) Preoperative photograph of a patient who underwent the LADE technique. (*B*) Postoperative photo 1 year after LADE.

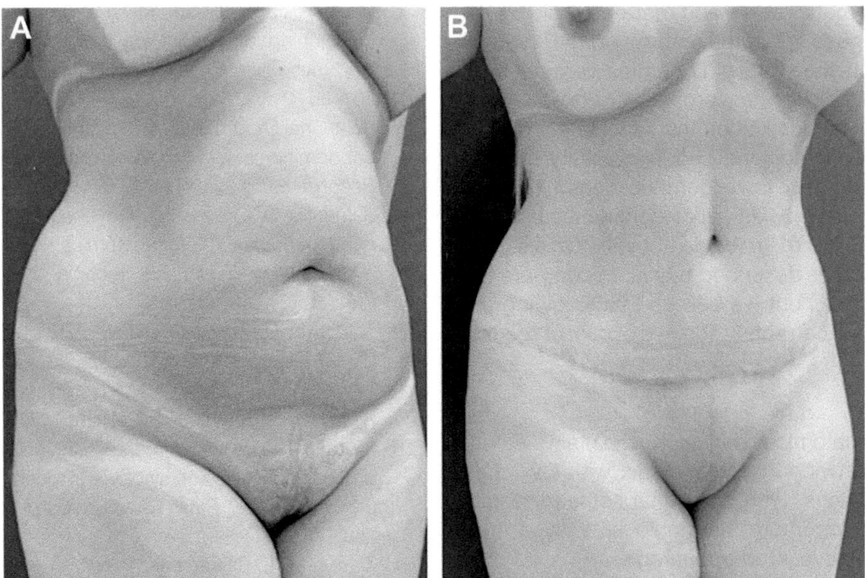

Fig. 16. (*A*) Preoperative photograph of a patient who underwent the LADE technique. (*B*) Postoperative photo 1 year after LADE.

As previously mentioned, the scope of the definition depends on numerous factors, such as the patient's BMI, skin quality, local muscle mass, the existence of intrinsic abnormalities, and/or deformities of the abdominal wall.

It is important to inform our patients that not everyone will achieve high definition; in fact, most will get moderate or even low definition. The definition of the abdominal region generates a better esthetic result, but when there is a greater risk of flap damage or multiple secondary procedures, we prefer to perform less aggressive, selective liposuction, without compromising the aforementioned anatomical safety.

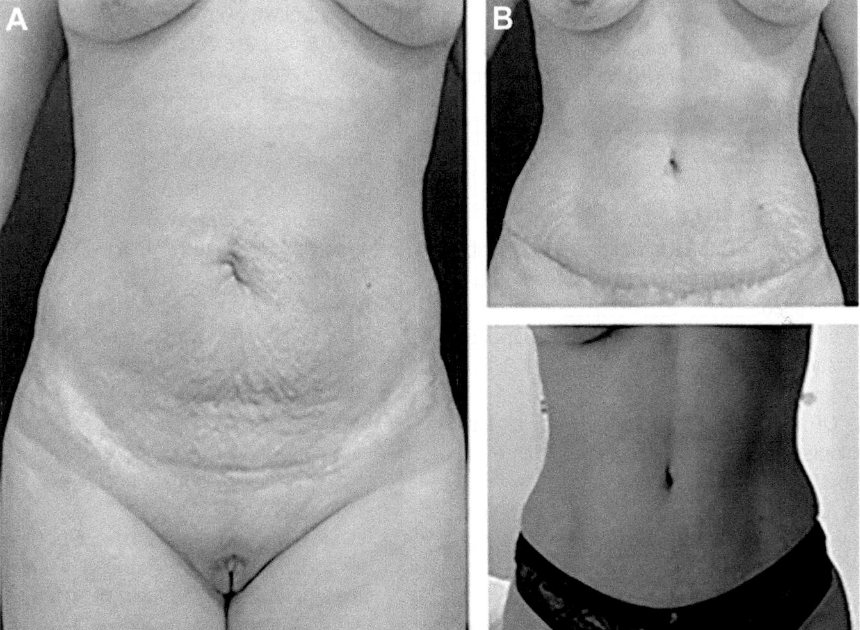

Fig. 17. (*A*) Preoperative photograph of a patient who underwent the LADE technique. (*B*) Postoperative photo 3 months after LADE.

In a systematic review and meta-analysis by Xia and colleagues[33] on the safety of LAP versus abdominoplasty, a total of 17 studies were selected from 483 eligible articles, providing data on 14,061 patients.[22] The publication tests the safety of LAP compared with traditional abdominoplasty, statistically demonstrating fewer complications in the LAP group (relative risk, 0.85; 95% confidence interval, 0.74–0.97; $P = 0.017$). We do not yet have a similar number of cases described by Xia, to compare the results of LADE, but we believe that following the technique, we can safely achieve excellent results.

SUMMARY

LAP with anatomical definition, maintains safety standards provided by LAP alone, with low rates of complications, with additional esthetic results that are much more harmonious, with a true abdominal rejuvenated appearance.

CLINICS CARE POINTS

- An adequate selection of the patient, a rigorous surgical marking, and respecting the liposuction areas are a guarantee of a more optimal result.
- Avoid excessive release in the midline to avoid compromising the irrigation of the flap.
- Preserve the Scarpa fascia to decrease associated morbidity.
- When performing omphaloplasty, the star technique is ideal to avoid retraction or closure of the new navel.

REFERENCES

1. Saldanha OR, Pinto EB, Matos WN Jr, et al. Lipoabdominoplasty without undermining. Aesthetic Surg J 2001;21(6):518–26.
2. Saldanha OR, Federico R, Daher PF, et al. Lipoabdominoplasty. Plast Reconstr Surg 2009;124: 934–42.
3. Saldanha OR, Azevedo SF, Delboni PS, et al. Lipoabdominoplasty: saldanha's technique. Clin Plast Surg 2010;37(3). 469–8.
4. Illouz YG. Body contouring by lipolysis: a 5-year experience with over 3000 cases. Plast Reconstr Surg 1983;72:591–7.
5. Villegas F. Abdominoplasty without flap dissection, full liposuction, transverse infraumbilical plication and neoumbilicoplasty with skin graft. (T.U.L.U.A). Can J Plast Surg 2011;19(A):95.
6. Mentz HA 3rd, Gilliland MD, Patronella CK. Abdominal etching: differential liposuction to detail abdominal musculature. Aesthetic Plast Surg 1993;17: 287–90.
7. Saldanha O, Ordenes A, Goyeneche C, et al. Lipoabdominoplasty with anatomical definition. Plast Reconstr Surg 2020;146(4):766–77.
8. Saldanha O, Ordenes A, Goyeneche C, et al. Lipoabdominoplasty with anatomical definition – Na evolution on saldanha's technique. Clin Plastic Surg 2020;1–15.
9. Saldanha O, Salles AG, Llaveria F, et al. Saldanha CB - Predictive factors for complications in plastic surgery procedures – suggested safety scores. Rev Bras Cir Plást 2014;29(1):105–13.
10. Tourani SS, Taylor GI, Ashtom MD. Scarpa fascia preservation in abdominoplasty: does it preserve the lymphatics? Plast Reconstr Surg 2015;136(2): 258.
11. Xiao X, Ye L. Efficacy and safety of Scarpa& fascia preservation during abdominoplasty: systematic review and meta-analysis. Aesthetic Plast Surg 2017; 41(3):585–90.
12. Friedman T, Coon D, Kanbour-shakir A, et al. Defining the lymphatic system of the anterior abdominal wall: an anatomical study. Plast Rebuild Surg 2015;135(4):1027–32.
13. Har-Shai L, Hayun Y, Barel E, et al. [scarpa fascia and abdominal wall deep adipose compartment preservation in abdominoplasty - current clinical and anatomical review]. Harefuah 2018;157(2): 87–90.
14. Costa-Ferreira A, Marco R, Vásconez L, et al. Abdominoplasty with scarpa fascia preservation. Ann Plast Surg 2016;76(Suppl 4):S264–74.
15. Costa-Ferreira A, Rebelo M, Silva A, et al. Scarpa fascia preservation during abdominoplasty: randomized clinical study of efficacy and safety. Plast Reconstr Surg 2013;131(3):644–51.
16. Costa-Ferreira A, Rebelo M, Vásconez LO, et al. Scarpa fascia preservation during abdominoplasty: a prospective study. Plast Rebuild Surg 2010; 125(4):1232–9.
17. Ardehali B, Fiorentino F. A meta-analysis of the effects of abdominoplasty modifications on the incidence of postoperative seroma. Aesthetic Surg J 2017;37(10):1136–43.
18. Seretis K, Goulis D, Demiri EC, et al. Prevention of seroma formation following abdominoplasty: a systematic review and meta-analysis. Aesthetic Surg J 2017;37(3):316–23.
19. Nahai F, Brown RG, Vasconez LO. Blood supply to the abdominal wall as related to planning abdominal incisions. Am Surg 1976;42(9):691–5.
20. Fodor PB, Cimino WW, Watson JP, et al. Suction-assisted lipoplasty: physics, optimization and clinical verification. Aesthetic Surg J 2005;25:234–46.

21. Ruth Graf et al. Lipoabdominoplasty 2004.
22. Munhoz e cols. Lipoabdominoplastia 2006. Chapter 12 of lipoabdominoplasty. 1st ed. Rio de Janeiro: Di-Livros; 2006.
23. Saldanha O, Salles A, Ferreira M, et al. Aesthetic evaluation of lipoabdominoplasty in overweight patients. Plast Reconstr Surg 2013;132(5):1103–12.
24. Babaitis R. BOOK: Lipodefinition – 3rd Generation of Liposuction.
25. Swanson E. Comparison of limited and full dissection abdominoplasty using laser fluorescence imaging to evaluate perfusion of the abdominal skin. Plast Reconstr Surg 2015;136:31e–43e.
26. Huger WE Jr. The anatomical rationale for abdominal lipectomy. Am Surg 1979;45(9):612–7.
27. El-Mrakby H.H. and Milner R.H., The vascular anatomy of the lower anterior abdominal wall: a microdissection study on the deep inferior epigastric vessels and the perforator branches, *Plast Reconstr Surg*, 109, 2002, 539–547. discussion 544-547.
28. Rozen WM, Ashton MW, Le Roux CM, et al. The perforating angiosome: a new concept in the design of deep inferior epigastric artery perforating flaps for breast reconstruction. Microsurgery 2010;30:1.
29. Smith LF, Smith LF Jr. Safely combining abdominoplasty with aggressive abdominal liposuction based on perforating vessels: technique and Review of 300 consecutive cases. Plast Reconstr Surg 2015;35(5): 1357–66.
30. Gutowski KA. Evidence-based medicine: abdominoplasty. Plast Reconstr Surg 2018;141(2):286e–99e.
31. Husain TM, Salgado CJ, Mundra LS, et al. Abdominal etching: surgical technique and outcomes. Plast Reconstr Surg 2019;143(4):1051–60.
32. Danilla S. Rectus abdominis fat transfer (RAFT) in lipoabdominoplasty: a new technique to achieve fitness body contour in patients that require tummy tuck. Aesthetic Plast Surg 2017;41(6):1389–99.
33. Xia Y, Zhao J, Cao DS. Safety of lipoabdominoplasty versus abdominoplasty: a systematic review and meta-analysis. Aesthetic Plast Surg 2019;43:167–74.

Management of the Musculoaponeurotic Layer in Abdominoplasty

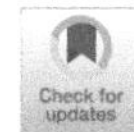

Fabio Xerfan Nahas, MD, PhD, MBA[a,*], Lydia Masako Ferreira, MD, PhD, MBA[b]

KEYWORDS

• Abdominoplasty • Rectus sheath • Technique • Plication • Rectus muscle • External oblique muscle

KEY POINTS

- The deformities of the myoaponeurotic layer of the abdomen are diverse.
- These deformities need specific techniques and should be identified.
- The knowledge of the local anatomy is paramount to understand and correct these deformities.
- Anatomical and histological conditions as well as the patient's age and amount of intraabdominal fat may limit the cosmetic result.

INTRODUCTION

The musculoaponeurotic layer of the anterior abdomen is an important layer of stabilization of the body, considered as the core of the body in physical exercises. It helps to balance the forces of the posterior abdominal wall, especially by the tension of the transverse muscle aponeurosis that keeps vertebral bones in place, avoiding nerve compression. A weak anterior abdominal wall may lead to back pain. For this reason, a patient with a lax abdominal wall with a large rectus diastasis may present an untreatable back pain by the traditional methods. This layer is also partially responsible for the cosmetic aspect of the abdomen. A lax anterior abdominal wall allows the projection of the abdominal organs forward and laterally.

It is paramount that plastic surgeons understand the histology and anatomy of muscles and fascias of the area as well as the available techniques to correct it. It is also relevant to know the types of suture that are more suitable for each technique and the possible repercussions of its correction both in the patient's pulmonary ventilation and in the venous flow of the lower limbs.

The idea of this article is to gather the most popular techniques available for the correction of these deformities and defects and to describe some of the scientific background behind them.

Histopathological Aspects

Fascias and muscles are the structures that provide support for the abdominal wall. In the body, the rib cage protects the lungs and heart, but in the abdominal region, its protection is made by muscles and aponeurosis only. These structures are very solid in the early ages, especially up to the 30th year of life. After that, there is an ageing process that changes its main structural fibers, the collagen.

In the aponeurosis, there are 2 types of collagen. Type I is the strongest fiber and keeps the aponeurotic resistance. Type III collagen is a more flexible fiber and is responsible for the abdominal movements and torsion. Each individual has a specific ratio between these fibers and that will determine the degree of laxity of the aponeurotic layer. It is known that patients who present direct hernias will have more type III fibers in the ratio as

[a] Adjunct Professor of Plastic Surgery, Federal University of São Paulo, UNIFESP, EPM, Av. Brasil 275, São Paulo, São Paulo 01431-000, Brazil; [b] Head and Full Professor, Federal University of São Paulo, UNIFESP, EPM, R. Napoleão de Barros, 715 – 4o. andar, São Paulo, São Paulo 04024-002, Brazil
* Corresponding author.
E-mail address: fabionahas@outlook.com

Clin Plastic Surg 51 (2024) 59–69
https://doi.org/10.1016/j.cps.2023.07.007
0094-1298/24/

compared to type I. Elderly patients will present an increase in type III collagen as compared to young patients. This condition will allow the abdominal wall to project, even if the patient has no rectus diastasis. These patients are more prone to develop recurrence of the deformity after plastic surgery. It is known that individuals who practice physical exercises will present less deformity and a more balanced ratio of collagen I/III.[1]

In the muscles, there are collagen I, III, IV, and V. In a study by Calvi and colleagues[2,3] in 2014, the amount of collagen I and III were significantly decreased in cadavers older than 30 years of age as compared to the younger group. This shows that the collagen structure not only of aponeurosis but also of muscles decrease with age as well. All these factors allow the diameter of the abdomen increase, independently of the adipose accumulation both in the abdominal cavity and in the subcutaneous.

Surgical anatomy

The main components of the surgical anatomy of the myoaponeurotic layer of the anterior abdominal wall are the recti muscles and the muscles of the flank (external oblique, internal oblique, and the transverse muscle) and the aponeurotic layer that imbricates all these muscles.

Each muscle of the flank has 2 aponeurotic layers that will extend toward the midline, forming the anterior and the posterior rectus sheath. Above the Arcuate Line, the external oblique aponeurosis and the part of the internal oblique aponeurosis will form the anterior rectus sheath, whereas the posterior rectus sheath will be formed by part of the internal oblique aponeurosis and the transverse muscle aponeurosis. Below the Arcuate Line, all the aponeurosis of the muscles of the flank will fuse and form the anterior rectus sheath. There is no posterior sheath below the Arcuate Line. This has a relevant impact in the thickness of the anterior rectus sheath in the lower abdomen, where any plication of this aponeurosis will be more reliable and less likely to present recurrence.

Usually, the wider area of postpregnancy diastasis is in the upper abdomen, close to the umbilicus. This is a very critical area to be corrected during plication and if there are hernias, they should be corrected. Some of these hernias are very small and not detected by ultrasound examination. This is why liposuction should be done with extreme care in the midline above the umbilicus. Some of these defects are virtual (between the decussation of the aponeurotic fusion form both sides) and the small tip of the cannulas will penetrate easily.

The normal separation between the recti muscles is between 1 and 1.5 cm.[4] When the plastic surgeon corrects the diastasis, it is important not to erase this fold. It can be erased by wide plications, when the approximation is done beyond the medial edges of the muscles. If this natural midline fold is erased, an abnormal contour of the abdomen is created.

The rectus diastasis is, most of the times, secondary to pregnancy and it has a fusiform aspect, with the muscles' insertion and origin close together in the midline. This is known by the general surgeons as epigastric hernia, which is a defect that does not have necessarily a hernia and was not recognized by plastic surgeons. This special condition is defined by a lateral insertion of the recti muscles at the costal margin and a specific technique should be done to correct it.

There is another aesthetic line that is located in the lateral aspect of the recti muscles. This corresponds to the projection of the semilunaris line. More modern techniques[5] make plications in these lines and in the midline so that the hypertrophy of the muscles will occur when patients exercise. Also, definition liposuction may be performed in these lines to highlight these areas.

It is also paramount to understand the anatomy of the muscles of the flank. There is a very loose connective tissue between the external and the internal oblique muscles. This allows a certain advancement of the external oblique muscle just by the plication of its aponeurosis, with no need for advancing them to improve the waistline in all cases.

The layer between the internal oblique and the transverse muscles is a much more difficult layer of dissection due to the presence of numerous vessels and nerves. These are motor nerves of the recti muscles and, if severed, there will occur a partial paralysis of this muscle.

In cases of extreme laxity of the abdominal wall, the balance between the anterior and the posterior abdominal wall is affected with a consequent compression of the nerves between the vertebrae. To reposition the vertebrae, it is necessary to exert traction in the lumbar fascia. The only muscle that surrounds the abdominal cavity completely is the transversus muscle. For this reason, some techniques have been described to correct low back pain by the traction of the transversus aponeurosis, which extends to the lumbar fascia.[6,7]

Evaluation/classification

A very easy way to evaluate the abdominal wall during surgery is to check first the diastasis and the insertion of the recti muscles. This is the first step to decide which technique to use. If the diastasis is fusiform (Type A), a plication approximating the medial edges of the recti muscles can be done. On the other hand, if there is a lateral insertion of the recti muscles in the costal margins (Type C), an advancement of the recti sheaths should be performed. The next step is to evaluate if there is still laxity after the plication of the recti muscles in Type A patients. In these cases, instead of making a more ample plication (that would erase the projection of the recti muscles in the abdomen), an "L" plication of the aponeurosis of the external oblique muscle should be done (Type B). The plastic surgeon can also indicate the advancement of the external oblique muscle associated with the plication of Type A patients, in more selective cases, if he judges that the patient needs a more marked waistline (Type D). This is a summary of the classification of the myoaponeurotic deformities[8] that will be described as follows (**Fig. 1**).

Type A

Deformity: These are patients that present a fusiform diastasis, in which the recti muscles are medially inserted in the costal margins.

Management: Plication of the anterior rectus sheath, approximating the muscle's medial edges (**Fig. 2**).

Scientific background: The plication in this type of patients is a very stable procedure. A series of prospective studies has proven using CT Scans that when 2-0 nylon sutures are used in a 2-layer fashion, it is stable for at least 6 months[9] and the same has been observed with 0-polydioxanone suture (PDS).[10] Two long-term studies have demonstrated that patients who had 2-0 nylon recti plications had no recurrence in an average follow-up of 7 years in a prospective study[11] and similar findings in a 4-year follow-up were observed when 0-PDS was used.[12] Another article has shown that rectus diastasis may resist pregnancy 2 years after the operation.[13]

Gama and colleagues (2017)[14] have compared 3 groups of 15 patients when different techniques were used. In one group, a 2-layer suture was used with no recurrence, in the second group, a Quill suture was used (and presented a 30% recurrence rate), whereas in the third group, a continuous suture was used and there was no recurrence rate with a statistically significant shorter time. Therefore, the last was very efficient and saved time.

Verissimo and colleagues (2014)[15] have used a triangular suture that corrects rectus diastasis and shortens the vertical elongation of the aponeurosis at the same time.

With these 2 last studies, we have changed our technique. We are currently doing 3 or 4 stitches in the infraumbilical using the triangular sutures (running from 2 to 3 cm vertically in the aponeurosis) and 3 more stitches in the supraumbilical area. A second layer of continuous suture is performed, locking every 2 or 3 passes.

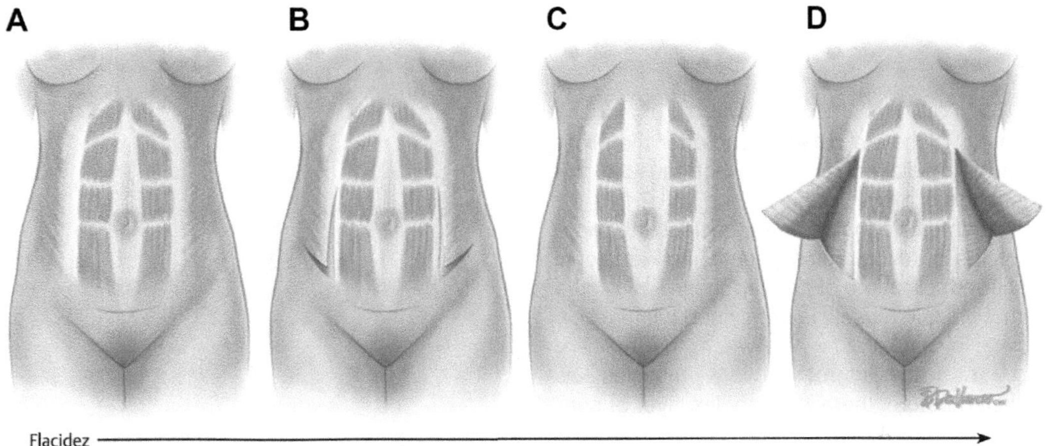

Fig. 1. Types of myoaponeurotic deformities: Type (*A*) –Rectus diastasis secondary to pregnancy; Type (*B*) – Rectus diastasis secondary to pregnancy not completely treated by the correction of diastasis. In this case, the "L" plication of the external oblique aponeurosis is indicated; Type (*C*) – Lateral insertion of the recti muscles (congenital rectus diastasis). In these patients, the advancement of the recti sheaths is indicated; Type (*D*) – Rectus diastasis secondary to pregnancy associated with a poor waistline. In these patients, the advancement of the recti sheaths is indicated. (*From* Aly A, Nahas F. The Art of Body Contouring: A Comprehensive Approach. Thieme; 2017; with permission.)

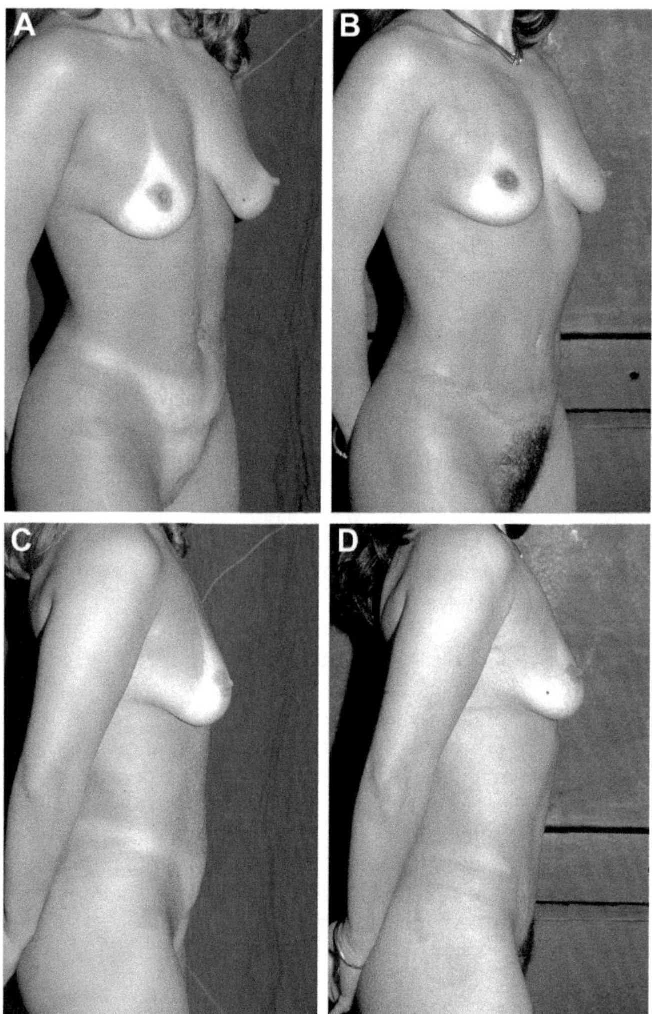

Fig. 2. This is the preoperative oblique view (*A*) and lateral view (*C*) of a 28-year-old female who presented rectus diastasis secondary to pregnancy; The postoperative oblique view (*B*) and lateral view (*D*) after a 2-layer plication was performed to correct rectus diastasis (Type [*A*] deformity).

Type B

Deformity: These are patients who after the plication of the medial edges of the recti muscles still present some laxity.

Management: In these cases, besides the plication of the anterior rectus sheath, an additional "L"-shaped plication of the aponeurosis of the external oblique muscle is performed bilaterally.

Scientific background: Between the external oblique and the internal oblique muscles, as mentioned before, there is a very lax layer of connective tissue, therefore the plication of the external oblique aponeurosis allows this muscle to slide over the internal oblique and there is a shortening between the origin and insertion of the muscle, thus optimizing its function. The horizontal branch of this plication shortens the vertical aspect of the anterior abdominal wall. As the deformity of the abdomen formed after pregnancy

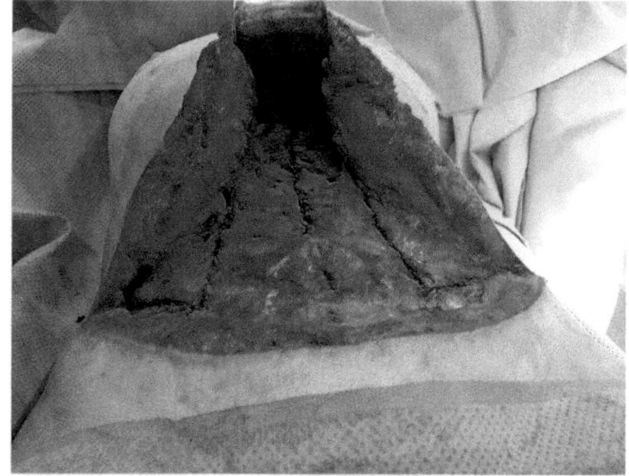

Fig. 3. Intraoperative aspect of the "L" plication of the external oblique aponeurosis.

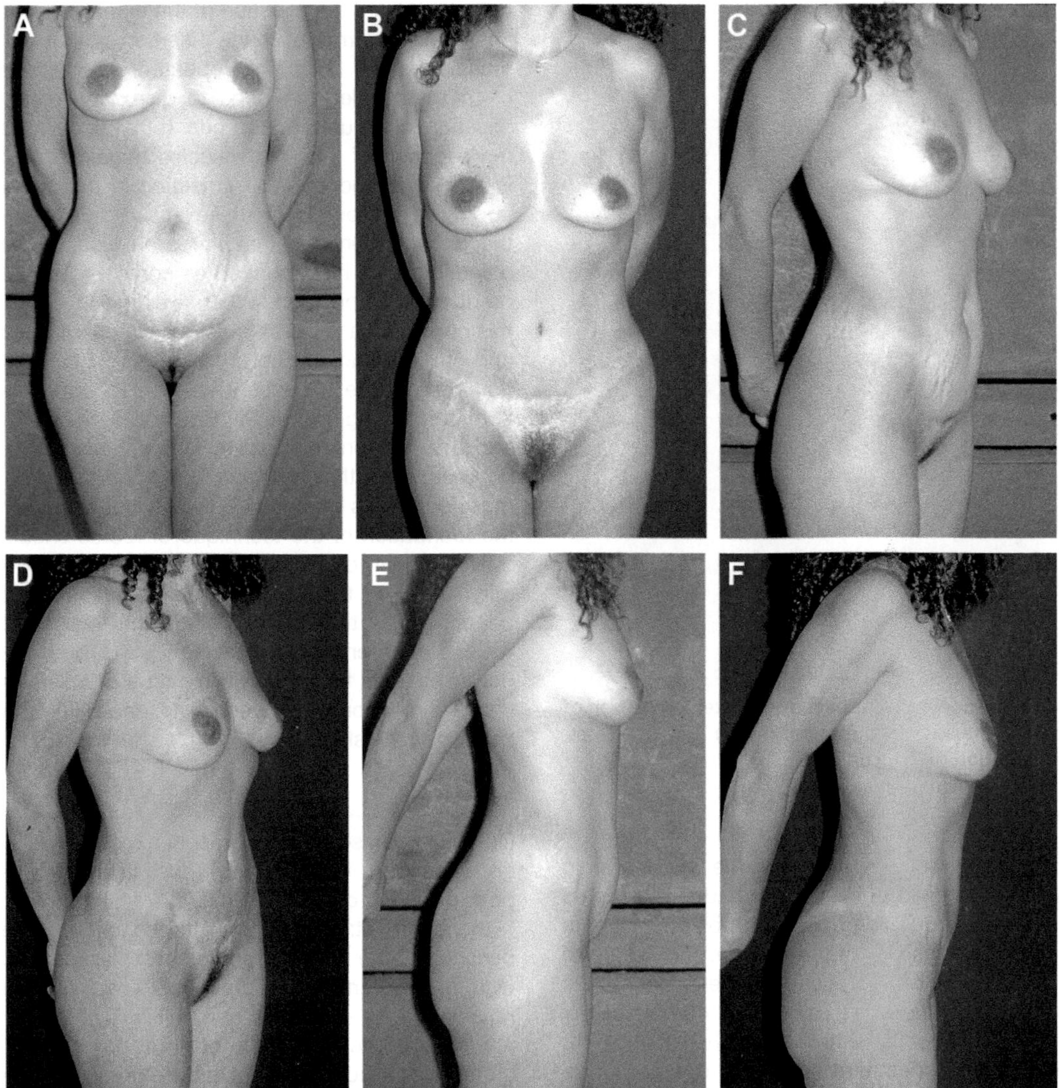

Fig. 4. Preoperative frontal (*A*), oblique (*C*) and lateral view (*E*) of a Type B deformity in a 32-year-old female. The patients presented persistent laxity after correction of rectus diastasis. For this reason, the "L" plication of the external oblique aponeurosis was performed and the result is observed on the frontal (*B*), oblique (*D*) and lateral view (*F*).

is multidirectional, a vertical associated to a horizontal shortening of the aponeurosis is desirable. The "L" plication of the external oblique aponeurosis helps to improve the fine contour of the abdomen, helping in the definition of this area. Plications should be placed between the muscles, where the natural folds and dimples of the abdomen are located. The midline fold in the upper abdomen is a typical example, created by the aponeurotic area between the recti muscles, the linea alba. Another natural fold is between the recti muscle and the external oblique muscle (semilunaris line), in the exact area where the vertical branch of the "L" plication is performed (**Fig. 3**). Sooudi and colleagues[16] have demonstrated that both of these lines, when visible, are the most significant signs of beauty in the abdomen.

The "L" plication also helps to increase waist definition, as the result of a medial inferior vector in the aponeurosis caused by this maneuver (**Fig. 4**).

Type C

Deformity: These patients present a lateral insertion of the recti muscles in the costal margin (**Fig. 5**). It is a congenital deformity and may be impaired after pregnancy.

Management: The advancement of the recti sheaths is performed. A longitudinal incision of

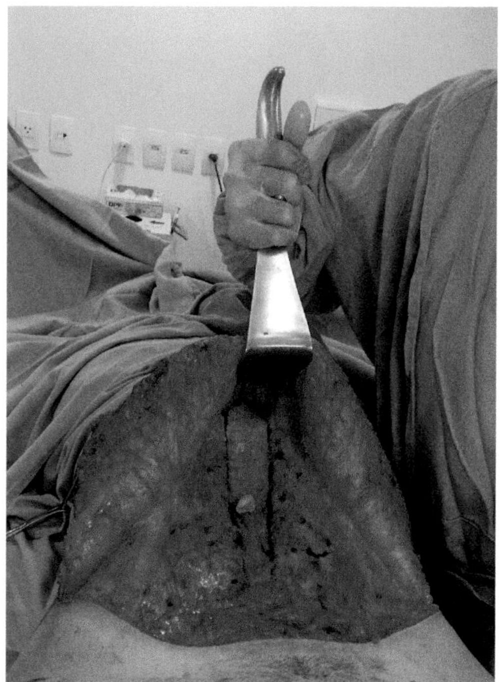

Fig. 5. Intraoperative aspect of the lateral insertion of the recti muscles in the costal margin. In such cases, the plication may recur.

the anterior rectus sheath from the costal margin inferiorly to the arcuate line is made. The rectus muscle is undermined from its posterior sheath to the lateral aspect of the muscle. A plication of the posterior rectus sheath is performed, thus invaginating the linea alba. To complete the advancement of the recti sheaths, the left and right anterior recti sheaths are sutured together in the midline (**Fig. 6**).

Scientific background: The lateral insertion of the recti muscles is a special congenital condition that will recur if the plication of the anterior rectus sheath is performed. As the insertion of the recti muscles is not confluent, repeated contractions of these muscles may lead to disruption of the plication in the upper abdomen. If that occurs, as the plication of the recti muscles remains intact in the lower abdomen, a projection of the upper abdomen will occur. In these cases, not rarely, the patient mentions that the projection of the epigastric area has impaired as compared to the preoperative condition. When we first identified this condition, a study in cadavers was performed and it has shown that there is a significant decrease in the necessary traction to bring the aponeurotic edges to the midline both in the upper and lower abdomen and in the anterior and posterior rectus sheath after the separation of the rectus muscle from its posterior sheath, what has been the foundation of the technique of rectus sheath advancement described to correct this deformity.[17,18] For this reason, this technique has been used in these cases since the year 2000 with no recurrence of diastasis (**Fig. 7**). The number of patients that present this type of diastasis varies from around between 8%[8] and 5%[19] according these studies.

Type D

Deformity: These patients present a rectus diastasis secondary to pregnancy associated with a poor definition of the waistline.

Management: These patients benefit from a plication of the anterior rectus sheath associated with the advancement of the external oblique muscles.

Scientific background: In our previous study in cadavers, the advancement of the external oblique muscles has a greater impact in the waistline as compared to the plication of the anterior rectus sheath.[20]

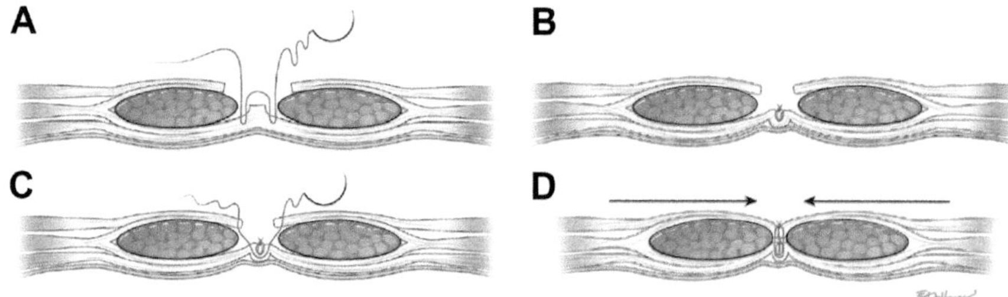

Fig. 6. This illustration shows how the advancement of the recti sheaths is done. (*A*). The first step is to make a vertical incision along the anterior rectus sheath, close to the linea alba to grant access to the posterior rectus sheath that is plicated. (*B*). The linea alba is plicated and invaginated. (*C*). A second suture is placed in the anterior rectus sheath and it is attached to the posterior sheath in the midline. (*D*) As the knot is tied, it brings the anterior aponeurosis attached to the rectus muscle toward the midline. (*From* Aly A, Nahas F. The Art of Body Contouring: A Comprehensive Approach. Thieme; 2017; with permission.)

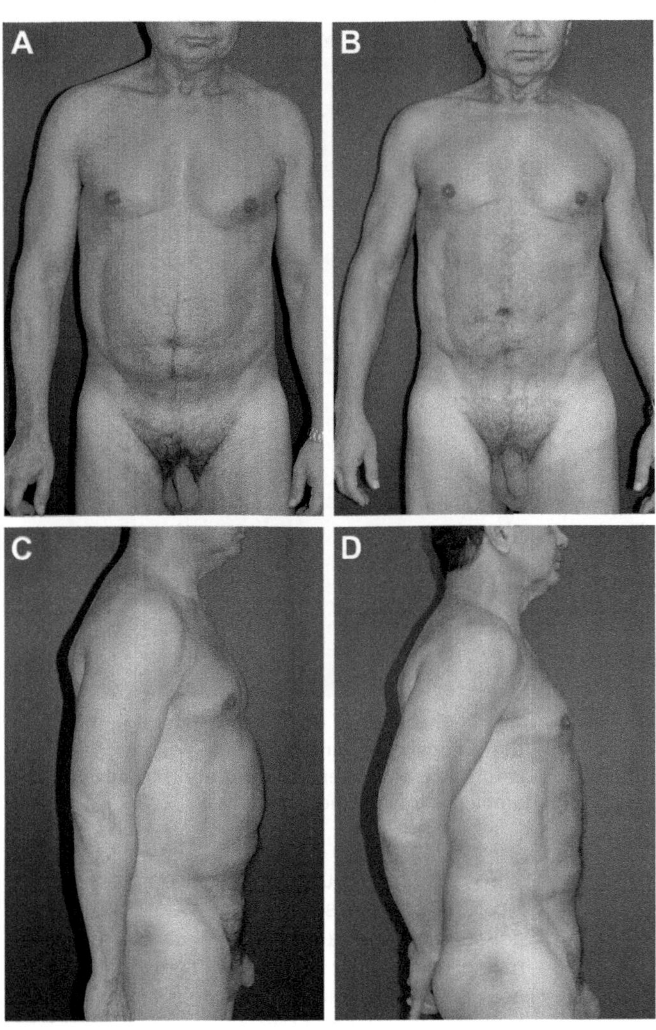

Fig. 7. This is the preoperative frontal (*A*) and lateral view (*C*) a Type (*C*) deformity in a 68-year-old male who presented a projected upper abdomen since his childhood, however, it has progressively impaired with age. He presented a lateral insertion of the recti muscles and the advancement of the recti sheath has been performed, correcting the projection of the upper abdomen and also bringing the semilunaris line more medially as seen on the frontal view (B) and on the lateral view (*D*).

Other Types of Plications

Several types of plication of the recti muscles have been described.

Tulua

Tulua is a technique created by Villegas and colleagues[21] in which a horizontal plication is performed including the area between the umbilicus and the pubis. It is performed with the operating table flexed to allow such a large plication. No skin undermining is performed. The skin is closed and the umbilicus is grafted in the ideal position. A vertical correction of the diastasis can be associated whenever necessary by dissecting a small tunnel over the linea alba and the medial aspect of the recti muscles. Although it is not a technique based on the correction of anatomical changes that occur after pregnancy, results are consistent. There are some issues that should be studied such as the possibility of inguinal and/or crural hernia formation due to the extreme traction exerted in the aponeurosis of the lower abdomen.[22]

Other Types of Plication–Indications

Many types of plications have been described, transverse, oblique, and horizontal, over the anterior rectus sheath and the external oblique aponeurosis.[23–26] In our view, these plications can be associated to the previous techniques described in specific deformities of the abdomen (**Figs. 8** and **9**).

Refinements–the Idea of Muscle Definition

The idea of not making any plications over the abdominal muscles allows natural results. This permits the natural projection of the muscles,

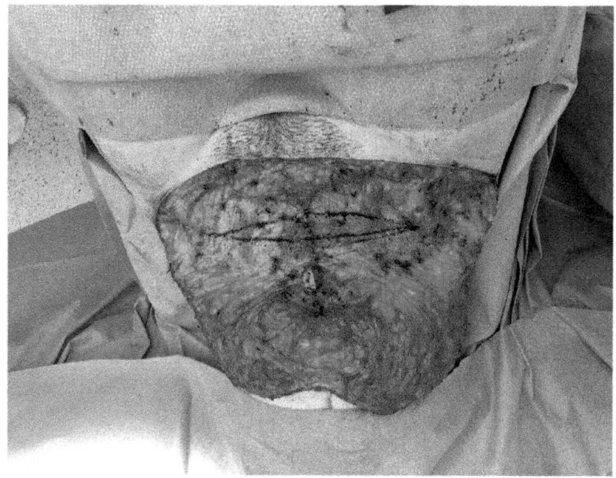

Fig. 8. An atypical horizontal plication in the aponeurosis. This patient, even after the plication, he still presented some laxity in the lower abdomen. A horizontal plication was performed to correct a localized deformity in that area. The horizontal plication also helps to bring the abdominal flap toward the pubis.

especially if the patient works out. Therefore, plications are always made in the areas of depression and folds in the anterior abdomen, such as over the linea alba and the semilunaris line.

Ample plications over the recti muscles, trying to correct the abdominal wall laxity may erase the fine contour of the abdomen, displacing these muscles.

If the local anatomy is preserved, when the patient exercises, muscle hypertrophy occurs as seen in **Figs. 3** and **10**. This will provide a long-lasting result.

Suture materials

The ideal suture for abdominal plication is either nonabsorbable 2-0 nylon or long-term absorbable material such as 0-PDS, which keeps its tensile force for 100 days and is totally resorbed in 180 days. For muscle advancement, a nonabsorbable suture is recommended such as 2-0 nylon. The use of short-term absorbable materials such as polyglactine (Vicryl®) is not indicated both in plications and muscle advancement.[27]

Postoperative care

The postoperative care described here is solely regarding the specific subject of this article, the correction of the myoaponeurotic layer.

Physical activities are started 1 month after the surgery such as walking and arms exercises with weight. However, patients who underwent plications should do abdominal sit ups and leg press only 45 days after the operation. Those with muscle advancements are allowed to do these types of physical activity 60 days after the operation.

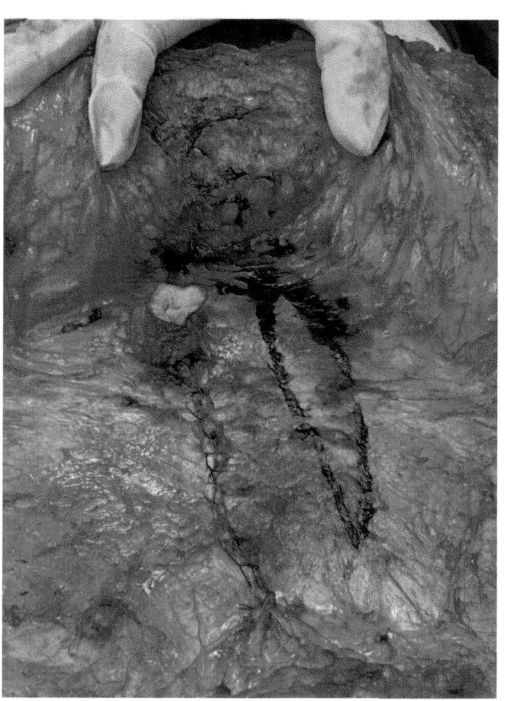

Fig. 9. This patient presented a lateral umbilicus in the preoperative. One of the ways to deal with that is to make a compensatory plication to advance the umbilicus toward the midline.

The use of regular compression garments is indicated for those patients who had muscle advancement for a period of 45 days. Those who had plications will use a very light compression garment for 3 weeks.[28,29] It is relevant to mention that the use of compression garments may lead to the increase of the intraabdominal pressure[30] and decrease in blood velocity inside the femoral vein,[31] thus potentially increasing the risk of *deep vein thrombosis* (DVT) and pulmonary embolism.

Limits of the Procedure

The correction of the myoaponeurotic deformities of the abdomen has some limitations. The extent of the deformity is usually not the main problem when the surgical correction is performed. The most frequent factor that plays a relevant role in this operation is the quality of the myoaponeurotic layer, amount of intrabadominal fat, and patient's age.

As mentioned before, both the aponeurosis and muscle laxity are related to the amount of collagen type in these structures. Elderly patients and individuals with predominance of type III collagen are more prone to present the recurrence of the laxity, as mentioned before, whereas younger patients will have a more stable result with time. The decrease of the amount of collagen types I and III in the recti muscles due to ageing, may also have a negative impact on the abdominal contour. We know that the abdominal wall in composed not only of muscles covered by fascia but also muscles with thin fascias or even without these structures. If this change in muscle composition occurs in all abdominal wall muscles, it is possible that muscles without strong fascias, such as those of the lumbar region, will get less tense with age and the abdominal diameter will increase.

Another factor that can be a key point in the outcome of the correction of these deformities is the intra-abdominal fat. Patients with this condition should be warned about the limitations of the result, as there is not an easy way to deal with this intra peritoneal adipose tissue. Removal of the epiploon has not been very successful in changing the abdominal contour. Radical fascial advancement of this type of patients is not effective either, as a more aggressive correction in some areas, such as the midline, may lead to a very projected waistline.

These conditions can be partially modified by losing weight and physical exercise. There is an interesting study by Rodrigues and colleagues,

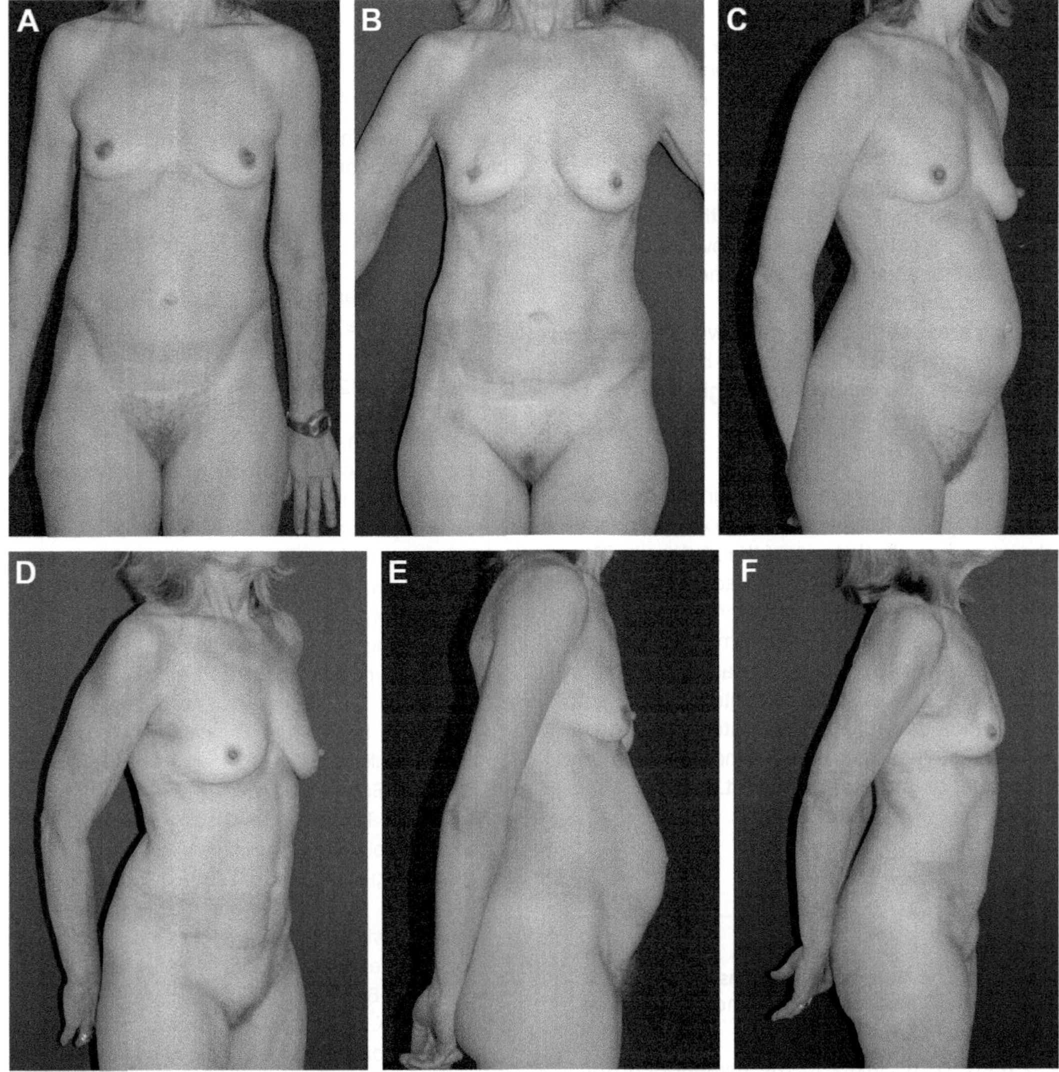

Fig. 10. This is the frontal (*A*), oblique (*C*) and lateral view (*E*) of a 38-year-old female who presented a very projected abdomen with a large rectus diastasis. Besides the correction of diastasis, an "L" plication was performed. These plications were done in the areas where there were folds and no muscle projection. The postoperative pictures at the frontal (*B*), oblique (*D*) and lateral view (*F*) are shown 22 years postoperative, when the lady was 60 years old. The plications lasted and it did not prevent the hypertrophy of the abdominal muscles, as the patient exercised.

2015[32] that has demonstrated that there is a positive correlation after the correction of rectus diastasis between the width of diastasis and the increase in the intra-abdominal pressure. This means that patients do not have similar myoaponeurotic tissue strength. A correction of a 4 cm diastasis in different patients, considering comparable body proportions, will not determine a similar increase in the intra-abdominal pressure. The differences in the myoaponeurotic collagen composition are fundamental in the success of this operation, as the whole myoaponeurotic laxity is more important than the width of the diastasis itself.

Complications

The main complications secondary to the myoaponeurotic corrections are recurrence and bulging deformities secondary to stronger corrections in certain areas.

Recurrence can be related to the no recognition of the insertion of the rectus abdominis muscle in the costal margin (type C) and, in these cases, a reoperation as extensive as the previous abdominoplasty is indicated with advancement of the recti sheaths, as described previously.

Bulging areas should be treated with the release of the overdone plications or/and by performing compensatory plications in the bulging areas.

SUMMARY

Most patients who present abdominal wall deformities will benefit from the correction of the laxity of the myoaponeurotic layer of the abdomen. Theses corrections should be done according to the patient's myoaponeurotic deformity. The knowledge of the local anatomy is paramount to correct these deformities. Complications are not common if the procedure is well indicated taking into consideration the limits of the anatomical and histological conditions as well as the patient's age and amount of intra-abdominal fat.

CLINICS CARE POINTS

- Identify the type of rectus diastasis. If it is a congenital diastasis, the advancement of the recti sheaths is indicated.
- If there is still laxity in the myoaponeurotic layer after the correction of the rectus diastasis, an "L" plication of the external oblique aponeurosis should be performed.
- Do use triangular sutures when correcting rectus diastasis secondary to pregnancy. The deformity of the myoaponeurotic layer is multidimensional and this type of suture promotes a vertical shortening of the aponeurosis by 8%.
- When doing procedures to correct the myoaponeurotic deformities as described in this article, very subtle increase of the intrabdominal pressure occurs. However, it is important to avoid tight compression garments, which may increase the intraabdominal pressure and decrease blood speed in the femoral vein, thus increasing the risk of complications.
- Diagnosis of the myoaponeurotic deformity is relevant so that an adequate specific treatment can be performed.

DISCLOSURE

None of the authors have any conflict of interests related to the content of this article.

REFERENCES

1. Nahas FX, Barbosa MV, Ferreira LM. Factors that may influence failure of the correction of the musculoaponeurotic deformities of the abdomen. Plast Reconstr Surg 2009;124:334 [author reply: 334-335].
2. Calvi EN, Nahas FX, Barbosa MV, et al. Collagen fibers in the rectus abdominis muscle of cadavers of different age. Hernia 2014;18(4):527–33.
3. Calvi EN, Nahas FX, Barbosa MV, et al. An experimental model for the study of collagen fibers in skeletal muscle. Acta Cir Bras 2012;27(10):681–6.
4. Barbosa MVJ, Dias AL, Bauti I, et al. The normal width of the linea alba in cadavers – a parameter to define rectus diastasis. Anatomy 2021;15(2):132–6.
5. Nahas FX, Ferreira LM. Concepts on correction of the musculoaponeurotic layer in abdominoplasty. Clin Plast Surg 2010;37(3):527–38.
6. Toranto IR. The relief of low back pain with the WARP abdominoplasty: a preliminary report. Plast Reconstr Surg 1990;85(4):545–55.
7. Nahas FX. Commentary on: improvement in back pain following abdominoplasty: results of a 10-year, single-surgeon series. Aesthet Surg J 2020;40(12):1316–8.
8. Nahas FX. An aesthetic classification of the abdomen based on the myoaponeurotic layer. Plast Reconstr Surg 2001;108(6):1787–95 [discussion: 1796-1787].
9. Nahas FX, Augusto SM, Ghelfond C. Should diastasis recti be corrected? Aesthetic Plast Surg 1997;21(4):285–9.

10. Nahas FX, Augusto SM, Ghelfond C. Nylon versus polydioxanone in the correction of rectus diastasis. Plast Reconstr Surg 2001;107(3):700–6.
11. Nahas FX, Ferreira LM, Augusto SM, et al. Long-term follow-up of correction of rectus diastasis. Plast Reconstr Surg 2005;115(6):1736–41 [discussion: 1742-1733].
12. Nahas FX, Ferreira LM, Ely PB, et al. Rectus diastasis corrected with absorbable suture: a long-term evaluation. Aesthetic Plast Surg 2011;35(1):43–8.
13. Nahas FX. Pregnancy after abdominoplasty. Aesthetic Plast Surg 2002;26(4):284–6.
14. Gama LJM, Barbosa MVJ, Czapkowski A, et al. Single-layer plication for repair of diastasis recti: the most rapid and efficient technique. Aesthet Surg J 2017;37(6):698–705.
15. Verissimo P, Nahas FX, Barbosa MV, et al. Is it possible to repair diastasis recti and shorten the aponeurosis at the same time? Aesthetic Plast Surg 2014;38(2):379–86.
16. Sood R, Muhammad LN, Sasson DC, et al. Development and initial validation of a novel professional aesthetic scale for the female abdomen. Plast Reconstr Surg 2022 Sep 1;150(3):546e–56e.
17. Nahas FX, Ishida J, Gemperli R, et al. Abdominal wall closure after selective aponeurotic incision and undermining. Ann Plast Surg 1998;41(6): 606–13 [discussion: 613-7].
18. Nahas FX, Ferreira LM, Mendes Jde A. An efficient way to correct recurrent rectus diastasis. Aesthetic Plast Surg 2004;28(4):189–96.
19. de Castro EJ, Radwanski HN, Pitanguy I, et al. Long-term ultrasonographic evaluation of midline aponeurotic plication during abdominoplasty. Plast Reconstr Surg 2013;132(2):333–8.
20. Nahas FX. Advancement of the external oblique muscle flap to improve the waistline: a study in cadavers. Plast Reconstr Surg 2001;108(2):550–5.
21. Villegas FJ. A novel approach to abdominoplasty: TULUA modifications (transverse plication, no undermining, full liposuction, neoumbilicoplasty, and low transverse abdominal scar). Aesthetic Plast Surg 2014;38(3):511–20.
22. Nahas FX. Commentary on: TULUA lipoabdominoplasty: no supraumbilical elevation combined with transverse infraumbilical plication, video description, and experience with 164 patients. Aesthet Surg J 2021;41(5):595–7.
23. Marques A, Brenda E, Pereira MD, et al. Abdominoplasty with two fusiform plications. Aesthetic Plast Surg 1996;20(3):249–51.
24. Abramo AC, Casas SG, Oliveira VR, et al. H-Shaped, double-contour plication in abdominoplasty. Aesthetic Plast Surg 1999;23(4):260–6.
25. Yousif NJ, Lifchez SD, Nguyen HH. Transverse rectus sheath plication in abdominoplasty. Plast Reconstr Surg 2004;114(3):778–84.
26. Sozer SO, Agullo FJ. Triple plication in miniabdominoplasty. Aesthetic Plast Surg 2006;30(3):263–8.
27. Nahas FX, Faustino LD, Ferreira LM. Abdominal wall plication and correction of deformities of the myoaponeurotic layer: focusing on materials and techniques used for synthesis. Aesthet Surg J 2019; 39(Suppl_2):S78–84.
28. Martins MRC, Moraes BZF, Fabri DC, et al. Do abdominal binders prevent seroma formation and recurrent diastasis following abdominoplasty? Aesthet Surg J 2022;42(11):1294–302.
29. Fontes de Moraes BZ, Ferreira LM, Martins MRC, et al. Do compression garments prevent subcutaneous edema after abdominoplasty? Aesthet Surg J 2023;43(3):329–36.
30. Rodrigues MA, Nahas FX, Gomes HC, et al. Ventilatory function and intra-abdominal pressure in patients who underwent abdominoplasty with plication of the external oblique aponeurosis. Aesthetic Plast Surg 2013;37(5):993–9.
31. Berjeaut RH, Nahas FX, Dos Santos LK, et al. Does the use of compression garments increase venous stasis in the common femoral vein? Plast Reconstr Surg 2015;135(1):85e–91e.
32. Rodrigues MA, Nahas FX, Reis RP, et al. Does diastasis width influence the variation of the intra-abdominal pressure after correction of rectus diastasis? Aesthet Surg J 2015;35(5):583–8.

Maximizing the TULUA Abdominoplasty with Oblique Flankplasty

Dennis J. Hurwitz, MD[a,b,*], Dani Kruchevsky, MD[a]

KEYWORDS

• Oblique flankplasty • TULUA • Transverse plication • Lower body lift • Abdominoplasty

KEY POINTS

- Oblique flankplasty creates smooth deep flanks, substantial long-lasting elevation of the buttocks and lateral thighs, small hip prominences, and transverse tightening of the abdomen.
- TULUA allows extensive fat removal from deep and superficial layers in the abdominal wall to deliver high-definition liposculpture on a flat, tight abdomen.
- Oblique flankplasty integrates well with TULUA for a 360° torso reshaping.
- Optimal candidates for TULUA alone or TULUA/oblique flankplasty tend to be male, muscular, but overweight patients desiring high-definition contouring.

INTRODUCTION

Since the first dermolipectomy reported by Demars and Marx in 1880,[1] abdominoplasty techniques have been constantly improving. The advent of liposuction-assisted abdominoplasty by Illouz[2] and the subsequent modifications have dramatically enhanced the esthetics.[3]

However, wound healing complications due to reduced vascularization caused by wide undermining, aggressive liposuction, and high-tension wound closure beset early adopters thereby retarding acceptance. With the advent of limited midline supraumbilical dissection with preservation of epigastric perforators and no superficial liposuction, lipoabdominoplasty was safer and gained acceptance.[4]

With the recent enthusiasm for abdominal etching, the question is how much liposuction is appropriate. Even as an isolated procedure, etching by liposuction can be complicated by burns and excessive scarring.[5–7] Furthermore, limited undermining of the epigastric flap leaves all transverse laxity, which may result in a midline dome-like redundancy after diastasis recti plication. Alternatively, a midline vertical excision as in a Fleur-de-lis pattern leaves an undesirable midline scar, blunting of esthetic contours, and a significant rate of delayed healing.

Posterior transverse lower body lift treats lower posterior trunk skin laxity and buttock ptosis.[8,9] Either this lower body lift or belt lipectomy[10] extends the lipoabdominoplasty for 360°. Unfortunately, both not only fail to eliminate flank excess but may also unmask mid-torso bulging surrounded by depressed scars. Moreover, these lower body lifts are often followed by high rate of complications, loss of desirable hip prominence, flattening of the buttocks, uneven descent of the transverse scar with deepening lateral gluteal depressions, recurrent skin laxity, and saddlebags.

TULUA: AN ALTERNATIVE LIPOABDOMINOPLASTY

TULUA modified lipoabdominoplasty, an acronym for transverse plication, no undermining, full liposuction, neoumbilicoplasty, and low transverse abdominal scar, was created by Columbian plastic surgeon Francisco Villegas and published in

[a] Hurwitz Center for Plastic Surgery; [b] University of Pittsburgh, 3109 Forbes Avenue #500, Pittsburgh, PA 15213, USA
* Corresponding author. 3109 Forbes Avenue #500, Pittsburgh, PA 15213.
E-mail address: Drhurwitz@pghplasticsurgery.com

Clin Plastic Surg 51 (2024) 71–80
https://doi.org/10.1016/j.cps.2023.06.012

2014.[11] Avoiding undermining of the epigastric flap and performing a broad low transverse plication of the lower rectus abdominis fascia flattens the central abdomen and relieves tension on the skin closure.[11,12]

Transverse plication facilitates closure of the suprapubic to the umbilicus excision and limits the risk of skin retraction and necrosis.[13] TULUAs great advantage is reduction of the risks of aggressive fat removal from both deep and superficial layers of the abdominal wall during abdominoplasty.[13] The ideal patient is either male or female with lipodystrophy and moderate redundant skin after weight loss without diastasis recti.

OBLIQUE FLANKPLASTY: AN ALTERNATIVE LOWER BODY LIFT

Since introduced in 2014, oblique flankplasty with lipoabdominoplasty (OFLA) creates smoothly transitioned deep flanks, suspends the buttocks and lateral thighs, defines smaller hip prominences, and facilitates transverse tightening of abdominal skin.[14,15] All attributes compliment TULUA.

Patient satisfaction was high with minimal secondary deformity and complications.[16] These outcomes were not routinely achieved by traditional lower body lifts performed by the senior author during the prior 25 years.

Primary healing along the entire flankplasty is consistent, because of minimal undermining, multilevel blood supply, and secure closure with running barbed sutures in multiple layers. Furthermore, as the closures lie within lumbar recesses, they are not subjected to bony prominences or shearing forces.[17–20]

The oblique flankplasty closures along the thoracic 11th and 12th dermatomes usually lead to flat, thin, and pale scars. The position of the lower posterior trunk side lying L-shaped closure is consistent with theories of optimal elective excision placement.[21] Our salutary scar experience is important because we reject the dogma of leaving the skin closure within lower underwear.

In contrast, lower body lift closures often experience delayed healing because of competing stretch forces, tissue pressure caused by underlying augmentation flaps, and sacral and posterior iliac bone crest prominences.

MAXIMIZING TULUA LIPOABDOMINOPLASTY AND OBLIQUE FLANKPLASTY

In the absence of posterior lower torso skin laxity and adiposity, TULUA is adequate esthetic surgery for the lower body. However, undesirable posterior torso laxity and adiposity with blunting of the flanks beg for a complimentary oblique flankplasty. TULUA esthetically transitions into oblique flank excisions to deepen the waist with smooth transitions from costal margins to hips. With the posterior rotation advancement of the superior flap, the still horizontally loose epigastrium is adequately horizontally tightened to better reveal muscular etching.

SURGERY

Preoperative markings are made on the standing patient for correcting skin laxity and adiposity with highlighting superficial muscles. Depending on patient desires, there will be strategic liposuction of bulging adipose and emphasizing borders of the pectoralis major, latissimus dorsi, rectus abdominis, external oblique, serratus anterior, and gluteus maximus muscles. Also, the iliac crest, inguinal ligaments, and lower lumbar concavity can be accentuated.[11,12,22]

The marking starts with TULUA abdominoplasty by Villegas (Case 1, **Fig. 1**). The superior incision is level at or just inferior to the umbilicus. The inferior incision is drawn horizontally along the groins and mons pubis placed conservatively superior, allowing for an intraoperative further inferior horizontal resection, depending on the inferior descent of the epigastric flap after the transverse plication.

For the umbilicoplasty, we have used three methods. One is tunneling of the umbilical stalk to exit through small epigastric flaps. Two is an H-shaped flap umbilicoplasty. Three is a full-thickness skin graft with a U-shaped superior base umbilicoplasty.

The two TULUA horizontal markings end along the mid-lateral trunk hip and lateral gluteal regions. The width between these transverse lines is from 5 to 25 cm, depending on the lateral buttock and thigh laxity. The flankplasty incision lines of incision end at these lines.

The width of the obliquely oriented flank resection considers flank redundancy and buttock laxity.[16] A line is drawn along the crest of the flank bulge. At the middle of this line, the redundant tissue is gathered, allowing marks for the width of resection equal distance from superior and inferior to the crest marks. With the lateral hemi-buttock and upper thigh pushed superiorly as much as possible, the excision pattern of flank redundancy is continued to the previously marked lateral torso extension markings of the abdominoplasty (see **Fig. 1**). The posterior rotation advancement of the upper flap is systematically marked at 10-cm intervals along both the superior and inferior incision lines. These hatch marks guide for a smooth and symmetrical posterior advance of the epigastric flap to the inferior buttock closure.

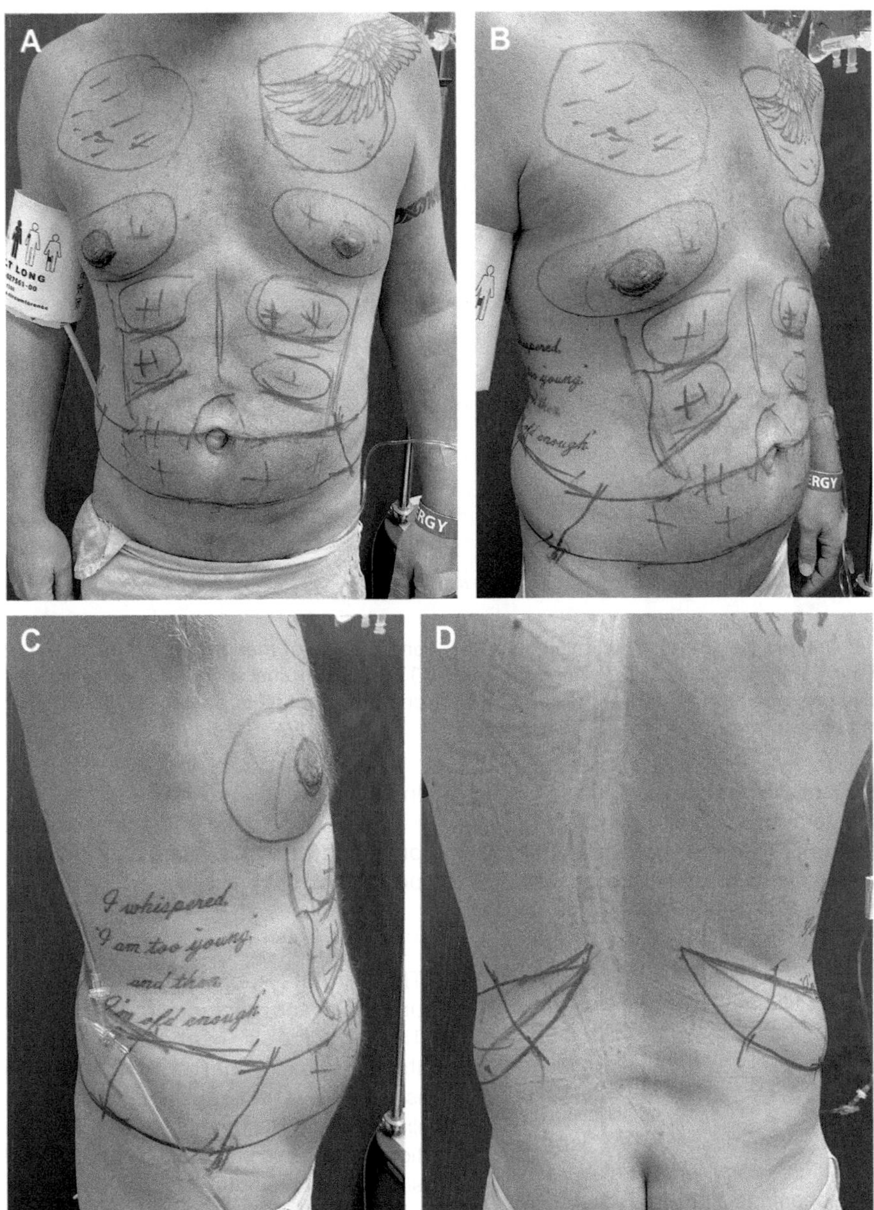

Fig. 1. *Case 1*: Combined modified TULUA and oblique flankplasty markings as well as correction of gynecomastia, by liposuction and direct gland removal, and lipografting of pectoralis major muscle. Four preoperative views. The markings from the umbilicus to mons pubis laterally ascend over his posterior iliac spines centered directly over the greatest projection of his flank roll to mark the oblique flankplasty as described. Anterior (*A*), right anterior oblique (*B*) , right lateral (*C*) and posterior (*D*) peroperative views.

Generally, the lower flap limb exceeds the upper limb by 1.2 to 1.5 times; it is compensated by the excessively long superior line in the usual abdominoplasty.

Posterior Operation

After the induction of general anaesthesia, the patient is turned prone onto two large gel rolls placed under the anterior costal margins and upper anterior thighs to allow for posterior advancement of the abdominal skin on closure of the flankplasty (Case 2, **Fig. 2**A). Because the anchor line is at the superior incision, the inferior incision is made first. After the buttock/upper thigh flap incision is completed, it is advanced using a towel clip to the proposed superior incision, which may be adjusted. Although no direct undermining is

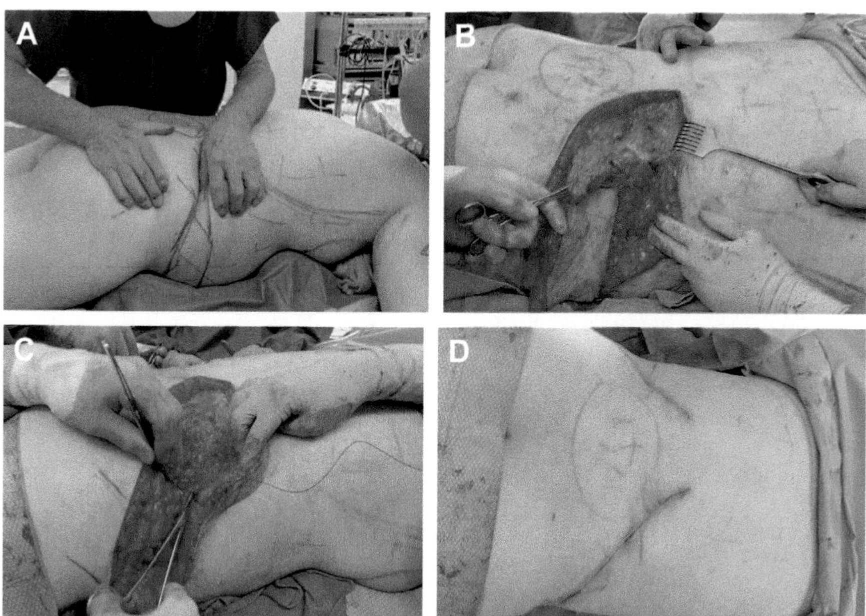

Fig. 2. *Case 1*: Oblique flankplasty operative course. (*A*) Confirmation of markings using pinch test. (*B*) Excising the marked and confirmed tissue without undermining. (*C*) The sub-cutaneous wound edges are approximated using #2 polydioxanone barbed suture including bites of underlying muscular fascia. (*D*) Oblique flankplasy incisions after closure in layers.

performed along the buttocks and thighs, oversized upper lateral thighs are liposuctioned. The superior incision is made to the latissimus dorsi muscle. Starting medially, the tissue between the two incisions is electrosurgically excised leaving a thin layer of areolar adipose tissue over muscle and fascia (**Fig.** 2B). The superficial fascial system (SFS) of the buttocks and lower back, including a third small bite of lumbodorsal fascia, is approximated using #2 polydioxanone (PDO) Quill (Surgical Specialties, Inc, Wyomissing, PA.) (**Fig.** 2C). Intradermal running 2-0 Quill Monoderm (Surgical Specialties, Inc, Wyomissing, PA) intradermal closure and skin glue complete the closure except for the lateral openings that lead to the TULUA lipoabdominoplasty (**Fig.** 2D). Small aliquots of liposomal bupivacaine (Exparel; Pacira Pharmaceuticals, USA) can be injected before closure for posterior 11 and 12 intercostal nerve blocks. The patient is then turned supine for TULUA.

TULUA

Through stealth access incisions in torso and arms, tumescent infiltration of 30 mL 1% lidocaine and 1 mL of epinephrine per liter saline for Vibration Amplification of Sound Energy at Resonance (VASER)lipo (Solta Medical–Bausch Health Companies, Inc, Bothell, WA) is followed by power-assisted liposuction (MicroAire Surgical Instruments, LLC, Charlottesville, VA) (Case 2, **Fig.** 3A). A thorough abdominal deep liposuction proceeds the abdominoplasty, whereas the superficial etching follows.[23,24]

Transverse Plication

The skin and subcutaneous tissue between the umbilicus and suprapubic is excised (**Fig.** 3B). The epigastric skin has been indirectly undermined through liposuction. Then, a wide horizontal ellipse is drawn over the exposed fascia from one anterior iliac spine to the other (**Fig.** 3C). Transverse plication of the rectus fascia is by running #2 PDO Quill suture in a horizontal mattress followed by a baseball stitch (**Fig.** 3D, E).

In cases where the stalk of the umbilicus is long enough to be transpositioned to the appropriate new location, we preserve it, in other cases, the umbilicus is amputated, and the opening is repaired with 0 polypropylene stitches. A narrow, short tunnel is dissected toward the appropriate location of the umbilicus if it is to be preserved, and umbilicoplasty is performed. Drainage is achieved using high-negative pressure internal therapy (Interi; IC Surgical, Grand Rapids, MI, USA).

The wound is closed in layers using no #2 PDO barbed suture (Surgical Specialties, Inc, Wyomissing, PA, USA) for the fascia and intradermal running 3-0 Quill Monoderm (Surgical Specialties,

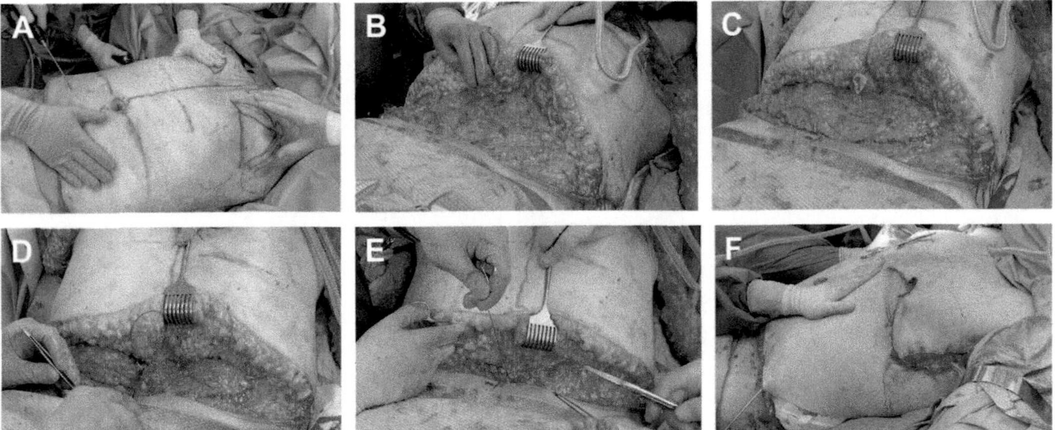

Fig. 3. *Case 2*: Modified TULUA lipoabdominoplasty operative course. (*A*) Fat emulsification using VASERLipo. (*B*) After removal of excess tissue according to the marking just above the level of the umbilicus. (*C*) Drawing of a horizontal ellipse for transverse plication. (*D, E*) Transverse plication is performed using no 2 polydioxanone barbed suture in two layers. Following, liposuction can be done over the flap to obtain an adequate and natural definition of the rectus abdominis muscles (*F*).

Inc., Wyomissing, PA, USA). Once the abdominal flap has been advanced, superficial liposuction obtains natural definition of the rectus abdominis muscles (**Fig. 3**F).

Neoumbilicoplasty

In case the umbilicus cannot be preserved and transpositioned, an X-shaped incision is made across the *linea alba* deep enough to reach the rectus abdominis fascia and with 60° superior and inferior opposite angles. Upper incisions must be 10 mm long and lower incisions 5 mm long. In consequence, four triangular flaps are made: superior, inferior, left, and right. The three lower flaps are sutured with a continuous subcuticular stitch and fixed upward to the abdominal fascia at the base of the upper flap. We use a gauze covered with antibiotics (as a shaper) to induce deep flap adhesion and depth. Alternatively, the Villegas described skin graft with U flap umbilicoplasty is performed.

Final Steps

After confirming adequate blood flow to the distal end of the epigastric flap, superficial liposuction with an etching sculpture of the borders of the flat superficial muscles is performed. Selective muscular lipoaugmentation by injection of processed harvest fat completes the operation.

All operations were performed in an outpatient surgical center. The patient is instructed to walk three times daily and resume limited activities within 1 week. Deep venous thrombosis chemoprophylaxis is prescribed according to risk.[25] When umbilical sutures are removed, swelling reduction therapies are started.[26] The patient wears elastic garments continuously for 4 weeks.

Since December 2020 we have combined TULUA with oblique flankplasty in 11 cases.

CASE 1: MODIFIED TULUA, OBLIQUE FLANKPLASTY, AND EXCISION CORRECTION OF GYNECOMASTIA

A 49-year-old man, 5′10, requested body contouring of his chest, abdomen, and back. After mild weight loss, he was embarrassed by sagging gynecomastia, abdominal pannus, and love handles.

Four preoperative views show the surgical markings of the single-stage combined TULUA and oblique flankplasty, repair of umbilical hernia, as well correction of gynecomastia, by liposuction and direct gland removal, and lipografting of pectoralis major muscle (see **Fig. 1**). The lipoabdominoplasty markings ascend over his posterior iliac spines centered directly over the greatest projection of his flank roll to mark the oblique flankplasty as described.

The patient had TULUA/oblique flankplasty in November 2022, with U flap neoumbilicoplasty with skin graft. The resection weight of the flanks was 345 g on the left and 364 g on the right. High-definition etching of the abdomen was performed. Each pectoralis muscle was lipografted with 115 mL of processed fat. The patient has postoperative lymphatic drainage. The Interi drain was removed 15 days after surgery. The postoperative course was uneventful, and the patient was satisfied with the result. His combined operations

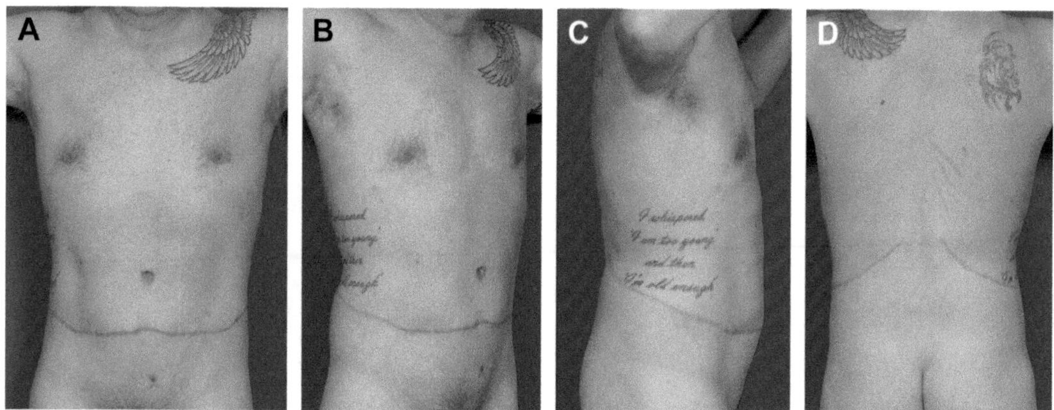

Fig. 4. *Case 1*: Seven months after, his combined operations replaced the bulging appearance of the torso, for a tight 360° wrap and masculine look. Anterior (*A*), right anterior oblique (*B*), right lateral (*C*) and posterior (*D*) postoperative views.

replaced the bulging appearance of the torso, for a tight 360° wrap and masculine look (**Fig. 4**). His androgynous body has become distinctly masculine with inconspicuous fading scars.

CASE 2: TULUA AND OBLIQUE FLANKPLASTY WITH BILATERAL BOOMERANG CORRECTION OF GYNECOMASTIA

Case 2 is a 20-year-old man, 6′1″, and 237 lb, with a stable body mass index (BMI) of 31.3. His highest weight was 250 lb. He is self-conscious of his generalized excess adiposity, which he feels is feminizing. His torso is broad, without definition of the waist or muscles. He has ptotic gynecomastia with well-defined inframammary fold (IMF).

The patient was marked for boomerang pattern correction of gynecomastia with a J-torsoplasty, a TULUA with umbilical transposition, oblique flankplasty, and lipografting to the pectoral and deltoid muscles (**Fig. 5**).[27,28]

In January 2021, his flank resection was 700 g per side, and the abdominal was 4900 g. Lipografting was performed using 170 mL of fat for each pectoralis muscle and 170 mL for each deltoid muscle (see **Figs. 2** and **3**).

Twelve days post-op, the patient presented with a surgical site infection treated with intravenous (IV) antibiotics and bedside incision and drainage of 150 cc of pus along the left groin closure. The patient continued antibiotic treatment as an outpatient with the resolution of the infection to continue otherwise an uneventful postoperative course.

At 2 months post-op, the patient was satisfied with the results. The breasts and flank rolls are gone, and the skin wrap is tight circumferentially around a masculinized torso, with inconspicuous scars that will continue to fade (**Fig. 6**).

His entire torso with prominent feminization was transformed to androgynous and distinctly masculine.

CASE 3: FEMALE HAD TULUA AND OBLIQUE FLANKPLASTY, LIMITED BUTTOCK PLASTY, AND THIGHPLASTY

A 58-year-old woman underwent gastric bypass surgery 15 years ago with a significant amount of weight loss. She is 5′8″ and 135 lb, with a stable BMI of 20.5. She was looking to treat the

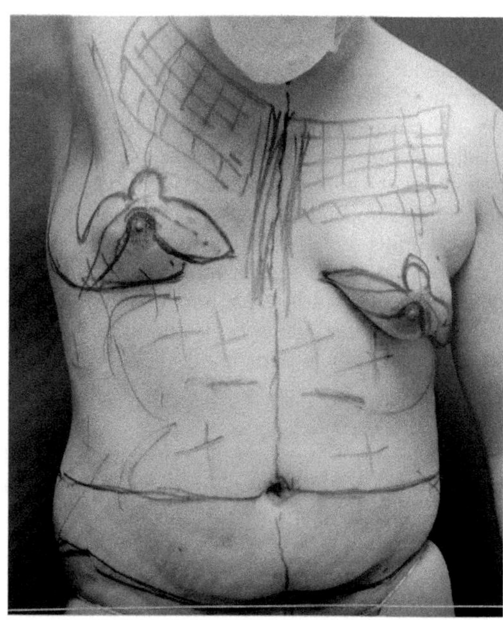

Fig. 5. *Case 2*: The patient was marked for boomerang pattern correction of gynecomastia with a J-torsoplasty, a TULUA high-definition lipoabdominoplasty, oblique flankplasty and lipografting to the pectoral and deltoid muscles.

generalized loose skin after weight loss that got worse over the years.

In May 2022, she was marked for TULUA, oblique flankplasty, limited buttock plasty, and thighplasty (**Fig. 7**). The volume of aspirated fat from each thigh was 200 mL and from the abdomen 600 mL.

The postoperative course was uneventful, and the patient was satisfied. The combined surgery replaced the loose skin with a tight 360° wrap that reveals the underlying muscularity and smoothly transition concave flanks (**Fig. 8**).

DISCUSSION

TULUA lipoabdominoplasty was developed to allow extensive fat removal from deep and superficial layers in the abdominal wall to deliver safe high-definition liposculpture on a flat abdomen. TULUA is indicated for mild to moderate skin laxity with moderate to severe subcutaneous adiposity and mild rectus fascia generalized laxity, especially in those seeking a better definition of superficial musculature. Hence, TULUA has a distinct advantage in overweight young athletic patients seeking body contouring. We have found that it performs less ideally in overweight females with poor body tone, as they often will have the relative contraindications of wide diastasis recti, obesity, or poor muscular development.

As early adopters, we have concerns about TULUA. There is the uncertainty of the short- and long-term retention of the low and wide transverse rectus fascia plication and lack of treatment of a widened linea alba. Studies have demonstrated some degree of relapse of a midline diastasis, and it is generally considered that women who give birth following a previous abdominoplasty are likely to have re-widened linea alba. It is hard to imagine that a low transverse plication, which will undergo constant abdominal stressors, will not have a relapse and this remains to be studied fully. Some of our patients have also complained of prolonged lower abdominal discomfort as the suture material likely invests into the muscular layer and may cause spasms. It is also difficult to predict the descent of the epigastric flap in relatively thin and minimally lax skinned patients.

In lipoabdominoplasty, the direct undermining of the upper midline at least as wide as the lateral trans-rectus perforators is a fundamental step in the release of the overlying flap for its descent to the pubis. Moreover, coupled with judicious

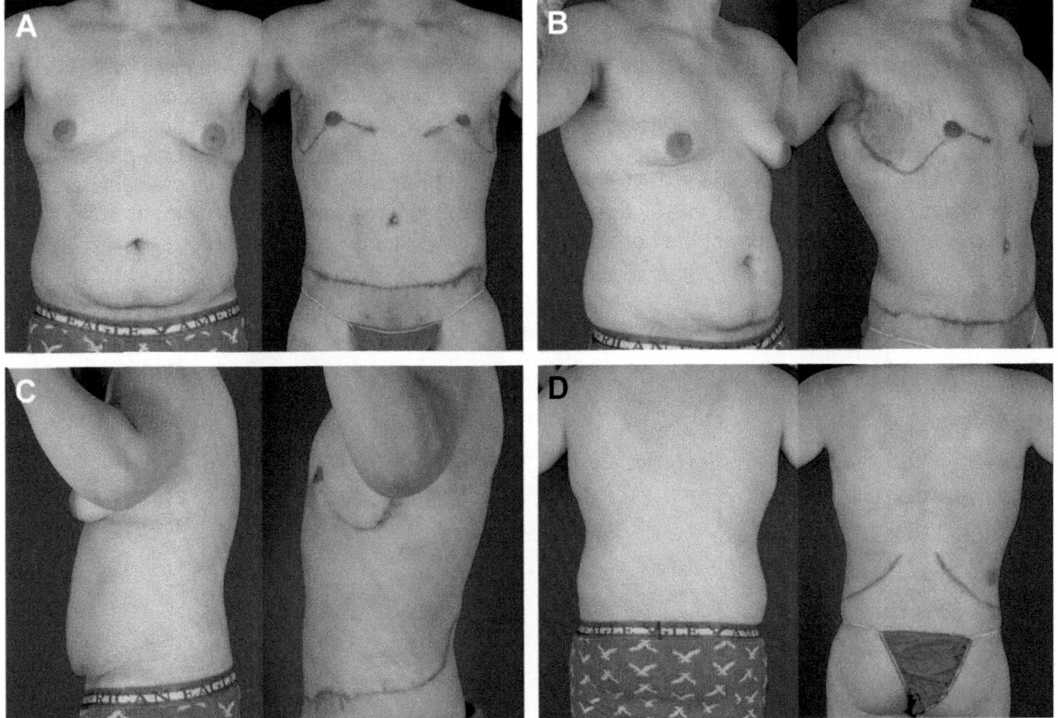

Fig. 6. *Case 2*: Two months post-op, his entire torso with prominent feminine features was transformed to androgynous and distinctly masculine. The breasts and flank roll are gone, and the skin wrap is 360° tight all over the torso. (*A*) Anterior view: *left*- preoperative, *right*- posoperative; (*B*) Right anterior oblique view: *left*- preoperative, *right*- posoperative; (*C*) Left lateral view: *left*- preoperative, *right*- posoperative; (*D*) Posterior view: *left*- preoperative, *right*- posoperative.

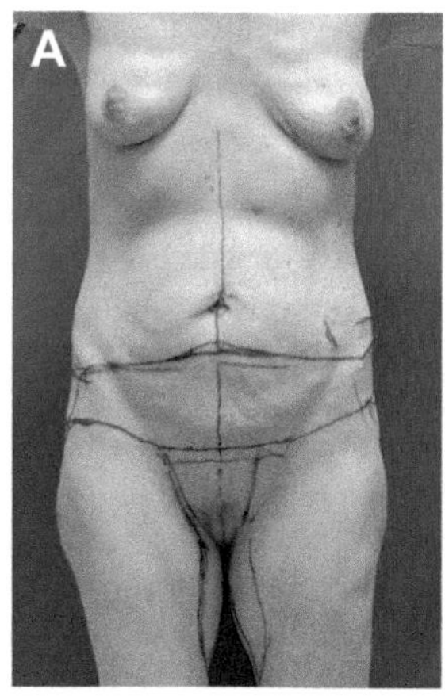
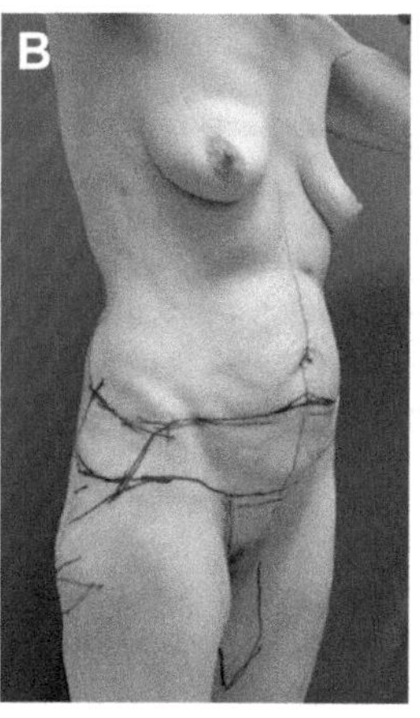
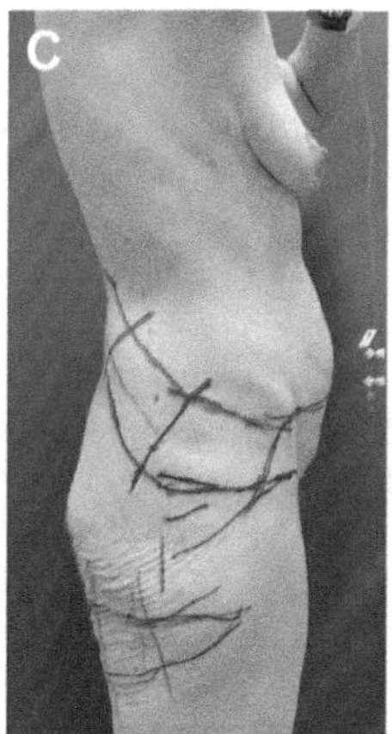
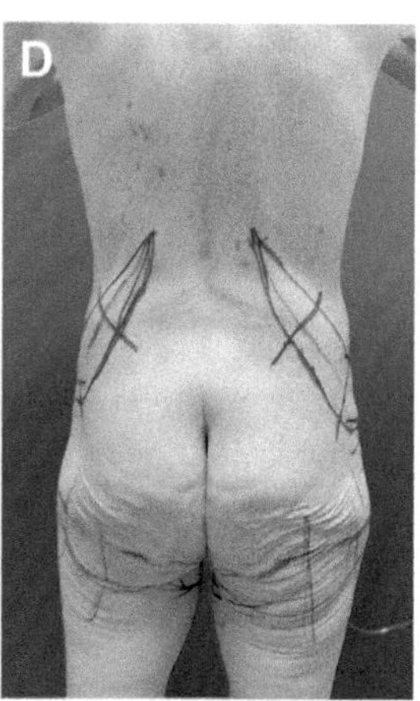

Fig. 7. *Case 3*: The patient was marked for modified TULUA lipoabdominoplasty, oblique flankplasty, limited buttock plasty, and thighplasty. Anterior (*A*), right anterior oblique (*B*) , right lateral (*C*) and posterior (*D*) peroperative views.

liposuction, the indirect undermining, which can be extended with spreading dissection with the LaRoe Undermining Forceps (ASSI, Westbury, NY, USA), leads to a generalized but limited redistribution of abdominal skin. Lately, lipoabdominoplasty proponents like Saldana have encouraged as safe more aggressive etching liposuction, especially when vertically oriented[29] (see article 5).

Although extensive liposuction and strong inferior pull of lower transverse closure favorably redistribute anterior mid and lower torso skin laxity, there is little reduction of horizontal laxity. The addition of a traditional lower body lift to treat lower torso skin laxity does not further correct anterior horizontal laxity. The more superiorly positioned belt lipectomy similar to Lockwood's high lateral tension abdominoplasty will partially correct the horizontal laxity but will not create an esthetically tight-skinned abdomen with a narrower waist. The oblique flankplasty was developed to facilitate smoothly transitioned narrow waists, superior rotation of lateral buttocks, improving the definition of the hips, and tightening of abdominal skin.

Since reviewing Villegas's article on TULUA for publication, 2 years ago, we have operated on 11 patients combining the modified TULUA with oblique flankplasty. All the patients expressed a high level of satisfaction. There were three minor complications: one surgical site infection at the groin closure requiring short hospital admission for IV antibiotics and bedside drainage; one patient had a seroma requiring percutaneous drainage; and one patient suffered from brief thrombophlebitis of the leg. No patients required revision surgery.

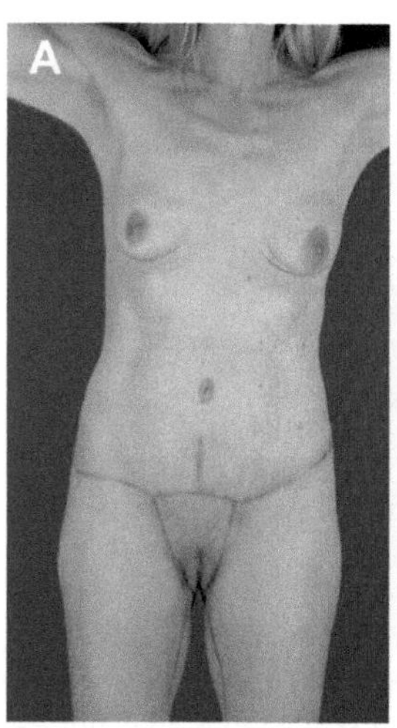
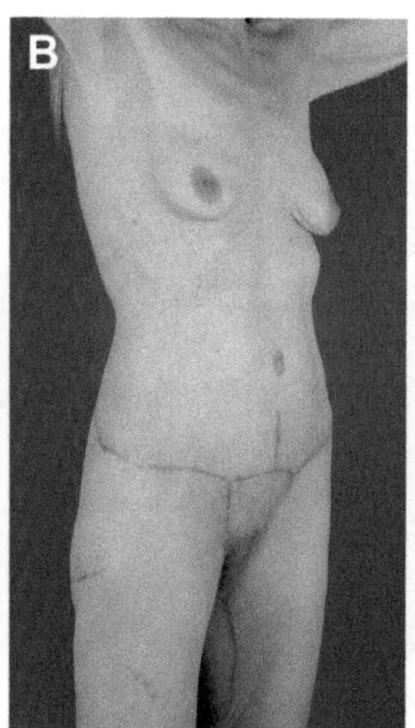
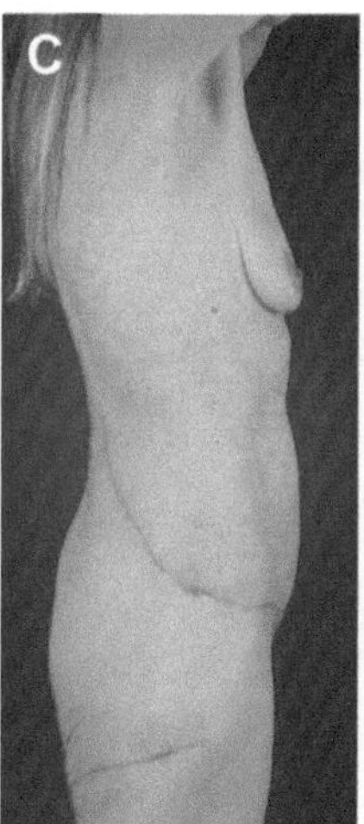
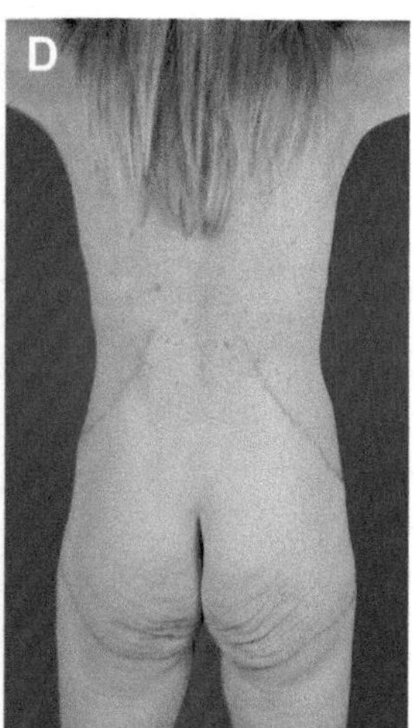

Fig. 8. *Case 3*: Three months after the surgery, the loose skin is replaced with a tight 360° wrap that reveals the underlying muscularity and enhanced flanks. Anterior (*A*), right anterior oblique (*B*) , right lateral (*C*) and posterior (*D*) postoperative views.

Oblique flankplasty complements TULUA as it provides direct contouring of the flanks, hips, and buttocks. Through naturally occurring minimal adherent lateral torso skin, flankplasty indirectly corrects the horizontal skin excess at the upper abdomen, which is not improved with an isolated TULUA. The flankplasty also follows the distinction of being a non-undermining procedure. Just as the TULUA allows for high-definition contouring of the abdomen, the flankplasty allows for powerful lipo-contouring of the back, hips, and buttocks without negatively impacting the results of the procedure. Finalizing the surgery with radiofrequency can safely be achieved in non-undermined fields. This complement of the oblique flankplasty TULUA combination treats a variety of challenging cases, with esthetic 360° torso reshaping.

Despite an exciting and formidable early experience, TULUA with oblique flankplasty are a paradigm shift for many surgeons and will remain a challenge to achieve consistent results. In our experience, the TULUA suffers from a difficult intraoperative decision-making process, where the amount of transverse tightening to be performed is not straightforward. A wide *linea alba* can be corrected visually with clear anatomic landmarks; however, the amount of transverse plication can be increased or decreased based on the laxity produced by table flexion. Overcorrection can also force the intraabdominal contents cephalad, and in patients who have had significant weight fluctuations or high BMI, flaring of the costal margin may worsen, leading to epigastric bulging. The flankplasty conversely can suffer from unfamiliar preoperative decision-making, with marking of the advancement rotation flap at proper intervals leading to improper flap positioning intraoperatively. Together, these complexities can result in challenging obstacles for newcomers. As always, a proper patient selection plays a role in all contouring surgery, and with an early experience, it is difficult to define the endpoints of candidacy for the procedures. Finally, despite Villegas' extensive experience, additional study is welcome from colleagues, particularly in determining the long-term sequelae of transverse plication.

Summary

We continue to apply TULUA alone or with oblique flankplasty to our considered optimal candidates, which tend to be male, muscular, but overweight patients desiring high-definition contouring. In cases in which these operations require further tightening, bipolar radiofrequency technology enhances the results without adding extra scars.

Despite our successes with TULUA, for most patients requesting 360° torso contouring, we continue to provide OFLA. We find vertical VASER etching and central undermining, assisted by discontinuous undermining through liposuction and application of LaRoe dissector, followed by central high tension through dermal advancement flap umbilicoplasty to be esthetically satisfying with rare complications.

CLINICS CARE POINTS

- Oblique flankplasty achieves smoothly transitioned deep flanks and substantial and long-lasting effect on raising the buttocks and lateral thighs, defines small hip prominences, and facilitates transverse tightening of abdominal skin.
- Placing of gel rolls placed under the anterior costal margins and upper anterior thighs while the patient is prone is important for suspending the loose-skinned abdomen which allows for unimpeded posterior advancement of the mid-torso skin during flankplasty closure.
- TULUA allows extensive fat removal from deep and superficial layers in the abdominal wall to deliver safe high-definition liposculpture on a flat abdomen.
- In cases, the navel stalk is long enough to be transpositioned and an umbilicoplasty can be performed, whereas for other cases, several techniques for umbilicoplasty exist.
- Optimal candidates for TULUA or TULUA/oblique flankplasty tend to be male, muscular, but overweight patients desiring high-definition contouring.
- In cases in which these operations require further tightening, bipolar radiofrequency technology enhances the results without adding extra scars.

DISCLOSURE

Dr D.J. Hurwitz was a paid investigator for InMode from 2010 to 2013, and received stock options. He has accepted $5000 in fees for lectures. He has received no editing or direct financial support for this article.

REFERENCES

1. Demars and Marx: In: voloir. opérations plastiques aus-aponévrotiques sur la paroi abdominale anterieure, Vol 1. Thèse, Paris, p 25. Vol 1. P.; 1960.

2. Illouz YG. A new safe and aesthetic approach to suction abdominoplasty. Aesthetic Plast Surg. 1992;16(3):237-245.
3. Matarasso A, Matarasso DM, Matarasso EJ. Abdominoplasty. Clin Plast Surg 2014;41(4):655–72.
4. Saldanha O. Lipoabdominoplasty without undermining. Aesthet Surg J 2001;21(6):518–26.
5. Danilla S, Babaitis RA, Jara RP, et al. High-definition liposculpture: what are the complications and how to manage them? Aesthetic Plast Surg 2020;44(2): 411–8.
6. Hoyos A, Millard J. VASER-assisted high-definition liposculpture. Aesthet Surg J 2007;27(6):594–604.
7. Blum CA, Sasser CGS, Kaplan JL. Complications from laser-assisted liposuction performed by noncore practitioners. Aesthetic Plast Surg 2013;37(5): 869–75.
8. González-Ulloa M. Belt lipectomy. Br J Plast Surg 1960;13:179–86.
9. Vilain R, Dubousset J. Technics and indications on circular lipectomy. apropos of 150 operations. Ann Chir 1964;18:289–300.
10. Aly AS, Cram AE, Chao M, et al. Belt lipectomy for circumferential truncal excess: the university of Iowa experience. Plast Reconstr Surg 2003;111(1): 398–413.
11. Villegas FJ. A novel approach to abdominoplasty: TULUA Modifications (Transverse plication, no undermining, full liposuction, neoumbilicoplasty, and low transverse abdominal scar). Aesthetic Plast Surg 2014;38(3):511–20.
12. Villegas Alzate FJ. A paradigm shift for abdominoplasty: transverse hypogastric plication without supraumbilical dissection, unrestricted liposuction, neoumbilicoplasty, and low placement of the scar (TULUA). In: Di Giuseppe A, Shiffman MA, editors. *Aesthetic plastic surgery of the abdomen.* Switzerland: Springer International Publishing; 2016. p. 171–93. https://doi.org/10.1007/978-3-319-20004-0_15.
13. Babaitis R, Villegas FJ, Hoyos AE, et al. TULUA male high-definition abdominoplasty. Plast Reconstr Surg 2022;149(1):96–104.
14. Hurwitz DJ. Aesthetic refinements in body contouring in the massive weight loss patient. Plast Reconstr Surg 2014;134(6):1185–95.
15. Hurwitz D. Body contouring surgery for women. In: Comprehensive body contouring. Springer Berlin Heidelberg; 2016. p. 63–179. https://doi.org/10.1007/978-3-662-46976-7_4.
16. Hurwitz DJ, Beidas O, Wright L. Reshaping the oversized waist through oblique flankplasty with lipoabdominoplasty. Plast Reconstr Surg 2019;143(5): 960e–72e.
17. Wilhelmi BJ, Blackwell SJ, Phillips LG. Langer's lines: to use or not to use. Plast Reconstr Surg 1999;104(1): 208–14.
18. On the anatomy and physiology of the skin. I. The cleavability of the cutis. (Translated from Langer, K. (1861). Zur Anatomie und Physiologie der Haut. I. Uber die Spaltbarkeit der Cutis. Sitzungsbericht der Mathematisch-naturwissenschaftlichen Classe der Kaiserlichen Academie der Wissenschaften, 44, 19. Br J Plast Surg 1978;31(1):3–8.
19. Kraissl CJ. The selection of appropriate lines for elective surgical incisions. Plast Reconstr Surg 1951;8(1):1–28.
20. Borges AF, Alexander JE. Relaxed skin tension lines, z-plasties on scars, and fusiform excision of lesions. Br J Plast Surg 1962;15:242–54.
21. Lemperle G, Tenenhaus M, Knapp D, et al. The direction of optimal skin incisions derived from striae distensae. Plast Reconstr Surg 2014;134(6):1424–34.
22. Hoyos AE, Perez ME, Castillo L. Dynamic definition mini-lipoabdominoplasty combining multilayer liposculpture, fat grafting, and muscular plication. Aesthet Surg J 2013;33(4):545–60.
23. Hoyos AE, Prendergast PM. Male abdomen and torso. In: High definition body sculpting. Springer Berlin Heidelberg; 2014. p. 95–107. https://doi.org/10.1007/978-3-642-54891-8_8.
24. Hoyos AE, Prendergast PM. Male torso and back. In: High definition body sculpting. Springer Berlin Heidelberg; 2014. p. 129–36. https://doi.org/10.1007/978-3-642-54891-8_11.
25. Griffin M, Akhavani MA, Muirhead N, et al. Risk of thromboembolism following body-contouring surgery after massive weight Loss. Eplasty 2015;15: e17.
26. Marxen T, Shauly O, Goel P, et al. The utility of lymphatic massage in cosmetic procedures. Aesthet Surg J Open Forum 2023;5. https://doi.org/10.1093/asjof/ojad023.
27. Hurwitz DJ. Boomerang pattern correction of gynecomastia. Plast Reconstr Surg 2015;135(2): 433–6.
28. Clavijo-Alvarez JA, Hurwitz DJ. J torsoplasty. Plast Reconstr Surg 2012;130(2):382e–3e.
29. Saldanha O, Ordenes AI, Goyeneche C, et al. Lipoabdominoplasty with anatomical definition. Plast Reconstr Surg 2020;146(4):766–77.

Finesse in Fleur-de-lis Abdominoplasty

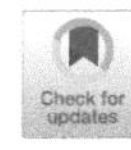

Flavio Henrique Mendes, MD, PhD*, Fausto Viterbo, MD, PhD, Weber Ribolli Moragas, MD

KEYWORDS

• Body contouring • Neoumbilicoplasty • Monsplasty • Massive weigh loss • Postbariatric

KEY POINTS

- Massive weight loss affects the entire superficial fascial system, and effective treatment demands both vertical and horizontal correction vectors in order to reestablish lower body contour.
- Abdominal approach should always be addressed by also considering the need for lifting and tightening of the adjacent structures in search of complete lower body contouring.
- Fleur-de-lis abdominoplasty is an effective indication especially for central body type patients, providing best waist definition and overall tissue readjustment.
- Technical refinements for neoumbilicus creation and monsplasty are essential to restore body contour and help to enhance the esthetic quality of surgical results.
- Advanced concepts of Fleur-de-lis abdominoplasty have recently achieved new and promising horizons by enhancing overall body contour providing unique and natural results.

 **Video content accompanies this article at http://www.plasticsurgery.theclinics.com.**

INTRODUCTION

Recent physiopathologic findings of body contour deformities following massive weight loss linked specific consideration of anatomic and biodynamic changes to improve results through best diagnosis and surgical planning for post–bariatric surgery patients. Surgeons had to shift some of the classic paradigms related to surgical strategies while performing regular contouring after pregnancy, aging, and mild weight variation.

It is very important to understand and keep in mind the difference between regular patients and the massive weight loss population. **Fig. 1** shows both previous defining morphologic distress, making it easier to figure that resulting deformities will follow different patterns, and that correction vectors will face and target different biodynamic situations.

As a fundamental concept, obesity and massive weight loss lead to extensive deformities with complex circumferential laxity that require a broader approach with modified correction vectors ruled by the continuity of concomitant affected areas. Although static images may not disclose such reality, **Fig. 2** shows a massive weight loss (MWL) patient treated by a conventional abdominoplasty and still presents residual laxity at the anterior and lateral aspects of the trunk. Therefore, it is advisable to not only evaluate just the abdomen but also consider the surrounding body elements for lifting and tightening indications. Very different from those of most conventional patients, MWL morphologic changes are not anatomically restricted to the anterior abdominal wall but closely related to the lower, lateral, and posterior aspects of the trunk, including the pubis, flanks, lateral thigh, and buttocks.

Besides, in order to achieve effective tissue readjustment in such patients, it may be necessary to treat both vertical and horizontal tissue excess, promoting not only lifting but also a tightening effect, which includes longitudinal resections over the

Botucatu Medical School, Paulista State University, Sao Paulo, Brazil
* Corresponding author. Rua Tomaz Antonio Gonzaga, 160 Jardim Ariano, Lins, São Paulo 16400-465, Brazil.
E-mail address: mendesmd@fhmendes.com.br

Clin Plastic Surg 51 (2024) 81–93
https://doi.org/10.1016/j.cps.2023.09.001

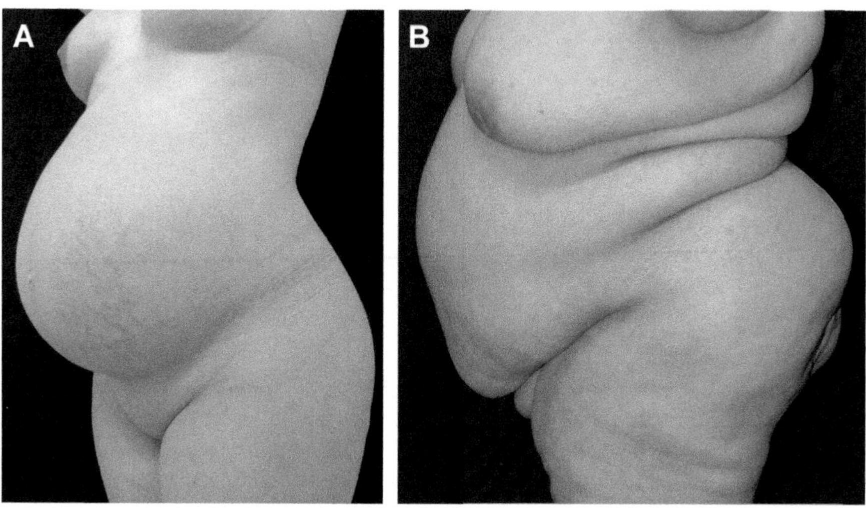

Fig. 1. Distinct patterns of previous morphologic distress: (*A*) pregnancy and (*B*) morbid obesity.

trunk and limbs.[1] Specifically on the central/lower body, those resections usually end up with anterior vertical scars seen on the Fleur-de-lis technique, with or without associated belt lipectomies.

LOWER BODY DEFORMITY

There is a constant fascia structure dividing superficial and deep fat compartments throughout nearly all of the trunk and limbs. In 1991, Lockwood[2] published new concepts that provided a better and more complete understanding of the entire 3-dimensional structure of connective tissue within subcutaneous fat, defining and popularizing the so-called superficial fascial system (SFS), which is specifically responsible for supporting the skin tegument (**Fig. 3**A). Large adipocytes accumulations by the obese patients create a generalized mechanical stretching effect in the SFS through volumetric increase of the whole subcutaneous space (**Fig. 3**B). Meanwhile, weight loss causes a massive adipocyte reduction reflecting volumetric deflation of the subcutaneous tissue without the retraction of its collagen network, which remains elongated and weak (**Fig. 3**C). Ultimately, SFS disability leads to significant looseness of the cutaneous covering as a whole.[3] Patients experience a generalized redundancy with great skin mobility, which directly influences body contour through general excess and localized descent of surrounding tissue. The zones of adherence promote a "selective limitation" in such mobility so that gravitational effect on different amounts of deflated tissue will determine different and individual contouring characteristics. In other words, the translational effect of mobile tissue in contrast to areas with greater deep fixation designs the contouring profile of post–bariatric surgery patients. This idea is the fundamental anatomic rule that defines body contour deformities in the MWL population, determining a completely different approach, targeting the new biodynamics of the involved tissues.[4]

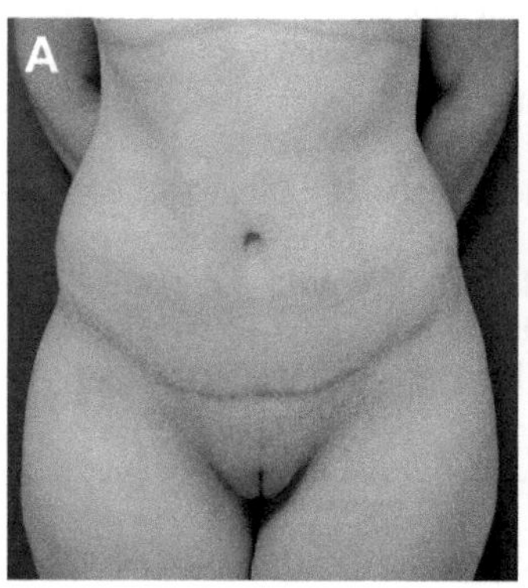

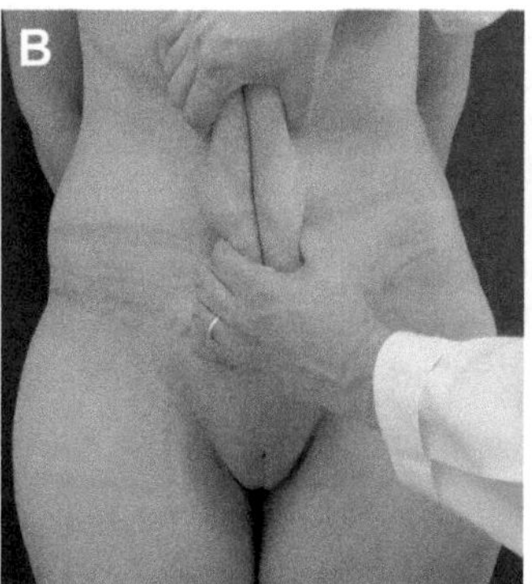

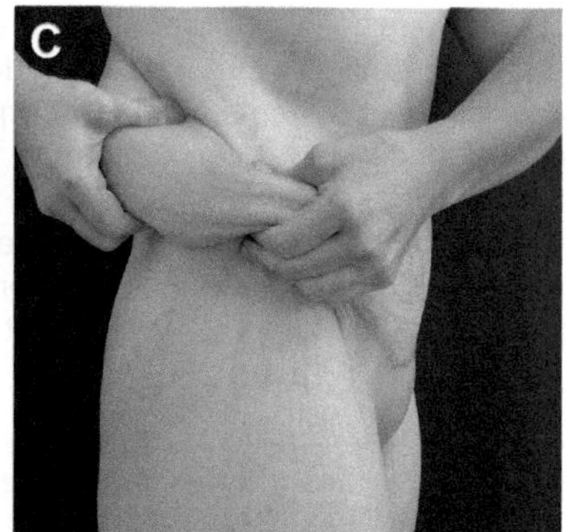

Fig. 2. Postoperative result of MWL patient treated by simple transverse abdominoplasty. (*A*) Static image, (*B*) anterior, and (*C*) lateral remaining excess tissue revealed by palpation.

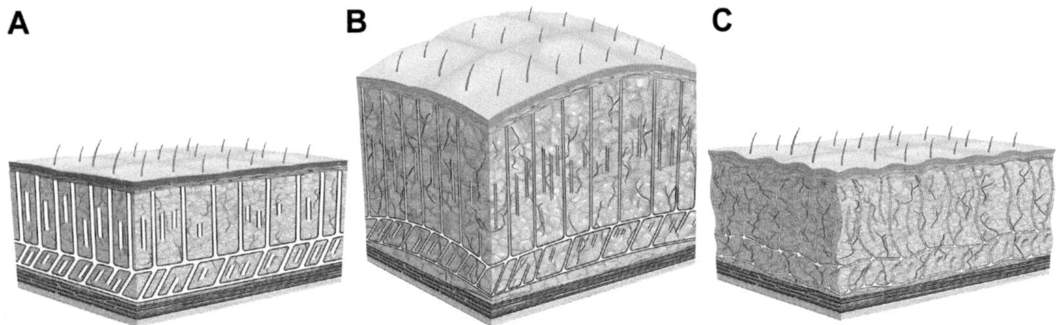

Fig. 3. Superficial fascial system. (*A*) Normal, (*B*) obese, and (*C*) massive weight loss.

PATIENT SELECTION

Physical examination of the lower body should begin with static inspection of the patient in a standing position, with the examiner seated on a swiveling stool to allow free movement all around. Wall mirrors will help the examiner to show and educate patients about their whole extent of tissue laxity (mobility) as well as the recommended vectors for best contouring readjustment. Orthostatic folds and sulci should be identified around the body, considering the physiopathology of MWL contour deformities. Vigorous palpation of the involved segments helps to simulate the effects to be obtained with tissue resection and potential correction vectors. Previous identification of scars and hernias at the abdominal wall is also essential for planning and safety of the proposed treatment. It is reasonable that post–bariatric surgery patients may demand not only lifting but also some extent of central body tightening, with vertical resections. **Fig. 4** shows a systematization of possible approaches to abdominoplasty after MWL, including anterior transverse (conventional), anterior combined (Fleur-de-lis), circumferential (belt), and circumferential combined (Fleur-de-lis + belt).[4]

Although the conventional (anterior transverse) abdominoplasty might be efficient to treat regular patients with excess tissue restricted to the anterior aspect of the lower trunk, this technique tends to be insufficient for treating general MWL circumferential laxity. In most cases, the anterior transverse approach alone does not correct horizontal excess tissue in the central/upper abdomen as well as lateral and posterior ptosis (thighs, flanks, and buttocks), leading to residual laxity that is extremely inconvenient when body contouring is evaluated as a whole (see **Fig. 4**A). The circumferential approach expands the anterior transverse resection of the lower abdomen to the flanks and lower dorsum, removing an actual belt of excess tissue to lift the anterior and lateral aspect of the thighs as well as the gluteal region but this technique alone still may not correct the horizontal excess in the upper abdomen and should result in greater or lesser levels of remaining anterior laxity (see **Fig. 4**B).

The *Fleur-de-lis* abdominoplasty combines longitudinal resection with the anterior transverse approach specifically to address the horizontal excess abdominal tissue, which is normally present in post–bariatric surgery patients (see **Fig. 4**C). This technique is mainly indicated for central body type patients, whereby fat is deposited above the waistline and significantly expands the whole abdominal circumference. Because these cases generally do not present excess tissue or notable fallen lateral and posterior structures of the lower body, a Fleur-de-lis approach can best provide proper adjustment of the body contour by obtaining the recommended vectors for the required correction. It is important to remember that although this technique can greatly improve contouring with good waist definition, it also leaves a visible and permanent median scar. It is up to the medical team to provide patients with detailed information about the pros and cons involved in this type of approach so they will help to choose their surgical planning.

Combining circumferential approach to the *Fleur-de-lis* abdominoplasty specifically addresses horizontal excess around the trunk, which is typically present in the post–bariatric surgery population, specially the gynecoid(pear) body type patients. It is mostly indicated for previous peripheral obesity and significant lower body deflation (below the waistline) but which also present some extent of central body circumferential laxity. Besides lifting lateral and posterior structures of the lower body, the combination with an anterior vertical resection can provide a tightening effect on the central body with the best contouring readjustment, by applying the most synergic vectors for the necessary corrections (see **Fig. 4**D). It is also important to consider the visible and permanent median scar that results from this

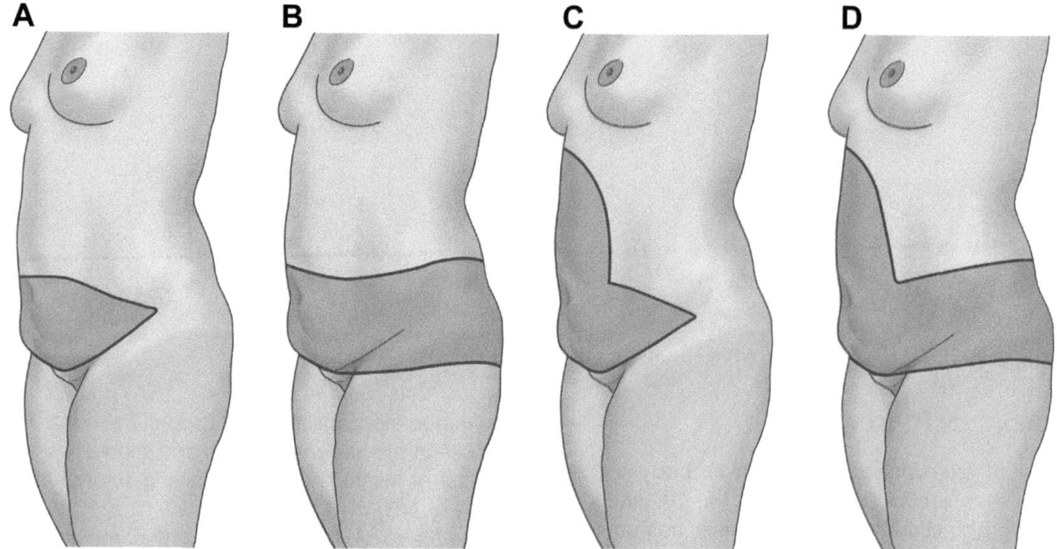

Fig. 4. Possible approaches for lower body readjustment. (*A*) Anterior transverse (conventional), (*B*) circumferential (belt), (*C*) anterior combined (Fleur-de-lis), and (*D*) circumferential combined (Fleur-de-lis + belt).

procedure. The patients should be very well informed about the limitations and possibilities of each approach in order to actively cooperate toward the best surgical option with an acceptable contour/scaring ratio.

VERTICAL RESECTION

Surgeons and patients must understand that, in many cases, just like it would happen to readjust old patients' clothes after massive weight loss, it will be necessary to provide not only horizontal but also vertical resections in order to properly fix the redundant skin around the body. It is important to establish that a Fleur-de-lis approach is not simply adding a vertical scar resection to a conventional anterior transverse abdominoplasty. The concept is completely different because we first aim an effective tightening of the whole central body with great waist definition by an aggressive anterior longitudinal resection (**Fig. 5**), which will be combined to some sort of transverse anterior resection or even circumferential belt lipectomy, in addition to promote the lifting of the ptotic structures such as pubis, lateral thighs, and buttocks.

Markings

After anterior and axillary midlines demarcation, patient is placed in the supine position to have a strong upward traction of the abdominal tissue to perform the lower horizontal marking 5 cm above the vulvar apex. With patient standing again, laterally continue the inferior horizontal line toward both flanks, usually until around the midaxillary line projection. Anteriorly, the Bury Test will determine the transversal extent of the vertical resection. This maneuver consists of pushing the medial aspect of one hand onto the anterior midline while the other hand equally grasps and moves both lateral tissue medially against each other and over the fixed midline skin. Burying midline tissue is an effective way to make sure that lateral borders will successfully and safely close after surgical resection. This maneuver seems to be more accurate and reliable than the "Pinch Test" that requires a safety margin to estimate the amount of tissue between then fingers.[5] The lower level of the vertical excision is usually placed below the umbilicus, being established by vigorous palpation sliding the central lower flap upward (pubis), under the sagging abdominal skin, toward each vertical line defining the turning point to start the upper horizontal marking, keeping this sliding check laterally to meet the ends of the previous lower lines. Markings of the neo umbilicus lateral flaps will be discussed ahead (Video 1).

Technique

In supine position, start the abdominal undermining through the inferior horizontal incision facing upward until the umbilical level. After completing skin incision of the right vertical limb, beveling cautery dissection is performed all the way through the subcutaneous tissue until the rectus sheath dissection plane. The same procedure on the left side joined both dissections at the central midline. During anterior tissue detachment, patients have the umbilical stalk isolated, clamped, and cut at

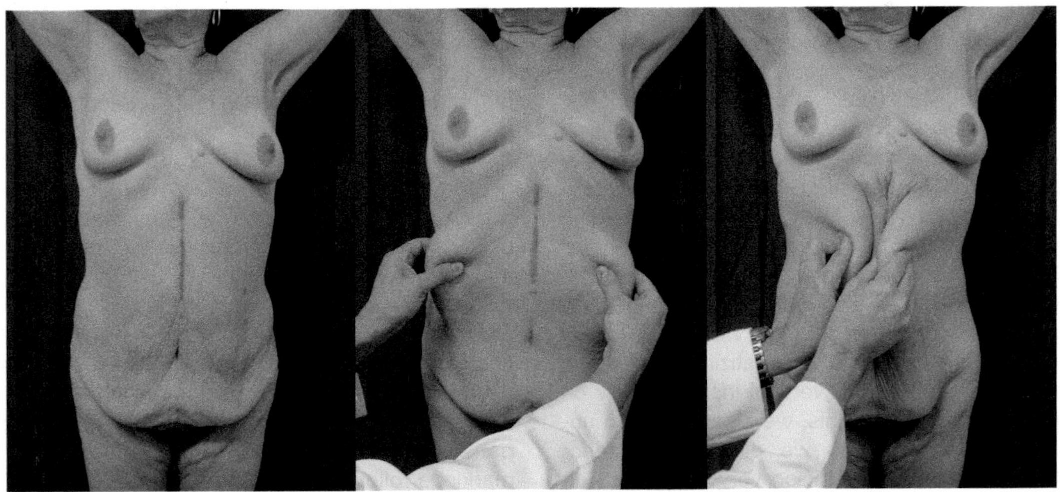

Fig. 5. Anterior longitudinal resection provides correction vectors that will promote effective tightening of the whole central body with proper waist definition.

its base, being finally resected along with the surgical specimen (Fig. 6A, B). A continuous closure suture with 2.0 nylon is performed at the amputated base just adjacent to the rectus sheath. Aponeurosis plication is performed as usual, whenever necessary.

Vertical flaps approximation is performed by a running spiral suture with vicryl 0 in the subcutaneous deep layer and 2.0 vicryl in the most superficial fat subdermal layer (see Video 2).

TECHNICAL REFINEMENTS

Previous subcutaneous infiltration with epinephrine along the incision lines and electrocautery dissection are some of the important technical points in order to reduce bleeding and trauma during surgery. MWL patients usually present enlarged vessels at the subcutaneous level, so that active and preventive hemostasis is essential. Plication of the anterior aponeurosis should be performed because it goes in conventional approach, considering prior distension by intra-abdominal fat during obesity or even previous pregnancies. Small and uncomplicated midline hernias may be simply corrected by plication but the use of alloplastic material (synthetic mesh) should be applied in complex cases (Video 2).

Although the observation and treatment of the whole circumferential lower body is mostly indicated for MWL patients, specifically for the Fleur-de-lis abdominoplasty both pubic and umbilical regions hold the key for making the highest impact toward outstanding lower body contour results.

PUBIS

The pubic region makes part of the lower body and requires a special attention in surgical planning as a fundamental element for overall contouring. As

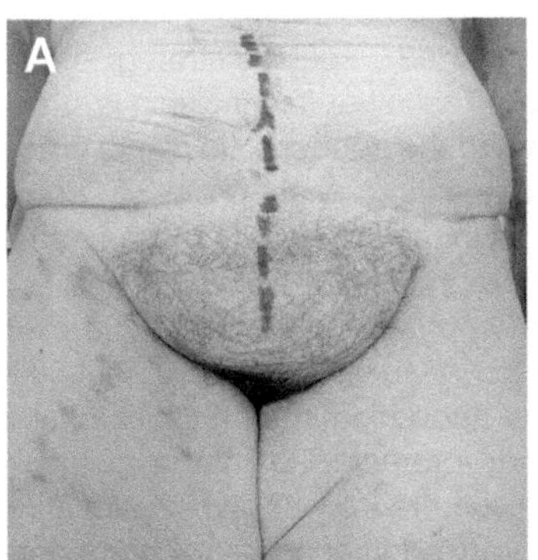

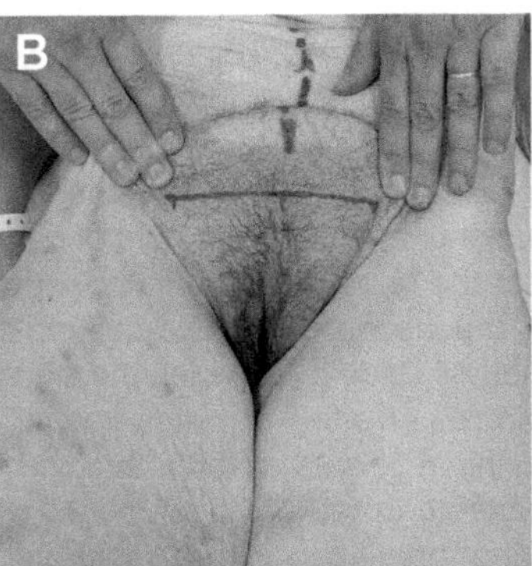

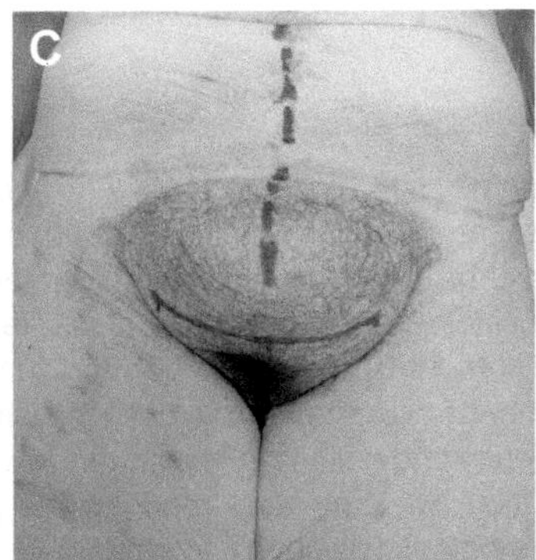

Fig. 6. (*A*) Horizontal dorsal decubitus, (*B*) cranial traction of the pubis with demarcation at 5 cm above the vulvar apex, and (*C*) final anterior lower marking.

with the navel, no esthetic result can be considered ideal if the pubic region is not balanced with the new abdominal contour. In general, massive weight loss significantly affects the mons pubis, which usually becomes redundant and ptotic in postbariatric patients. Literature presents several sorts of pubis resection techniques generally associated with lower body lifts and medial thigh reduction resulting in horizontal, vertical, and/or oblique final surrounding scars.[5–7,8,9–14]The continuity of those scars around the pubic area usually provides a "portrait" aspect that we must avoid for being extremely visible, stigmatizing, and unesthetic. Although medial vertical incisions may be hidden by the hairy pubis, we also find them unnecessary as long as we place the anterior abdominal horizontal incision very low, which allows proper resection and repositioning of the remaining ptosed tissue, as well as best restoring of the triangular shape of the new mons pubis.

Our treatment philosophy was derived from previous publications by Aly[5] and Kaluf[6], who already advocated a low incision in abdominoplasty procedures in combination with the pubic *lift*. The normal pubic area is shaped like an inverted triangle, and excess tissue following major weight loss is located on the highest portion corresponding to the base of this inverted triangle, by volumetric stretching in continuity with the abdominal wall during obesity.

Thus, if we place the low horizontal skin incision, just 5 cm above the vulvar apex, the entire contingent of the excess tissue should be removed along with the surgical apron. This would leave a new inverted triangle, which would be quite reduced and its base can be distributed and adjusted to the superior flap without the need for vertical resections. Regardless of the abdominal approach, that is, anterior transverse (conventional), anterior composite (Fleur-de-lis), circumferential (belt), or circumferential composite (Fleur-de-lis + belt), it will be possible to include the pubic region in the surgical planning of the lower body treatment.

Markings

As initially suggested by Aly[5], we consider it essential to perform this inferior marking at the level of the pubis, with the patients in the supine position because gravity facilitates the accomplishment of the upper traction maneuver, aiding in better distribution of tissues, with greater efficiency and uniformity. From this lower initial delimitation, we continued marking the patients in the orthostatic position, according to the previous planning of the resection (Fleur-de-lis, circumferential, and so forth).

Regardless of the intensity of pubic sagging and ptosis, the patients were initially placed in the horizontal dorsal decubitus position so that in the presence of vigorous cranial traction of all pubis, a first horizontal line of approximately 14 cm was then marked, with its central point 5 cm away from the vulvar rhyme (hairy) after marking the anterior midline. This is the new upper skin edge of the pubic region after apronectomy and flaps suturing. We call that "Lockwood Maneuver," which is tissue mobilization in search of the anchoring line, that is, the desired final position of the scars by moving the more fixed flaps' edges as opposed to the more mobile ones (**Fig. 6**). Following this initial delimitation, the patient is placed in the standing position, and the markings follow the needs and individual indications, with the planning of tissue resections in the anterior and or circumferential plane (**Fig. 7**, see Video 1).

Technique

Based on the preoperative observations, it is noted that most of the excess pubic tissue rests above this markings and will be eliminated along with the abdominal apron as part of the surgical resection. This can be observed clearly in **Fig. 8**. The intense structural disorder of the SFS allows for large dermo-adipose resections, with the possibility of primary closure only by approaching the flaps, without any detachment beyond the incised edges. With great viability and circulatory safety, this tissue redistribution corrects excesses and repositions structures with a greater contour harmony.

Because the edges to be approximated usually undergo great mobilization to reach their new position, especially in the Fleur-de-lis approach, where there is little or no undermining, there is a risk that the "inverted T-shape" region will have little subcutaneous tissue, thus causing excessive tension and local depression. To prevent this occurrence, we included 2 specific strategies during flap dissection. The lower flap incision is superiorly beveled toward the aponeurotic plane, with a subcutaneous angulation that provides some amount of deep fat in the upper pubic region, after the cutaneous incision (**Fig. 9**A). Thus, in addition to preserving the lymphatic circulation at this level, when the skin at the base of the pubic triangle migrates toward the abdominal flap, it slides over a fatty cushion that protects against a possible localized depression. Moreover, while elevating the upper flaps, an additional fatty component was also preserved in the corresponding central region for the same purpose[15] (see **Fig. 9**A).

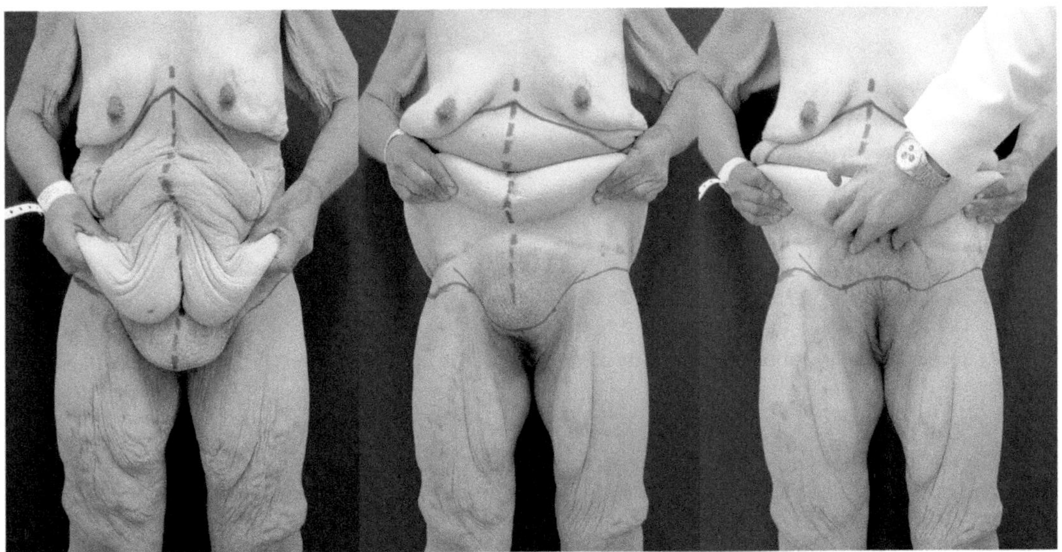

Fig. 7. Final markings for a circumferential combined approach (Fleur-de-lis + belt lipectomy). Note the lower position of the anterior pubic marking.

The central approximation of the flaps is initially performed by deeper sutures at the level of the SFS using simple vicryl 0, followed by spiral running sutures (fat/subdermal) using colorless vicryl 2.0 threads. It should be noted that because of the beveling of the upper region of the inverted triangle, we did not perform the aponeurotic fixation of the flaps but only the union of the subcutaneous tissue with deep sutures interesting the SFS (Fig. 9B). Such sutures followed laterally, distributing the tissues and reducing the tension for the closure of the skin.

At the time of flap approximation, if there are excess fatty tissues in the pubic cone already reduced by the low horizontal incision, we perform scissors lipectomy in a more superficial plane without liposuction or additional skin resection. We do not recommend resections of the deep fat at this level, since they tend to predispose to lymphatic complications, especially with the formation of prolonged edema and seromas in the postoperative period.

Figs. 10 and 11 present the final outcome of this approach in the patient that was previously presented in Figs. 6–8. This was a severe case with an extreme degree of tissue laxity after massive weight loss treated by lower body composite circumferential approach plus inner thigh reduction in a second operative time. Even in cases with an apparently less severe deformity, the pathophysiology of tissue laxity after a considerable weight loss requires to address the pubic region

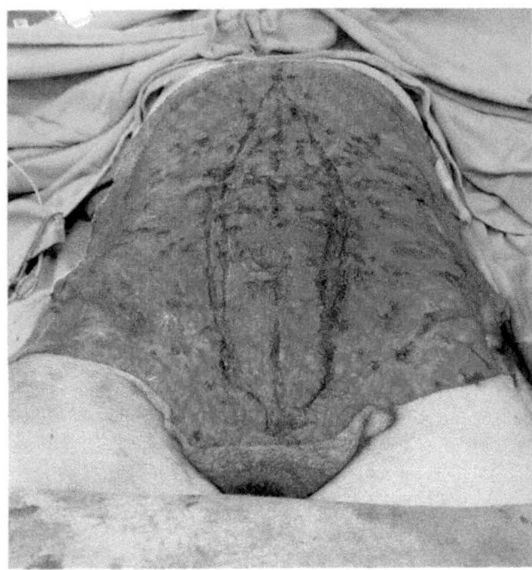

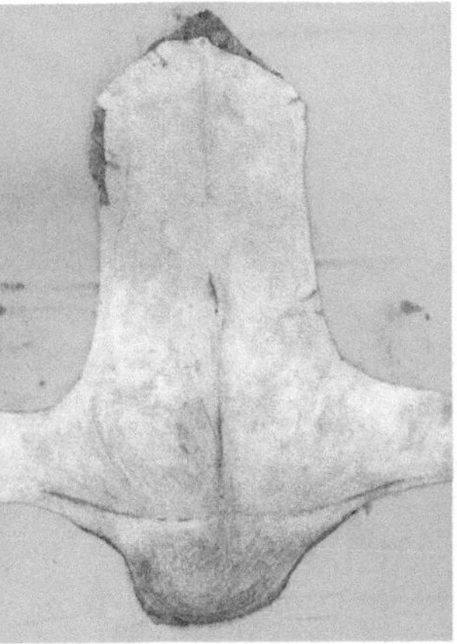

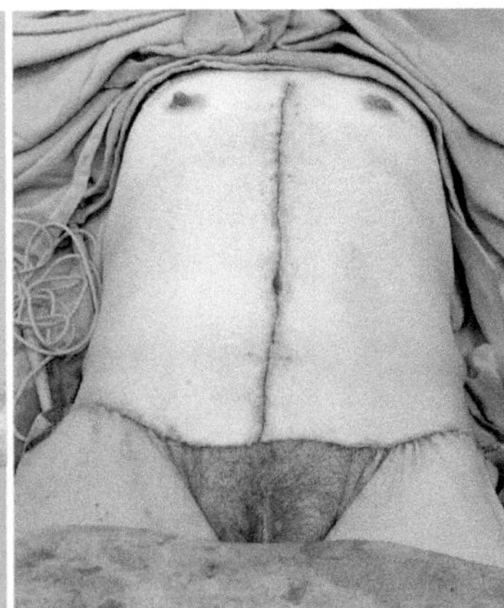

Fig. 8. Intraoperative view reconstructing the pubis with the abdominal contour. Note the great amount of pubic tissue resected along with the abdominal apron.

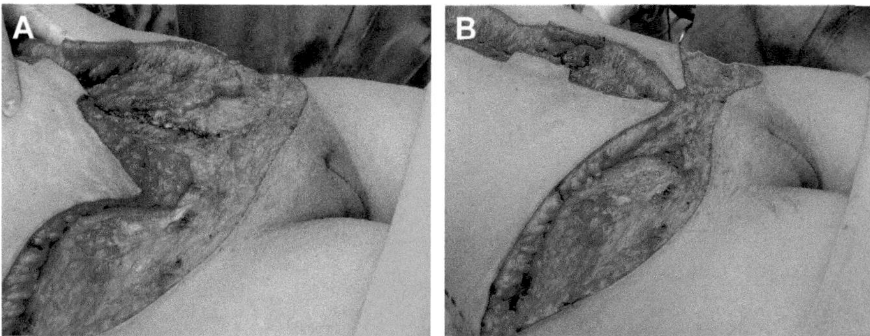

Fig. 9. (*A*) Beveled lower incision and extra fatty component at the upper flaps and (*B*) central deep sutures interesting the SFS.

along with the lower body to obtain more harmonious contour results (see Video 2).

NEO UMBILICUS

Although anterior vertical resections may provide enhanced lower body contouring for deflated patients, such indication have been restricted by visible and pathologic scaring usually with stigmatizing umbilical distortions. The presence of an "outer scar" around the umbilicus have been recognized as a source of several surgical complications that may lead to undesirable scaring with anatomic disarrangement and poor esthetic results, ultimately figured by stenosis or widening of the navel.

Rebuilding umbilical architecture following abdominoplasty is considered one of the most challenging tasks, especially for the massive weight loss patients that usually present with elongated umbilical stalks and critical tissue excess in both vertical and horizontal planes.[1] After the introduction of a "double lateral skin flap" to reconstruct the umbilicus within an anterior vertical scar,[16] several authors have also suggested similar approaches for creating a new umbilicus during the Fleur-de-lis abdominoplasty.[17–22] Donnabella[22] popularized such concept stating the importance of recreating all the umbilical anatomic landmarks (base, grooving, and ring) in search of natural results. Although conceptually comprehensive, those publications lack to standardize and fully describe technical steps. Following Donnabella's principles, we have suggested a specific and reproducible looping suture technique in order to anatomically recreate the new umbilicus.

Markings

Both vertical markings of the anterior resection includes the design of a lateral skin flap, 8.0 cm

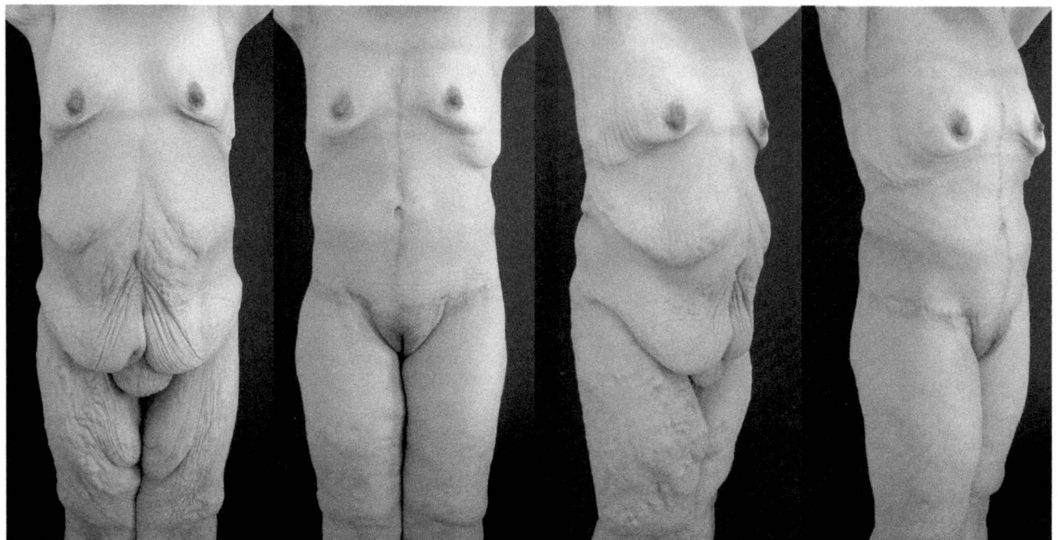

Fig. 10. Lower body readjustment: Preoperative and postoperative images of the composite circumferential approach (12 months) plus internal reduction of the thighs (6 months).

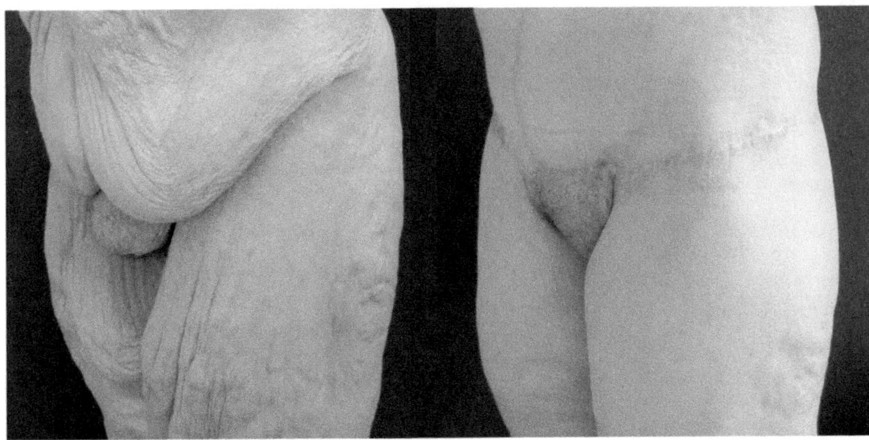

Fig. 11. Lower body readjustment: Final aspect showing the harmonious redefinition of the pubis in detail.

wide × 1.5 cm long, that will be undermined and preserved by its pedicle, apart from the resected surgical specimen (**Fig. 12**). We prefer to mark those lateral skin flaps initially wider than they will finally stand, in order to allow a greater range of possibilities for better establishing the umbilical final position, after moving and approximating abdominal remaining tissue[17] (see Video 1).

Technique

Although suturing the vertical edges, both parallel skin flaps (8.0 cm wide × 1.5 cm long) that were preserved by the Fleur-de-lis preoperative demarcation, were then intraoperatively redesigned into a proper size and position, at the iliac crest level, finally measuring approximately 2.5 × 1.5 cm. Rather than rectangular with sharp edges, the final shape of the flaps had a rounded design[22] (**Fig. 13**A, B). After removing excessive tissue and defatting the skin flaps, 3 nylon 2.0 sutures are placed in a looping technique in order to create a medial deep aponeurotic attachment, reconstructing the navel base (**Fig. 13**C1–3).

Umbilical Base: Looping Suture. (A) The looping suture needle initially enters the skin and transects the left flap exiting through the dermis, at 1.0 cm far from its edge; (B) It now enters the rectus sheet

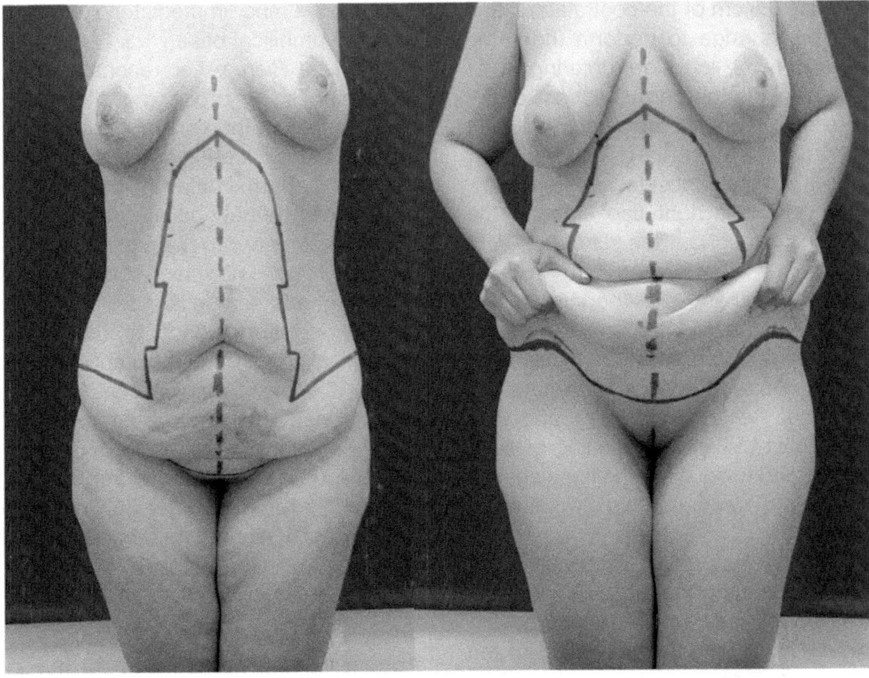

Fig. 12. Lower body readjustment: Fleur-de-lis approach.

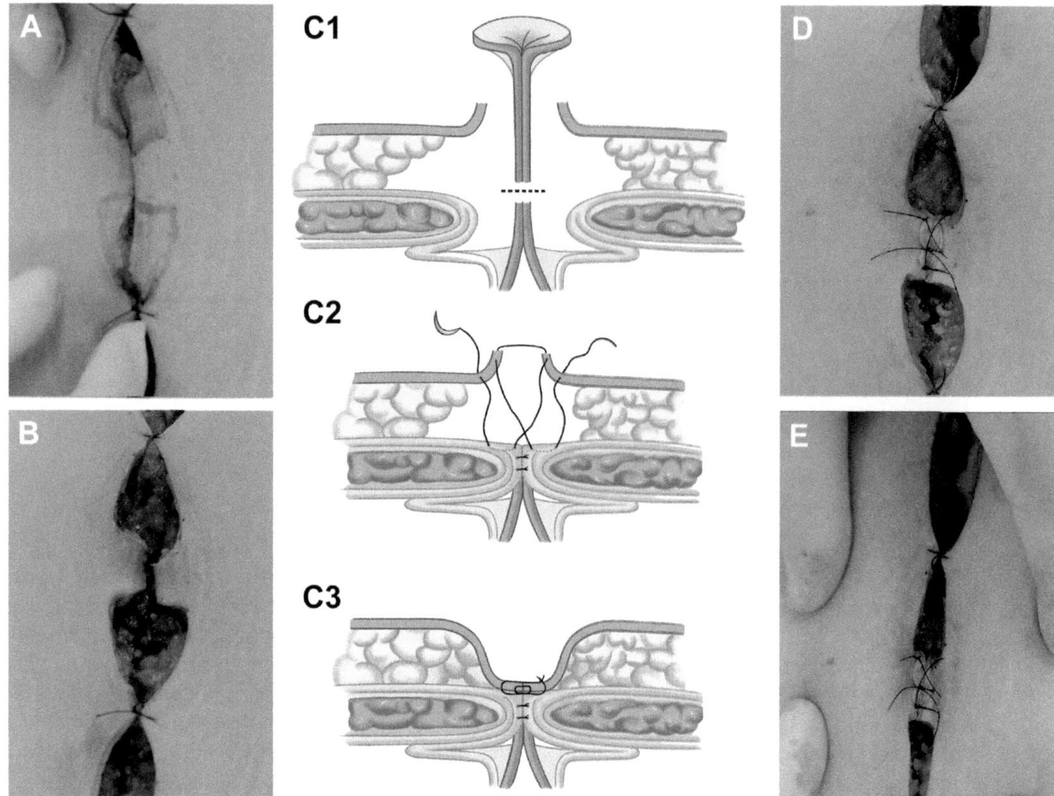

Fig. 13. Inner scar neo umbilicus: surgical sequence. (*A*) Innner flap positioning of the final neoumbilicus. (*B*) Final flaps after excessive skin ressection. (*C*) Umbilical Management. (*C1*) Umbilical amputation. (*C2*) Looping suture of the flaps into each other and the aponeurosis. (*C3*) Neo umbilicus sutured. (*D*) Looping suture of the flaps. (*E*) Neo umbilical formation while vertical edges are aproximated.

at the same side and runs immediately under it for 1.0 cm until exiting at the midline; (C) Then, the suture needle grasps 0.5 cm of the contralateral flap dermis exiting on its edge to perform the same 0.5 cm grasping on the left side, entering at its edge and exiting inside the dermal aspect of the flap; (D) The needle reenters the rectus sheet at the midline and runs immediately under it for 1.0 cm until exiting at the right side; and (E) Finally, the needle transects the right flap entering the dermis and exiting throughout the skin, at 1.0 cm far from its edge.

Three looping stiches are performed as mentioned above, one at the center and 2 others at superior and inferior borders of the flaps. Initial stiches were left loose in order to facilitate the accomplishment of the following ones, and they were all tightened at the end. Tightening of each looping suture helped to squeeze the flaps against each other into the deep midline aponeurosis (**Fig. 13**D, E).

Umbilical Grooving: Fat Suture. Because it is not possible to retract the umbilical base deeper than the aponeurosis level, the best umbilical grooving was achieved by increasing the projection of the surrounding areas. That was accomplished by two 2.0 Vycril sutures, with a long needle (4 cm), approximating lateral fat tissue into the midline right above and immediately under the reconstructed umbilical base.

Umbilical Ring. After reconstructing the base and establishing proper navel grooving, the 3-plane suture of the vertical edges helped to provide the ring configuration of the umbilicus because it approximates the covering tissue under and above the new navel. After all, deeply cutaneous attachment to the rectus sheet (base), surrounded by normal subcutaneous tissue (grooving) and scar less outer skin configures the natural ring appearance to the surface of the abdominal wall around the umbilicus (see Video 2).

Fig. 13 shows a surgical sequence of the umbilical reconstruction by the lateral skin flaps, and **Fig. 14** shows several results in detail.

The looping stiches are kept in place to be completely removed after 30 days, whereas the vertical incisions had absorbable internal sutures.

DISCUSSION

Abdominal approaches that do not include the correction of the pubis usually result in a bulky

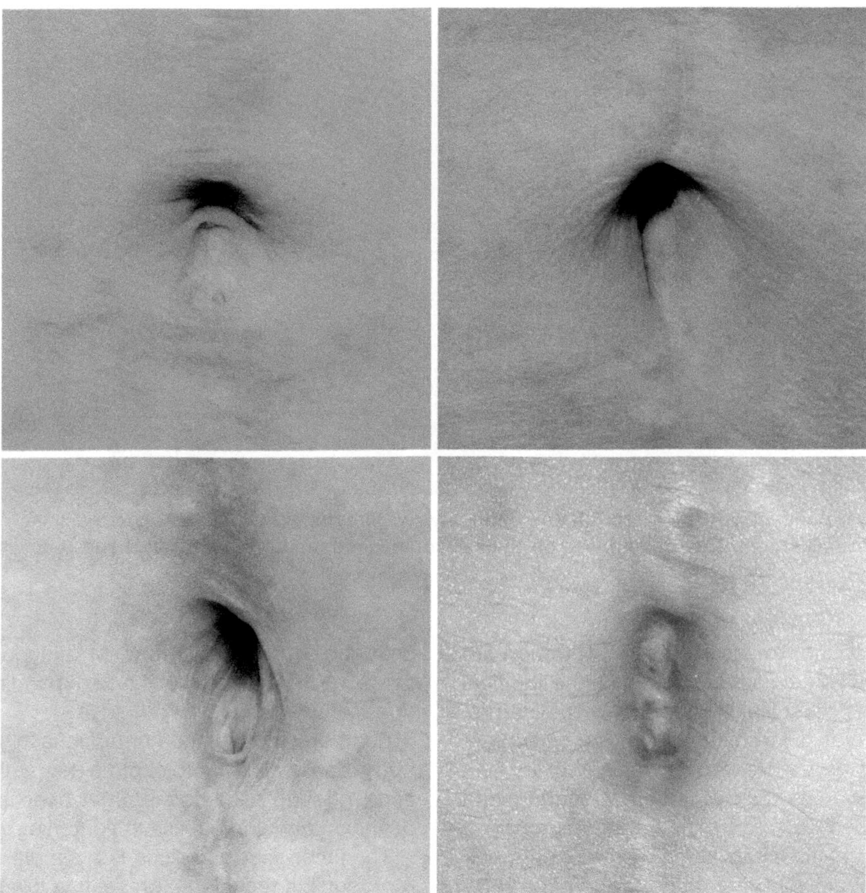

Fig. 14. Inner scar neo umbilicus: results.

and ptotic aspect, in disharmony with the new and improved abdominal contour. Similarly, possible attempts of isolated treatment of the pubic region will require more scars, with an unnatural aspect of the segment.

Small suture dehiscence and formation of localized seromas are the main adverse events reported with this approach, and the treatment is usually conservative with serial dressings and punctures, respectively. Other possible minor and major complications described in literature are related to postbariatric condition in general[23]; however, there is no evidence of a direct causal relationship with the specific approach of the pubic region. The production and approximation of fatty flaps in the lower central region, which corresponds to the upper limit of the new pubis, seem to be an important strategy to ensure optimal closure of the sutures without localized dimpling due to the great concentric migration of those flaps especially with their fixation to the aponeurotic sheet.

Low positioning of the anterior scar and the alignment of the flaps by specific anchoring at the SFS/Skin allow best harmonic contour of the pubic area in Fleur-de-lis abdominoplasty, without the need for additional resections and scars (**Fig. 15**). Quality evaluation of the results could and should be improved in future studies with the use of more objective and prospective criteria, with the participation of both patients and independent observers.

Normal umbilical appearance is fundamental in order to achieve harmonious body contouring with esthetically balanced abdominal results. The navel has been stated as the "*surgeon's signature*" and must receive appropriate attention during the approach because no surgical outcome will be considered completely favorable if it presents with problems regarding shape, size, position, and scaring. Despite our technique of inner scar umbilicus is always the same, resulting shapes may vary, even though getting to reconstruct the anatomic landmarks. Skin quality,

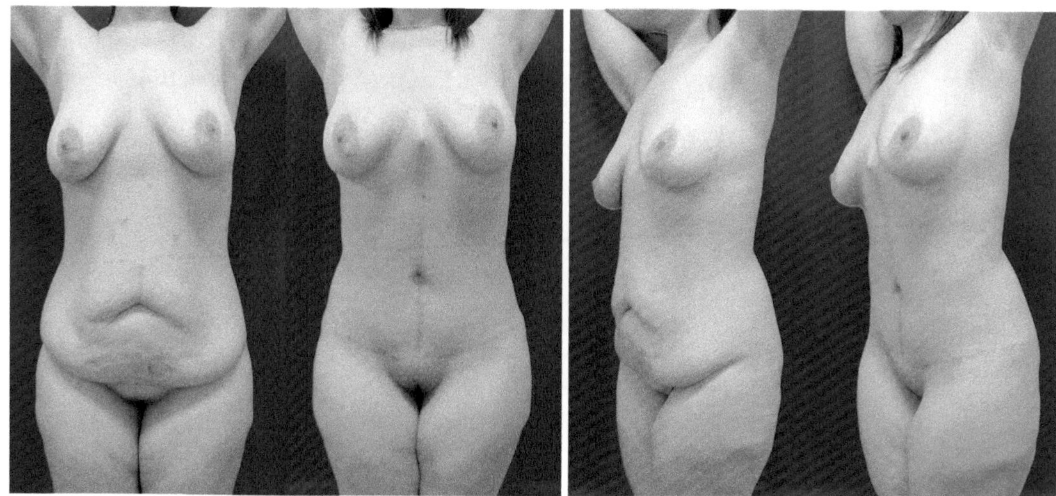

Fig. 15. Lower body readjustment: frontal and oblique views. Preoperative and postoperative image of a Fleur-de-lis approach (12 months) with emphasis on the harmonious redefinition of the navel and pubic region.

subcutaneous thickness, and scar retraction are some of the variables that may influence the final navel aspect, just as it happens in the nature, where several different umbilical shapes might develop to be considered normal, both in men and women. The lack of external scaring and the inner healing pattern of the new umbilicus also seem to help establishing a better scar quality for both superior and inferior abdominal vertical scars.[24] Local complications such as widening or stenosis are unlikely with this technique, and the results are natural and sustainable. Routinely building a new inner scar umbilicus in Fleur-de-lis abdominoplasties has completely changed our critical view of anterior vertical scars, reducing limitations and expanding indications for the procedure (Fig. 16).

Such predictable and harmonious lower/central body results allow us to explore new esthetic horizons, offering patients the great benefits of waist definition and vertical tissue tightening.

The inner scar umbilicus is a simple, safe, and reproducible technique, presenting low complication rates with sustainable, nice, and natural results. The high quality of navel tridimensional reconstruction makes it our first choice for Fleur-de-lis abdominoplasties, especially for post–bariatric body contouring.

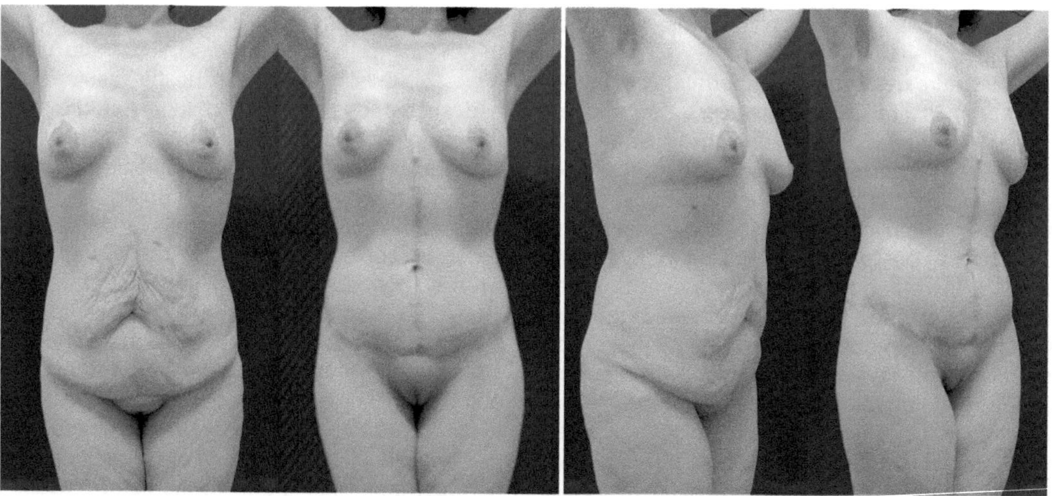

Fig. 16. Lower body readjustment: frontal and oblique views. Preoperative and postoperative images of a Fleur-de-lis + belt lipectomy (12 months) with emphasis on the harmonious redefinition of the navel and pubic region.

CLINICS CARE POINTS

- When planning MWL abdominoplasty, consider the surrounding complex circumferential laxity that requires a broader approach with modified correction vectors ruled by the continuity of concomitant affected areas.
- Vigorous palpation of the involved segments helps to simulate the effects to be obtained with tissue resection and potential correction vectors.
- The *Fleur-de-lis* abdominoplasty combines longitudinal resection with the anterior transverse approach specifically to address the horizontal excess abdominal tissue, which is normally present in central body type MWL patients.
- Low positioning of the anterior scar and the alignment of the flaps by specific anchoring at the SFS/Skin allow best harmonic contour of the pubic area in Fleur-de-lis abdominoplasty.
- The lack of external scaring and the inner healing pattern of the new umbilicus help establishing a better scar quality for both superior and inferior abdominal vertical scars.

DISCLOSURE

The authors have nothing to disclose.

SUPPLEMENTARY DATA

Supplementary data related to this article can be found online at https://doi.org/10.1016/j.cps.2023.09.001.

REFERENCES

1. Mendes FH, Viterbo F. Abdominoplasty after massive weight loss. In: Avelar JM, editor. New concepts on abdominoplasties and further aplications, 23. Springer; 2016. p. 356–88.
2. Lockwood TE. Superficial fascial system (SFS) of the trunk and extremities: a new concept. Plast Reconstr Surg 1991;87(6):1009–18.
3. Mendes FH, Viterbo F. Reajuste do corpo inferior: conceitos e filosofia de tratamento. In: Mendes FH, Viterbo F, editors. Cirurgia Plástica Pós-Bariátrica. Rio de Janeiro: DiLivros; 2016. p. 201–65.
4. Mendes FH, Donnabella A, Moreira ARF. Fleur-de-lis abdominoplasty and neo-umbilicus. Clin Plastic Surg 2019;46:49–60.
5. Aly AS. Belt lipectomy. In: Aly AS, editor. Body Contouring after massive weight loss. 1st edition. St Louis: Quality Medical Publishing; 2006. p. 71–145.
6. Kaluf R, Araújo GAZ, Martins DL, et al. Tratamento da regiao pubiana na abdominoplastia de pacientes apos grande perda ponderal. Rev Bras Cir Plast 2008;23(4):302–4.
7. Loeb R. Narrowing of the mons pubis during thigh lifts. Ann Plast Surg 1979;2(4):290–7.
8. Matarasso A, Wallach SG. Abdominal contour surgery: treating all aesthetic units, including the mons pubis. Aesthet Surg J 2001;21(2):111–297.
9. Hurwitz DJ. Single-staged total body lift after massive weight loss. Ann Plast Surg 2004;52(5):435–41.
10. Filho JM, Belerique M, Franco D, et al. Dermolipectomy of the pubic area associated with abdominoplasty. Aesthetic Plast Surg 2007;31(1):12–5.
11. Alter GJ. Management of the mons pubis and labia majora in the massive weight loss patient. Aesthet Surg J 2009;29(5):432–42.
12. El-Khatib HA. Mons pubis ptosis: classification and strategy for treatment. Aesthetic Plast Surg 2011;35(1):24–30.
13. Marques M, Modolin M, Cintra W, et al. Monsplasty for women after massive weight loss. Aesthetic Plast Surg 2012;36(3):511–6.
14. Tavares-Filho JM, Franco D, Franco T. Refinamentos na abordagem da regiao pubiana. In: Mendes FH, Viterbo F, editors. Cirurgia Plastica Pos-Bariatrica. Rio de Janeiro: DiLivros; 2016. p. 354–65.
15. Mendes FH, Viterbo F, Gabas JMC, et al. Revisiting postbariatric monsplasty. Rev Bras Cir Plást 2017;32(3):383–90.
16. Franco D, Medeiros J, Farias C, et al. Umbilical reconstruction for patients with a midline scar. Aesthetic Plast Surg 2006;30(5):595–8.
17. Silva FN, Oliveira EA. Neoonphaloplasty in vertical abdominoplasty. Rev Bras Cir Plast 2010;25:330–6.
18. Reno AB, Mizukami A, Calaes IL, et al. Neoomphaloplasty in anchor-line abdominoplasty performed in patients who have previously undergone bariatric surgery. Rev Bras Cir Plast 2013;28(1):114–8.
19. Cavalcante ELF. Neo-umbilicoplasty as an option in umbilical reconstruction in abdominal anchor dermolipectomy post gastroplasty. Rev Bras Cir Plast 2010;25(3):509–18.
20. Monte ALR. Treatatment of the umbilical stenosis in a vertical dermolipectomy patient. Rev Bras Cir Plast 2011;26(1):167–70.
21. Mizukami A, Ribeiro BB, Reno BA, et al. Retrospective analysis of 70 patients who underwent postbariatric abdominoplasty with neo-omphaloplasty. Rev Bras Cir Plast 2014;29(1):89–93.
22. Donnabella A. Anatomical reconstruction of the umbilicus. Rev Bras Cir Plást 2013;28:119–23.
23. Cavalcante HA, Lima EM Jr, Mendes FH. Eventos adversos em cirurgia plástica pós-bariátrica. In: Mendes FH, Viterbo F, editors. Cirurgia Plástica Pós-Bariátrica. Rio de Janeiro: DiLivros; 2016. p. 719–45.
24. Mendes FH, Viterbo F. Inner scar umbilicus: new horizons for vertical abdominoplasty. Plast Reconstr Surg 2018;141(4). 507e–16e.

Circumferential Surgical Contouring of the Upper and Lower Body

Joshua A. David, MD, Jeffrey A. Gusenoff, MD*

KEYWORDS

• Abdominoplasty • Body contouring • Buttocks • Circumferential • Lower body lift
• Panniculectomy • Staging • Thighs

KEY POINTS

- Deformities in the body contouring population are rarely isolated to 1 area, and procedures can be combined and/or staged to achieve optimal results while maintaining patient safety.
- While there is no formula for optimal surgical sequencing and timing, there are certain principles which–when applied appropriately–can yield results that are reliable, aesthetically pleasing, and aligned with the patient's desires and preferences.
- This article outlines our latest thinking in circumferential body contouring, and how to integrate the lower body lift with procedures of the abdomen, upper body, breasts, back, and arms, in order to achieve the complete 360° look.

INTRODUCTION

Since its inception, the field of body contouring surgery has undergone continuous evolution. Whereas early iterations during the late 19th century were preoccupied with the functional excision of adipocutaneous tissue, over the next century or so, there emerged an appreciation for the aesthetic implications of skin, fat and soft tissue removal.[1] Within this burgeoning discipline however, surgical advances were generally restricted to structures of the anterior trunk, using vectors of tissue movement in only a unidirectional, vertical plane. By the end of the 20th century however, landmark anatomical studies and conceptual developments in surgically reshaping the natural contours of the human body by pioneers such as Pitanguy, Lockwood, Illuouz, and Matarasso propelled the field into a new era. The resulting landscape, therefore, was seemingly primed for the body contouring revolution starting in the early 2000s, borne out of a precipitous rise of bariatric surgery. Addressing the many challenges of this novel massive weight loss (MWL) population and their diverse, unpredictable deformities required the integration of emerging concepts in fascial architecture and soft tissue resuspension, alongside real-time insights into the importance of adjacent anatomy and interactions with circumferential, multi-dimensional forces.

Today, our modern era continues to present new challenges and opportunities for the field of body contouring surgery. These include advancements in alternative fat-reduction technologies, shifting aesthetic and cultural trends, and lofty patient expectations fueled by social media. In this article, we present our most up-to-date perspectives and surgical approaches to circumferential body contouring, with a particular focus on integrating the lower body, abdomen, and upper body in order to achieve a comprehensive, 360° transformation.

PREOPERATIVE ASSESSMENT

Patient Selection

While the potential to help MWL patients achieve their desired physical transformation can be a

Department of Plastic Surgery, University of Pittsburgh Medical Center, 3550 Terrace Street, 6B Scaife Hall, Pittsburgh, PA 15261, USA
* Corresponding author.
E-mail address: gusenoffja@upmc.edu

Clin Plastic Surg 51 (2024) 95–110
https://doi.org/10.1016/j.cps.2023.06.003

deeply rewarding experience, it is important to recognize the added complexities and responsibilities involved in caring for this patient population. Ensuring patient safety is of paramount importance in the decision-making process for any body contouring procedure, and requires meticulous, individualized preoperative planning.

Prior to taking any patient to the operating room, a comprehensive preoperative consultation should be conducted, adhering to the standards established by Pitanguy nearly four decades ago.[2] This assessment should include detailed past and current histories of the patient's weight loss, personal or familial medical conditions, prior surgeries, functional status, lifestyle, nutrition, and any other relevant social issues. For MWL patients, is recommended to wait a minimum of 12-18 months after bariatric surgery, and ensure at least 3 months of weight stability, before proceeding with body contouring surgery. It is important to recognize that body mass index (BMI) may not be the best predictor of operative success or failure; while complications are certainly higher with increasing BMI, our studies have shown no evidence for a strict cutoff point.[3] Therefore, patients should be evaluated on an individual basis to identify their specific deformity, overall physical fitness, and personal goals to determine what can be offered to help them. Document any wound healing-related risk factors, such as smoking, diabetes, hypertension, nutritional deficiencies, and chronic steroid use. The identification of any inherited conditions or acquired (eg, medications) patient factors affecting coagulation is particularly important for body contouring procedures, since larger body surface area, longer surgery duration, and prolonged hypothermia substantially increase the risk of blood loss.[4] Remember that surgery is not a solution for every patient; familiarity with the ever-growing array of nonsurgical or minimally invasive options, such as high-intensity focused ultrasonic (HIFU) therapy, radiofrequency, and mesotherapy, is recommended.

Patient Expectations

In the context of post-MWL body-contouring surgery, it is critical to manage patient expectations effectively. Patients must be willing to trade significant functional and cosmetic improvements for significant scars, and should be well-informed regarding expected incision placement, the anticipated recovery process, and surgical complications–both broadly and procedure/anatomy-specific. These include bleeding, infection, scarring, seroma, delayed healing, need for additional surgery, as well as malposition or loss of the umbilicus or nipple areola complex for abdominal/breast procedures, and loss of sensation along the medial arm for brachioplasty. Patients should also be made aware that certain circumferential or extremity procedures can result in lifelong complications such as lymphedema. Anesthesia-related risks should be discussed as well, including venous thromboembolism, reactions to medication, or even death. Nonetheless, patients can be reassured that, while complications following body contouring procedures are relatively common, they are typically minor, and able to be managed in the outpatient setting.

Surgical Setting/Team

When determining the appropriate surgical setting for body contouring procedures, several factors must be taken into consideration. For instance, while an outpatient surgical center may be suitable for healthy patients, restrictions on liposuction volume or length of surgery may limit the scope of procedures that can be performed. For patients with significant comorbidities or other operative risks, a hospital setting may be more appropriate. The extent of operative intervention that can be provided to a patient will depend on the surgeon's experience with various body contouring procedures and their level of comfort in performing lengthier cases. When available, team members such as dedicated physician extenders, residents, or a second co-surgeon can broaden the available surgical options. At our center, we have established a large, coordinated team consisting of a senior surgeon, a dedicated body contouring surgical fellow, plastic surgery residents, and physician extenders. This allows us to facilitate efficiency in the operating room and reduce the total number of surgeries. Surgeons without these resources may require four or five stages to achieve the desired results.

Intra-operative Considerations

For the most part, the intra-operative risks for body contouring surgery mirror those for surgery in general. The use of peri-operative antibiotic and pharmacologic venous thromboembolism (VTE) prophylaxis is controversial, although we generally utilize both for body contouring. It is worth reiterating several factors that require extra vigilance in the MWL patient, such as body temperature and avoidance of hypothermia, fluid balance, and positioning. While seemingly self-evident, failure to properly attend to any one of these can have disastrous consequences. Making sure to have a contingency plan in place at all times is a prudent approach to mitigating potential harm.

SURGICAL PLANNING

Rating Deformities

Classification systems are instrumental in describing clinical features, but their utility is limited without correlation to appropriate surgical interventions or specific outcomes. Until recently, attempts to systematically organize or quantify the deformities associated with MWL fell short of this objective. Most often, they were either too limited in scope to be useful for a diverse patient population, or had been repurposed from older rating systems that were inadequate in accounting for the distinctive deformities observed in the MWL population.

To address this need for a comprehensive and organized approach to patients undergoing body contouring surgery, a team from our institution previously developed the Pittsburgh Rating Scale.[5] This validated instrument offers a systematic evaluation and classification system for the specific deformities and anatomical regions most associated with laxity and ptosis after MWL, and corresponding surgical interventions tailored to the level of deformity present. Since its initial publication nearly 2 decades ago, we have found the Pittsburgh Rating Scale to be a valuable tool not only for patient counseling, but also for analyzing our surgical outcomes and further characterizing deformities of the breasts,[6] outer thighs,[7] and abdomen.[8]

Combining and Staging Procedures

Given the extent and severity of post-MWL deformities, it is rare that a single procedure can adequately address all of the patients functional and cosmetic concerns. Fortunately, procedures can often be combined and/or staged in a way that aligns with the patient's goals and available resources.

In the field of body contouring, performing more than 1 procedure in a single stage has several advantages. For instance, combining procedures reduces the total number of operations patients must endure, which can be physically taxing and require long recovery periods. From a financial perspective, not only does this equate to less time taken off work, but minimizes anesthesia and facility fees as well, especially if an abdominal procedure is involved since these are often already covered by the patient's insurance. In our practice, more than 40% of our body contouring cases involve multiple procedures.[9] Combining procedures may also provide benefits with regard to long-term weight distribution; more extensive procedures and a greater number of anatomic areas treated have been correlated with the duration and magnitude of weight loss achieved over time.[10] Patients should be counseled that, although complication rates are higher in multiple-procedure cases, the per-procedure complication rate remains the same.[9,11]

With appropriate planning, surgeons can assist most patients accomplish their body contouring objectives within 1 or 2 stages. Occasionally, we will add a third and final stage for neck or facial rejuvenation. While there is no standard algorithm for combining or staging procedures, there are several key principles–illustrated in **Table 1**, **Fig. 1**–that should be considered. Most importantly, as will be discussed in more detail later, it is essential to account for the vectors of pull generated by the distinct, anatomically conserved suspensory and anchoring properties of the superficial fascial system (SFS).[12] Staging procedures are a valuable strategy for avoiding simultaneous distraction of opposing tension vectors.

The staged approach to body contouring surgery provides an opportunity to address any unexpected contour irregularities resulting from skin relaxation, offering a "second chance" for achieving optimal results. In the MWL population, this phenomenon can be particularly drastic and unpredictable–so much so, that we have added a section to our surgical consent forms emphasizing the possibility of suboptimal cosmetic outcomes necessitating surgical revision. Additional stages can also be useful for addressing any minor wound complications, scars, or performing any ancillary or cosmetic procedures.

From a patient safety standpoint, staging surgery can minimize uninterrupted operative time and blood loss, or reduce postoperative recovery time and hospital stay.[9] Additionally, multiple, shorter operations is a safe alternative for higher-risk patients who may not tolerate lengthy, combined procedures with multiple position changes. For surgeons, staging can mitigate fatigue that often arises during long and technically demanding procedures. With regard to the ideal timing between staged operations, evidence is scarce. We recommend waiting at least three months before performing any additional procedures or necessary revisions, at which point the tissues usually have sufficiently settled to allow for accurate assessment of any residual skin laxity.

During the preoperative consultation, we ask patients to prioritize the anatomical regions of highest concern. We then discuss various safe surgical options based on their preferences and desires, including anticipated scar placement, recovery times, and their available social networks. During this discussion, it is important to provide a thorough explanation of the surgical reasoning

Table 1
Combining body contouring procedures: pearls & common pitfalls

Procedure A	Procedure B	Pearls/Pitfalls
LBL	VTL	Keep incisions medial to the inguinal crease to prevent scar descent or migration onto the anterior thigh over time
	UBL	Avoid opposing vectors of tension, as this may result in webbing or suboptimal skin excision
Abdominoplasty	Mastopexy	Utilizing a FDL for the abdominal procedure can result in the suboptimal medialization of the IMF
Mastopexy	Brachioplasty	While mild to moderate back excess can be pulled in, suboptimal pleating may occur and must be considered
UBL	Mastopexy	When performing a UBL prior to breast auto-augmentation, preservation of the lateral chest roll tissues is critical
	Brachioplasty	Extending the brachioplasty inferiorly onto the lateral torso can lead to a confluence of scars (ie, T-point) susceptible to breakdown
Brachioplasty	VTL	Surgical recovery for multiple extremities can be challenging, and requires adequate patient support

Select combinations of procedures preferred by the authors, along with pearls and common pitfalls to consider during surgical planning.

Abbreviations: FDL, fleur-de-lis (abdominoplasty); IMF, infra-mammary fold; LBL, lower body lift; UBL, upper body lift; VTLS, vertical thigh lift.

process, as patient expectations may not always align with the optimal staging and combination design.

LOWER BODY

Inferomedial descent of skin and soft tissues within the thigh and gluteal regions has remained a central focus of functional and aesthetic concerns across time and despite evolving gender norms and cultural trends. Stigmata of massive weight loss include buttock deflation with a loss of volume and projection, as well as descent of the lateral thighs, leading to the development of saddlebags. Historically, these areas were treated as independent units, and attempts to address lower body deformities were plagued by high complication rates, poor outcomes, and unreliable scarring. With time–and strongly influenced by developments from Lockwood and his contemporaries–surgeons came to appreciate the importance of treating the outer thighs and buttocks as part of a larger anatomic subunit which includes the abdomen.[13] Subsequent advances in our understanding of the mechanical properties of circumferential skin excision have enabled the application of significantly greater levels of tension without fear of lateral skin redundancy (ie, a standing cone deformity). These principles underlie several common techniques used to correct lower body deformities.

The lower body lift (LBL) is a dynamic procedure in the body contouring surgeon's arsenal. When performed alone, it can produce a significant impact on the lower torso, buttocks, and thighs, while combined with other procedures, it can provide a transformative effect on patients' lives. However, the term has been erroneously applied to any circumferential procedure of the lower body; a true LBL necessitates scar placement that is sufficiently caudal to directly impact the lower buttock region, including the contours of the lower gluteal fold and outer thigh region. Furthermore, a LBL allows for concomitant gluteal auto-augmentation, if desired, using well-vascularized adipose flaps based on reliable gluteal artery perforators. Scars can typically be concealed by standard underwear, shorts, or bathing suits (**Fig. 2**). Techniques such as the belt lipectomy or oblique flankplasty are based too superiorly to achieve any meaningful effect on the lower buttocks or lateral thigh. Ideal LBL design, while based on these fundamental principles, does not follow anatomic landmarks but is rather tailored to the specific needs of each patient. This approach allows for the LBL to be effectively combined with an inner thigh lift (Lockwood Type 1) or abdominoplasty (Lockwood Type 2) to achieve a comprehensive body contouring outcome.

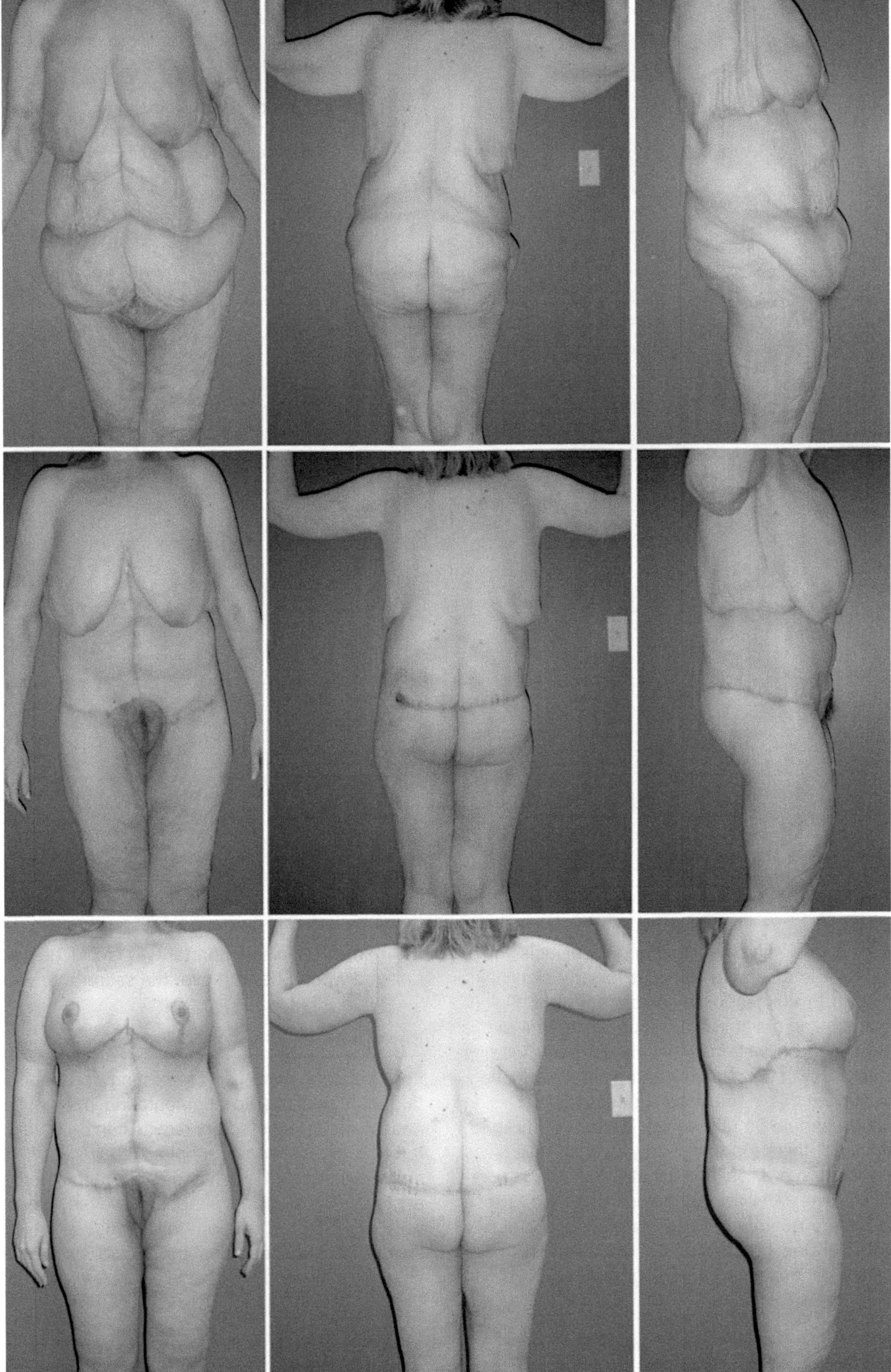

Fig. 1. Illustrates a typical body contouring combination/staging strategy. Preoperative views (*top row*) demonstrate upper and lower body deformities in a female patient following massive weight loss. Stage I (*center row*): postoperative views taken 5 months after her first surgery, consisting of a fleur-de-lis abdominoplasty, lateral

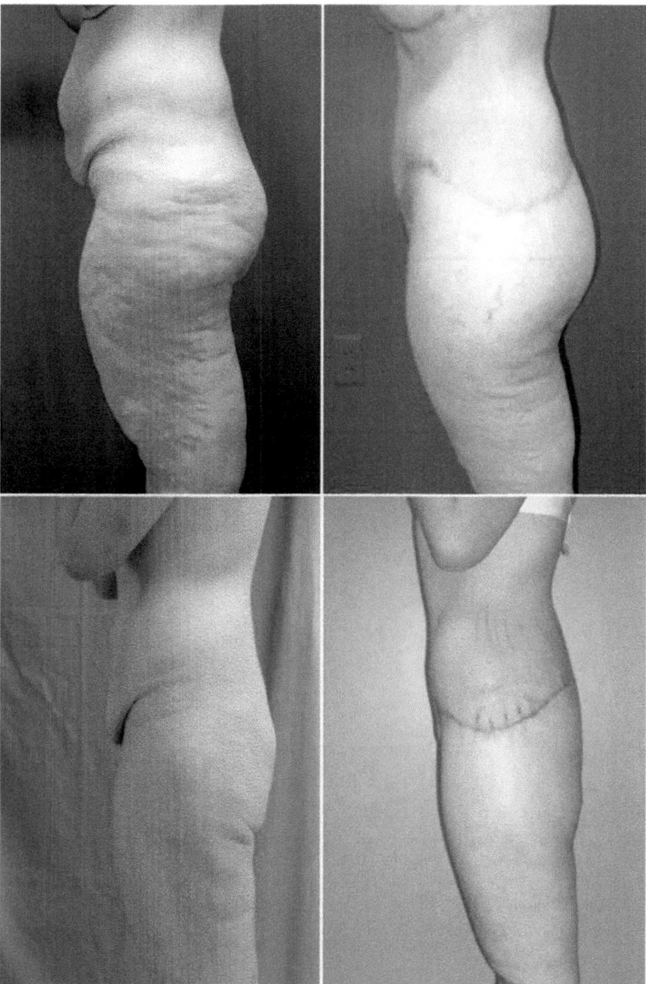

Fig. 2. Pre (*left*) and postoperative (*right*) images of 2 patients who underwent lower body lift, one of whom included buttock auto-augmentation (*top row*). Note the striking difference in buttock contour and projection.

When designing the upper and lower incisions of a LBL, it is crucial to account for any significant laxity in the gluteal or lower back region. Failure to do so can result in erroneous placement of the lower incision well into the gluteal cleft, leading to limb length discrepancy and gluteal elongation. To prevent this, a "gullwing" upper incision design pattern should be utilized, as illustrated in **Fig. 3**. Although this approach may result in excess midline tissue or bulging initially, this typically resolves over time as the tissues descend. These temporary postoperative deformities are typically well-tolerated but should be discussed with the patient in advance. Avoiding over-resection in the midline is also important to avoid areas of delayed wound healing over the sacrum.

Buttocks

For patients with a preexisting pronounced buttock "shelf," auto-augmentation may not be necessary, as satisfactory results can be obtained through excision-only techniques. Over time, the excised tissues will relax and conform to a normal, aesthetically pleasing shape. However, patients with significant deflation following weight loss should be cautioned about the possibility of gluteal volume loss and flattening with excision-only

thigh/buttock lift, and brachioplasty. Stage II (*bottom row*): postoperative views taken 9 months after her second surgery, which consisted of dermal suspension and parenchymal reshaping mastopexy, upper back lift, and vertical medial thigh lift. This staged approach also provided an opportunity to address the small area of dehiscence that had developed along the left lateral buttock incision.

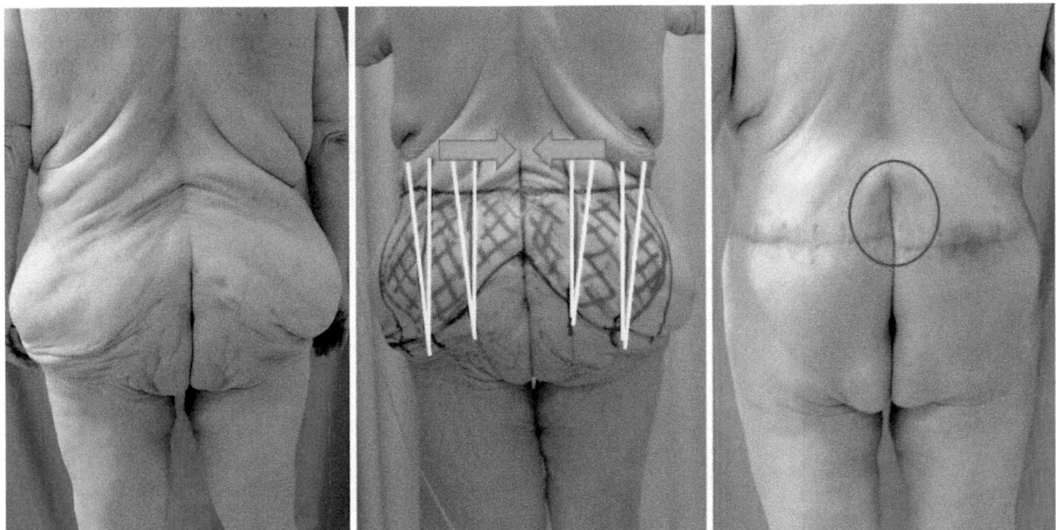

Fig. 3. Left panel: patient presenting with marked skin laxity of the lower back. The center panel demonstrates suboptimal preoperative markings; note the substantial discrepancy in upper and lower incision lengths, and malalignment of the orientation lines (*yellow lines*). This manifested postoperatively (*right panel*) as uneven tissue distribution across the closure and an elongated gluteal cleft. This could have been avoided by incorporating a gullwing pattern into the upper incision (*solid blue lines*), which helps transmit forces toward the midline (*blue arrows*). Gluteal elongation is demonstrated with the (*red circle*).

techniques. Interestingly, surgeons tend to find auto-augmented buttocks more aesthetically pleasing, whereas patients report similarly high levels of satisfaction regardless of whether they underwent augmented or nonaugmented procedures.[14]

Challenges of gluteal auto-augmentation include designing an appropriate excision pattern and the need to commit to both upper and lower incisions simultaneously. However, the likelihood of suboptimal outcomes can be curtailed with judicious patient selection and meticulous preoperative marking, as illustrated in **Fig. 4**. Patients should be counseled that buttock augmentation carries a higher risk of complications compared to nonaugmentation techniques, with wound dehiscence being the most common. In cases of acute dehiscence, prompt management with local anesthetic, irrigation, and re-closure over a penrose drain is recommended. Wounds that have been open for an extended period should be managed conservatively with regular dressing changes; any attempts to close primarily should be performed in a delayed fashion, and only once the wound is clean and surrounding tissues have sufficiently softened.

If skin laxity is not a significant concern, the use of fat grafting for buttock augmentation can moderately enhance projection and help contour the lower back and flanks. However, it is important to manage patient expectations, as multiple rounds of fat grafting may be necessary to achieve the desired outcome, particularly given ongoing controversy and safety concerns surrounding pulmonary fat emboli. Additionally, the deflated skin, prominent cellulite, and poor-quality residual fat typically observed in the MWL population renders them less-than-ideal candidates for the transfer of de-vascularized, free adipose grafts. For surgeons, harvest, and processing of large volumes of fat can be physically taxing, costly, and time-consuming.

Thighs

The lateral thigh deformity at the level of the inferior gluteal fold–colloquially known as the saddlebag–can range from a slight protrusion of the outer thigh to a more extensive pannus extending down the leg. Females tend to exhibit more severe saddlebag deformities than males owing to the preferential accumulation of adiposity in the hips and thighs, as typical of the gynecoid fat distribution.

Addressing the saddlebag deformity remains one of the most significant challenges encountered by the body contouring surgeon, owing to the need for a low, unattractive scar when performing large excisions, the tendency to reveal new deformities and for scar migration, and high

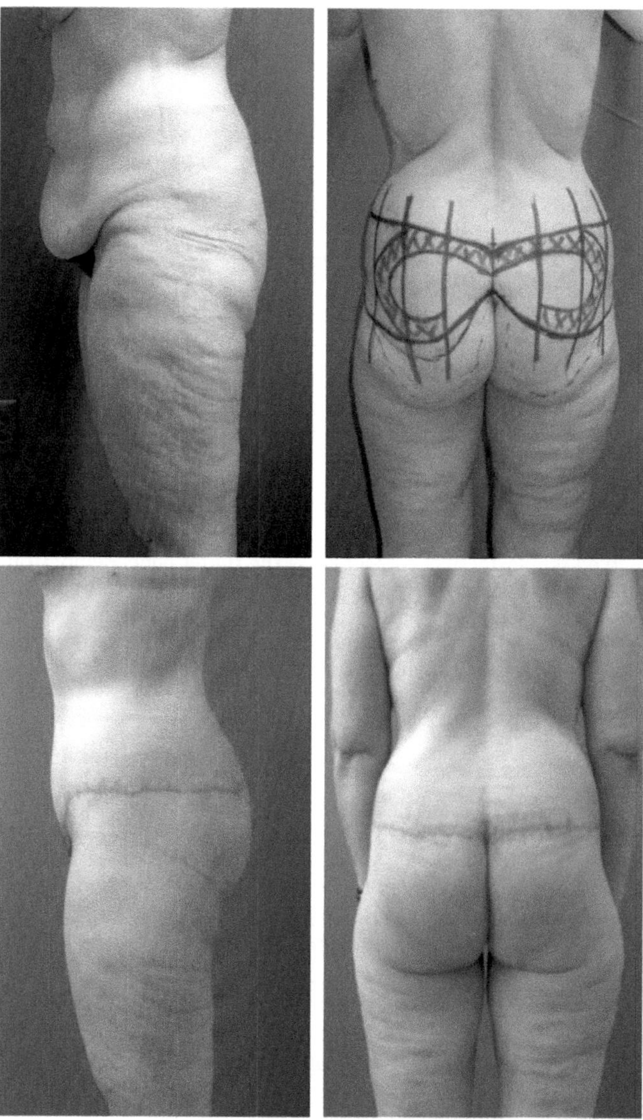

Fig. 4. Gluteal flap auto-augmentation. Top row: preoperative views and our lower body lift markings, which feature a gentle gullwing pattern and relatively equal upper and lower incision lengths. Postoperative results (*bottom row*) demonstrate nice buttock projection without gluteal elongation.

recurrence rates (**Fig. 5**).[7] Although a LBL can successfully improve lateral thigh deformities in the short-term, its effect on the medial thigh is minimal. Therefore, satisfactory correction requires individualized treatment of each affected area. We prefer a staged approach, in which only the lateral thighs are addressed during the first stage with an LBL. The lateral thigh tissues are then allowed to descend and rotate inferomedially, at which point the residual skin deformity can be addressed with a second stage medial thigh lift.

Two distinct procedures have been described for contouring the medial thigh: the vertical excision and the horizontal excision. Despite the appeal of a transverse-only incision, the benefits of this approach are limited to the most superior portion of the thigh. In our experience, suspensory forces of the transverse lift are not transmitted to the distal portion of the medial thigh, even when tissues are anchored to Colles fascia. Conversely, over-aggressive transverse lifts can lead to both cosmetic and functional issues and should not be considered a substitute for a vertical thighplasty, when indicated.

The vertical excision, in contrast, offers more reliable outcomes for addressing both proximal and distal skin laxity of the medial thigh. However, it is important to account for the vectors of pull generated with this technique, and how they might interact with other areas being treated. For

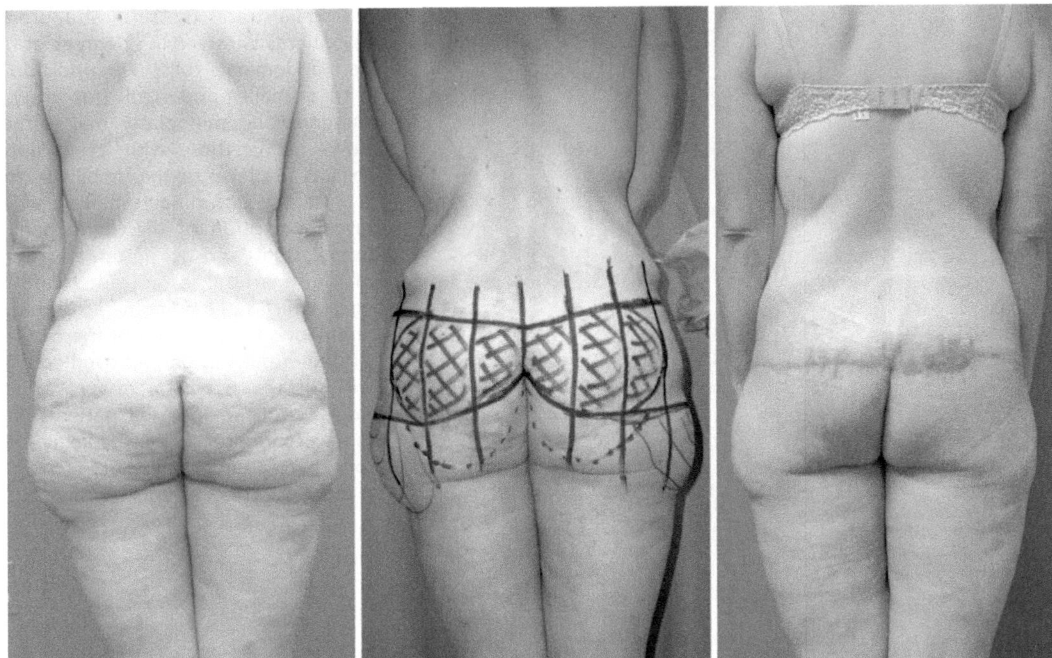

Fig. 5. Preoperative view (*left*) of a massive weight loss patient who sought a lower body lift to enhance the appearance of the buttocks and outer thighs. Despite a large skin excision (*red hashmarks*), wide undermining using a Lockwood dissector (*dotted lines*), and liposuction (*black hashmarks*), the patient experienced recurrence of her saddlebag deformity (*right image*).

instance, a vertical thigh lift can pull down loose abdominal tissue, so when addressing both areas, we typically perform the abdominal procedure first and address the inner thighs only once abdominal tension has been secured, or at a later stage. Similarly, a vertical thigh lift can exacerbate a thigh gap by pulling forward lax tissue of the posterior thigh and buttocks. Simulating these forces in the office can help identify patients who may benefit from addressing the buttocks first, or simultaneously with a LBL.

Abdomen

Abdominal contour deformities vary widely, ranging from minor panty girdle lines or a limited pannus to the presence of multiple rolls over the anterior abdomen or those extending laterally to the posterior trunk. Most patients seeking abdominal contouring after MWL present with high-grade abdominal deformities, necessitating more aggressive surgical intervention–often in conjunction with other procedures–to achieve the desired outcome.[8]

The preoperative abdominal assessment typically begins with the pannus. The points at which the pannus terminates laterally along the mid-axillary lines should be identified and are a useful landmark for illustrating the anticipated scar length to patients. For patients for whom this point is not well-defined, re-positioning them in a bent over "diver's pose" can help accentuate the natural endpoint of their skin excess. It is vital to mark this point preoperatively with the patient standing, as identification becomes considerably more difficult once the patient is supine in the operating room. Failure to recognize the true lateral endpoint will undoubtedly result in a dog ear deformity, which patients often mischaracterize as residual fat. Following the examination of the pannus, the central abdomen is evaluated for adiposity and residual laxity. To assess the potential benefit of a rectus plication, patients are asked to suck in their gut, although those with significant intra-abdominal fat may experience minimal improvement. When performing the abdominoplasty, sufficient undermining is necessary to allow for abdominal wall plication up to the level of the xiphoid. Failure to do so results in a residual upper abdominal bulge.

Multiple abdominal rolls of varying size and shape, caused by abnormal areas of aberrant fascial thickening, are common in the MWL population, and require surgical correction that is tailored to the specific deformity (**Fig. 6**). For isolated minor rolls situated around the umbilicus,

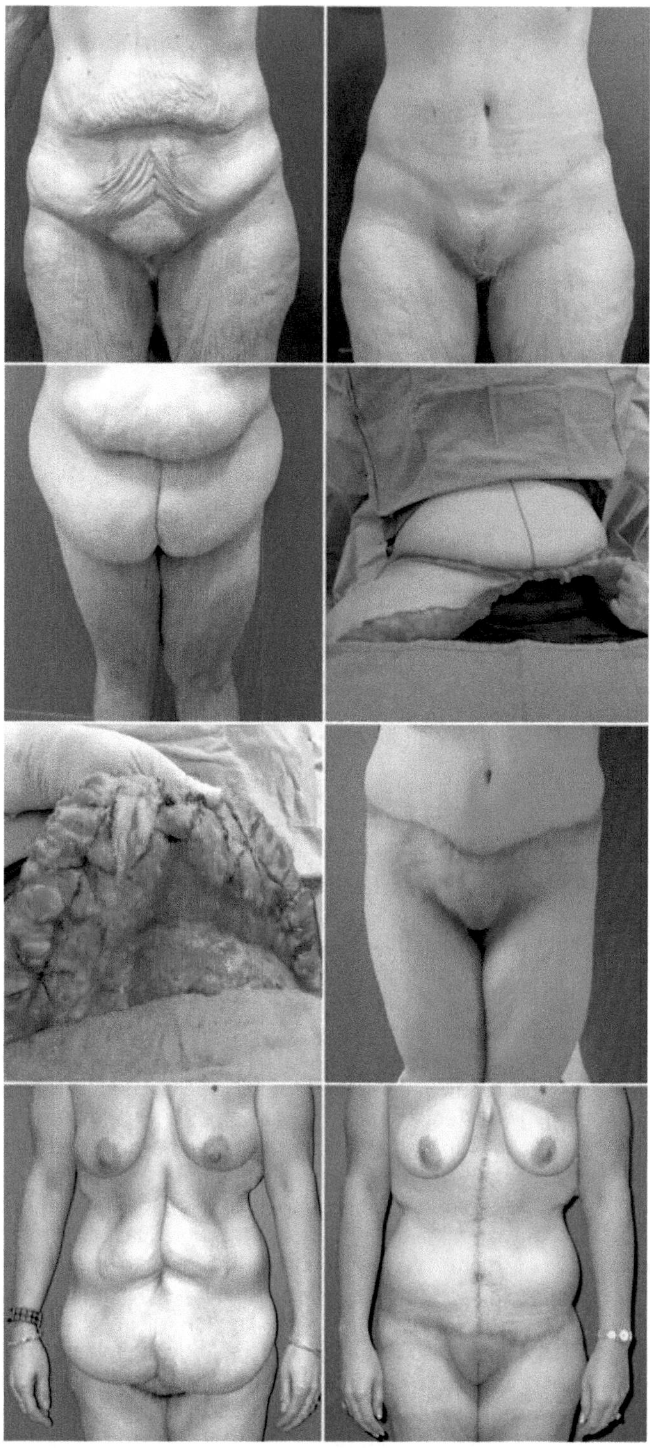

Fig. 6. Illustrates the surgical approach to patients with varying degrees of upper abdominal rolls. For individuals with a smaller upper roll (*top row*), a standard abdominoplasty may suffice. However, for those with larger upper rolls at the level of the umbilicus (*row 2, left*), the unfurling technique–which involves excision of the lower pannus (*row 2*, right) and "X" patterned scoring of the superficial fascia (*row 3, left image*), which releases tight fascial bands and allows for unfurling of the fat. This strategy results in an improved contour without the need for a vertical scar (*row 3, right image*). For patients with more pronounced epigastric laxity (*bottom row*), a fleur-de-lis (FDL) technique is the most effective approach.

standard abdominoplasty procedures may suffice. For larger single or double rolls however, an unfurling technique involving the cauterization of the superficial fascial system along its length may be necessary, in addition to excision of residual sub-scarpal tissues and skin to achieve a smooth, uniform contour. This procedure is particularly suitable for patients with a significant upper-roll

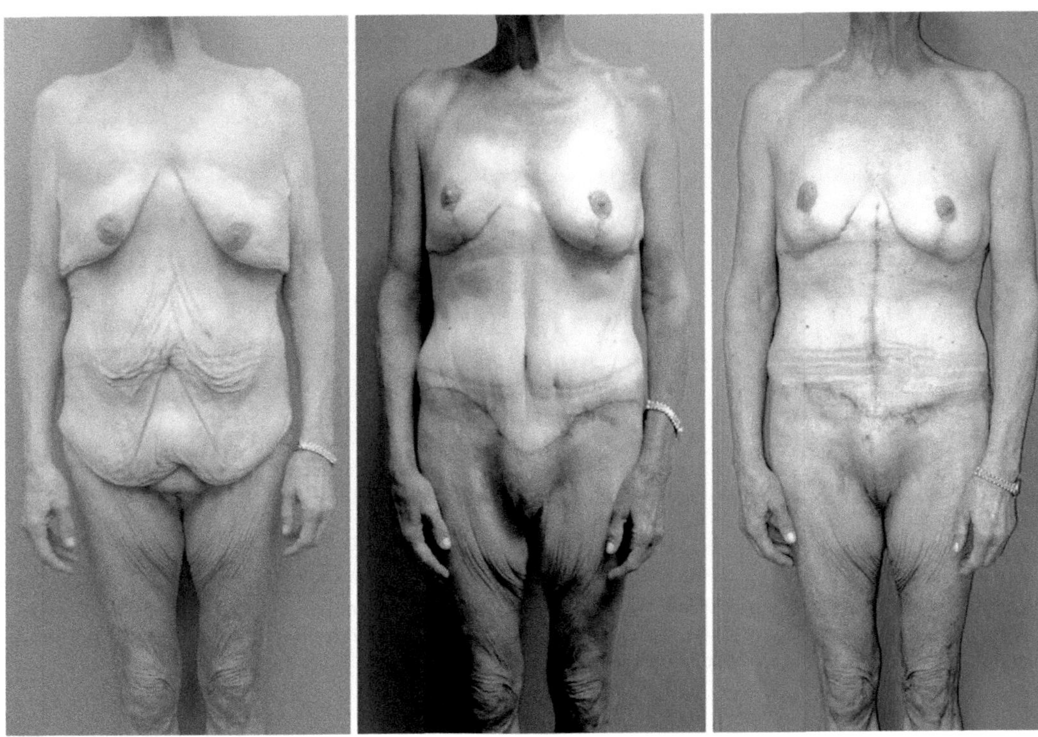

Fig. 7. This patient with mid-epigastric rolls and upper abdominal laxity was initially hesitant to commit to a vertical scar. Following standard abdominoplasty (*center*), she was unhappy with the appearance of the abdomen, and elected to undergo a fleur-de-lis abdominoplasty eight months later with vertical scar and rectus plication (*right*).

deformity who do not wish to undergo a vertical incision. For patients with significant epigastric laxity or a high roll that does not extend around the back, a fleur-de-lis (FDL) extension may be required to achieve satisfactory epigastric narrowing and lateral undermining. Note that these patients have often experienced a greater change in BMI with their weight loss, and are at high risk for postoperative complications such as fat necrosis and T-point dehiscence.[15] To manage these cases safely, a functional panniculectomy followed by a staged, cosmetic FDL at later date is our preferred approach. This is also a viable option for patients who are not be willing to commit to a vertical scar at the first stage (**Fig. 7**).

Abdominal deformities rarely exist in isolation, and attempts at surgical correction without the consideration of the surrounding anatomy will result in suboptimal or deficient results. For example, as demonstrated in **Fig. 8**, an attempt at the correction of this high upper abdominal roll with FDL abdominoplasty alone resulted in a residual deformity. However, the astute body contouring surgeon can preempt this suboptimal outcome by recognizing that this anterior-only approach won't address the excess upper roll tissues extending posteriorly to the back. An integrated approach to abdominal contouring may range from a corset-type or extended abdominoplasty to an upper body lift (UBL, discussed later in discussion). In fact, the vertical FDL excision may even worsen a high double or triple roll deformity by advancing excess upper lateral tissue toward the midline. In these cases, one can consider performing the UBL first to eliminate the need for a vertical component during the subsequent abdominal stage.[16] Alternatively, for female patients, this excess tissue can be used for breast auto-augmentation (discussed later in discussion). Finally, flank liposuction is another safe and effective adjunct for improving abdominal contour, particularly in patients with flank lipodystrophy. These additional procedures also provide ample opportunities for addressing the lower body as well, but remember to consider the counteracting forces generated by the abdomen and the anterior thigh during planning, as previously discussed.

Regardless of the abdominal contouring strategy undertaken, it is important to address mons laxity or fullness, and in most cases, the umbilicus should be transposed and preserved. Preoperatively, the patient's midline should be marked on

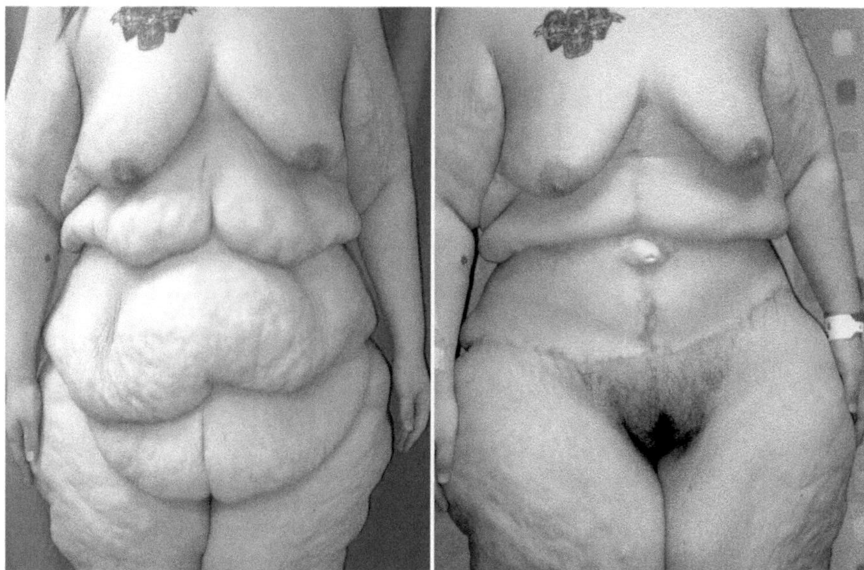

Fig. 8. For severe triple or mega-roll deformities, a fleur-de-lis abdominoplasty alone may be insufficient to achieve optimal results, as seen in this patient who exhibited a residual high upper roll postoperatively. In these challenging cases, an upper body lift or corset procedure can help refine body contours.

both the abdominal wall and mons, as these are often not vertically aligned. If an off-centered umbilicus is identified, it can be shifted intraoperatively using differential plication. However, in patients with a high BMI or low-set umbilicus, transposition attempts may lead to inferior skin flap ischemia or wound dehiscence, in which case umbilical sacrifice may be necessary. Delayed umbilical reconstruction can be performed later via a number of local flap techniques.

When addressing pubic descent, achieving uniform thickness between the mons and the abdominal flap is critical for preventing a step-off deformity. **Fig. 9** demonstrates our method of assessing upper flap thickness and using this measurement to set the mons. Liposuction is another modality that can be helpful for thinning the mons region, although prolonged edema can result. If narrowing of the mons region is desired, lateral wedge excision can be performed. This technique is most utilized in combination with thighplasty procedures.

UPPER BODY

As in the lower body and abdominal region, patients with MWL exhibit characteristic patterns of tissue redundancy and skin laxity in the breast, mid- and upper back, and arms. The addition of an upper body component to a lower body or abdominal procedure can be transformative in improving a patient's overall contour. Although various techniques and approaches have been developed to address these deformities, the fundamental body contouring principles of surgical planning and staging remain constant.

A traditional LBL has limited ability to address laxity in the upper back due to a strong midline zone of adherence, which dampens any forces

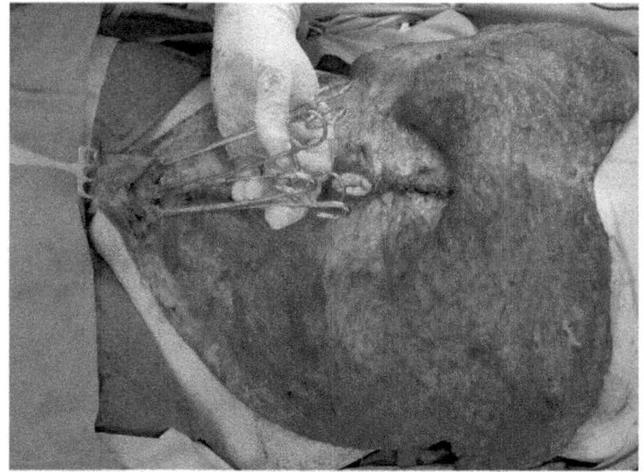

Fig. 9. Illustrates our preferred method for restoring the mons pubis. After marking the appropriate thickness, 3 Aliss clamps, and a facelift rake are used to separate the mons tissue from the excess tissue to be resected. The mons is then re-suspended with 1 to 2 sutures. It is critical to ensure equal thickness of the mons and upper abdominal flaps in order to prevent a step-off deformity.

applied across this region. Therefore, a separate surgical intervention is usually required for correcting deformities of this region. A range of techniques exist for addressing upper back rolls, and these include transverse excision along the upper back, bilateral longitudinal or oblique scars over the lateral chest, as well as a circumferential approach.

A UBL can both reshape the breast and eliminate epigastric and mid-back rolls via a transverse, near-circumferential scar that can be hidden within the brassiere line (**Fig. 10**). It is useful to have the patient wear a commonly used bra on the day of surgery to assist with markings. We mark the bra pattern with a dotted line (representing the anticipated upper incision) and apply gentle tension to verify that it will remain well-concealed. The lower incision can then be estimated via pinch test. As with a brachioplasty or thighplasty, tissue resection is performed with "precision excision," whereby undermining proceeds from the committed upper incision in the inferior direction, making sure to periodically confirm your location with towel clamps.

UBL are more commonly performed at a second stage after addressing the abdomen, although there are circumstances in which it can be advantageous to perform the UBL first, as discussed above (eg, high double or triple rolls). However, insurance coverage remains a significant obstacle to this strategy. Attempts to lift the upper and lower body simultaneously generate opposing forces, leading to an unsightly web-like effect of the lateral torso. Characteristic widening of the transverse back scar over time is another significant drawback, and can become visible even if the scar is initially well-hidden in the bra-line. Patients should be cautioned regarding this potential outcome beforehand.

Breasts

Numerous techniques have been developed for addressing the wide range of breast deformities observed after MWL, which include high-grade breast ptosis, nipple-areola complex medialization, and extension into lateral chest rolls.[6] Any approach to correcting the deflated breast in this population must consider the entire aesthetic unit and should ideally recycle the excess tissue of

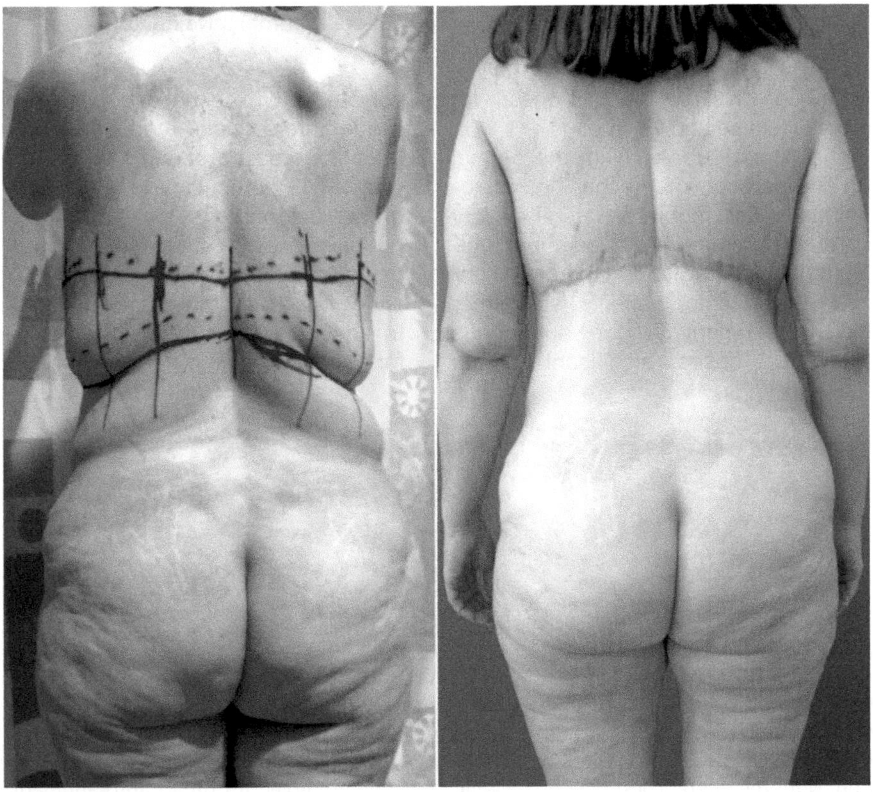

Fig. 10. When marking the upper body lift (*left*), ensure that the resulting scar is concealed within the bra line. It is important to anticipate the widening of the transverse scar (*right*) due to opposing forces along the back, even when performed as an isolated procedure.

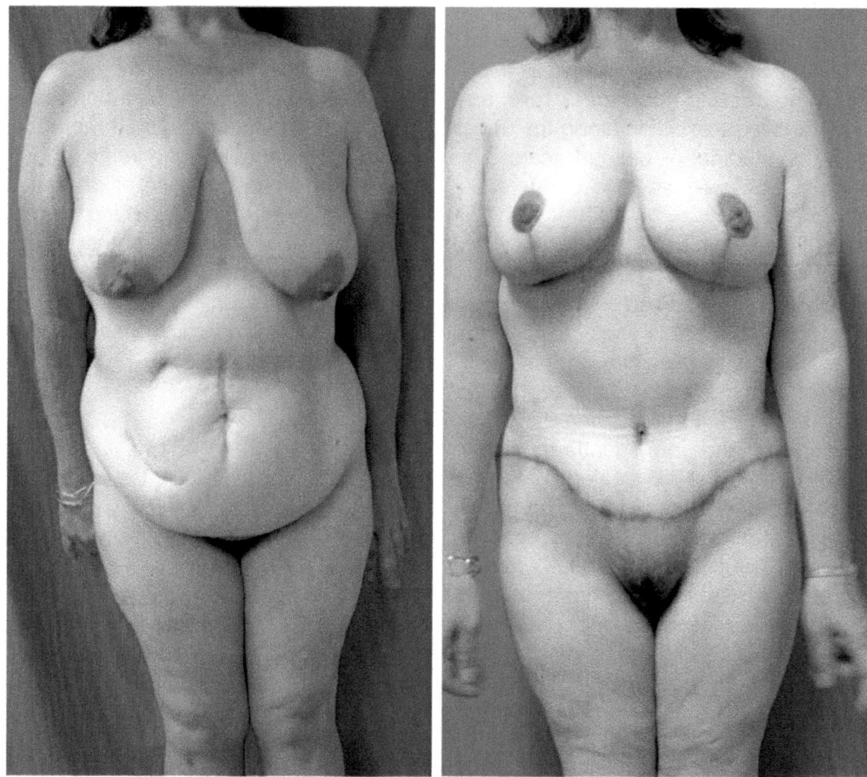

Fig. 11. The mastopexy/abdominoplasty combination can achieve transformative results for the entire torso.

the upper abdomen and lateral chest for enhancing breast shape and volume.

We have had great success with the dermal suspension and parenchymal reshaping mastopexy technique, which mobilizes lateral axillary rolls into the breast mound to augment volume.[17–19] In contrast, traditional augmentation/mastopexy is reserved for patients who either lack sufficient parenchyma for autologous reconstruction or desire significant breast volume that exceeds capabilities of their own tissue. Interestingly, reduction mammaplasty is often the breast procedure of choice for patients with MWL, particularly those with higher-grade breast deformities. However, this finding may be biased by cost considerations, given that breast reductions are often covered by insurance; it is likely that some patients are willing to accept smaller, ptotic breasts in exchange for lower cost.

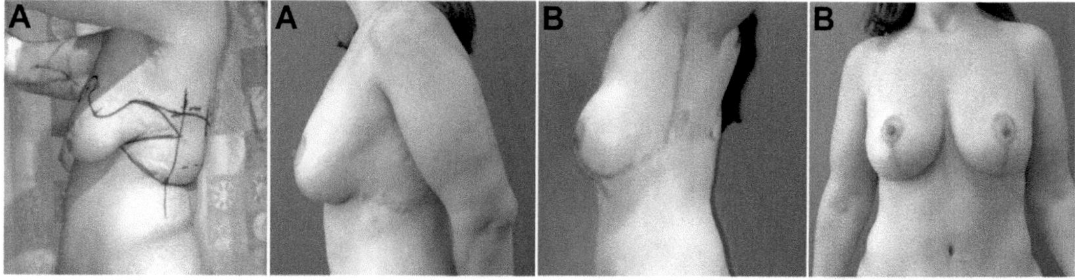

Fig. 12. Markings and postoperative results (*A, B*) for a patient who underwent dermal suspension and parenchymal reshaping mastopexy with extension onto the back for incorporating into an upper body lift in a single incorporation. Note the lateral chest wall tissue which must be preserved for breast auto-augmentation. When this patient subsequently returned for a brachioplasty, we were able to incorporate the previous scar into our new incision (center right). However, be aware that this technique can lead to a confluence of scars that is prone to breakdown.

In our practice, it is rare for a MWL patient to undergo an isolated mastopexy without opting to include any additional contouring procedures. Specifically, the synergistic effects of an abdominoplasty and mastopexy can be dramatic (**Fig. 11**). However, it is critical to assess inframammary fold (IMF) stability before deciding whether to perform the breast and abdominal components concurrently or sequentially, since abdominal tightening can lower the IMF. If any IMF movement is anticipated, we prefer to stage the breast reshaping until the abdominal portion has been completed to avoid these competing vectors of pull. If performed concurrently, we recommend performing the abdominal portion first to allow for the re-evaluation of the new IMF position and adjustment of markings as necessary. We will also stage breast procedures in patients undergoing FDL abdominoplasty for practical reasons; IMF medialization and abducted upper extremity positioning on the operating table causes varying degrees of breast distortion, complicating the effort to achieve optimal shape and symmetry.

The versatility of the dermal suspension and parenchymal reshaping mastopexy technique is highlighted by the various modifications available for addressing adjacent anatomic regions, incorporating other upper body procedures, or minimizing scar burden (**Fig. 12**). For example, the lateral breast flap incision can be extended onto the back as part of a UBL. Similarly, by curving the incision up toward the axilla, it can be merged with a brachioplasty incision, with the added benefit of correcting mild back rolls. Merging the IMF incisions with the brachioplasty can also help pull mild amounts of back tissue while avoiding the bra line incision, although this can result in the pleating of the lateral chest wall that can persist for some time before settling down.

Arms

Brachioplasty is infrequently performed as a standalone procedure in the MWL population,[20] and is often combined with an LBL given the relative distance between the 2 regions. If considering combining arm contouring with a UBL however, avoid extending the brachioplasty onto the lateral chest–the resulting confluence of incisions in a T-point is very prone to wound breakdown. Liposuction is a valuable adjunct for addressing any focal lipodystrophy of the posterior arm, an area that most excisional brachioplasty techniques do not target. We have found this technique to be safe and effective for achieving a natural and smooth contour, particularly in patients with thicker arms.[21]

When combining brachioplasty with other procedures, patients must be appropriately counseled and emotionally equipped to face the many challenges and restrictions imposed by simultaneous surgical recovery of the upper and lower extremities. This is especially true for patients who do not have a strong social support system, given how difficult the surgical dressings and functional impairments are to manage without assistance.

SUMMARY

Here, we summarize our experience with circumferential body contouring surgery. With thoughtful and methodical planning, the optimization of patient selection and safety, and an emphasis on integrated, anatomical design, it is possible to achieve a comprehensive 360° result from head to toe.

CLINICS CARE POINTS

- An integrated approach to the surgical treatment of the body contouring patient and the diverse, unpredictable range of deformities seen in the massive weight loss population requires a 360° approach to adjacent anatomy, fascial architecture, soft tissue resuspension, and circumferential, multi-dimensional forces.
- Wait a minimum of 12-18 months after bariatric surgery, and 3 months of weight stability, before proceeding with body contouring surgery
- Managing patient expectations are as important for optimal outcomes as the surgery itself.
- In addition to the typical surgical considerations, extra attention should be paid to patient wound-healing risk factors and intraoperative body temperature, fluid balance, and positioning on the OR table.
- The Pittsburgh Rating Scale is a validated instrument for characterizing the unique deformities and anatomic considerations of the body contouring population and can assist with surgical planning.
- A single procedure will rarely be able to achieve all functional and cosmetic goals in the massive weight loss population. Numerous strategies for combining and/or staging body contouring procedures exist and should be individualized to the patient.
- The outer thighs, buttocks, and abdomen function as an integrated anatomic unit, and should be treated as such for surgical planning purposes.
- Lower body lift markings should account for laxity in the gluteal or lower back regions to

avoid gluteal cleft elongation. This can be further assisted by a "gullwing" design for the upper incision, and attention to equal upper and lower incision lengths.

- Satisfactory correction of circumferential thigh deformities may require a staged approach, in which the lateral thigh/saddlebag deformity is addressed initially with a lower body lift, followed by a delayed vertical thigh excision once tissues have settled.
- High-grade abdominal deformities–especially those with high double or triple-rolls–often require treatment of adjacent anatomic regions for optimal correction.
- Have the patient wear a commonly used bra on the day of surgery to assist with markings and ensure that the resulting scar will be well-hidden within the brassiere strap.
- Breast auto-augmentation takes advantage of excess upper abdominal and lateral chest tissues to correct the deflated breast.

DISCLOSURE

- Authors' contributions: Both authors (J.A. David, J.A. Gusenoff) made substantial contributions to the conception and design of the study and performed data acquisition, data analysis, and interpretation, and provided administrative, technical, and material support.
- Availability of data and materials: N/A.
- *Financial support* and sponsorship: None.
- Conflicts of interest: All authors declared that there are no conflicts of interest.
- Ethical approval and consent to participate: N/A. All patient photographs are de-identified.
- Consent for publication: N/A.

REFERENCES

1. Rubin JP, Jewell ML, Uebel CO, et al. Body contouring and liposuction. London: Saunders; 2013.
2. Pitanguy I, Ceravolo MP. Our experience with combined procedures in aesthetic plastic surgery. Plast Reconstr Surg 1983;71:56–65.
3. Coon D, Gusenoff JA, Kannan N, et al. Body mass and surgical complications in the postbariatric reconstructive patient: analysis of 511 cases. Ann Surg 2009;249(3):397–401.
4. Coon D, Michaels Jt, Gusenoff JA, et al. Hypothermia and complications in postbariatric body contouring. Plast Reconstr Surg 2012;130:443–8.
5. Song AY, Jean RD, Hurwitz DJ, et al. A classification of contour deformities after bariatric weight loss: the Pittsburgh Rating Scale. Plast Reconstr Surg 2005; 116:1535–44 [discussion: 45-6].
6. Pang JH, Coombs DM, James I, et al. Characterizing breast deformities after massive weight loss: utilizing the pittsburgh rating scale to examine factors affecting severity score and surgical decision making in a retrospective series. Ann Plast Surg 2018;80:207–11.
7. Dreifuss SE, Beidas OE, Rubin JP, et al. Characterizing the saddlebag deformity after lower body lift. Aesthetic Surg J 2018;38:1115–23.
8. Zammerilla LL, Zou RH, Dong ZM, et al. Classifying severity of abdominal contour deformities after weight loss to aid in patient counseling: a review of 1006 cases. Plast Reconstr Surg 2014;134. 888e-94e.
9. Coon D, Michaels J, Gusenoff JA, et al. Multiple procedures and staging in the massive weight loss population. Plast Reconstr Surg 2010;125:691–8.
10. Wiser I, Heller L, Spector C, et al. Body contouring procedures in three or more anatomical areas are associated with long-term body mass index decrease in massive weight loss patients: a retrospective cohort study. J Plast Reconstr Aesthetic Surg 2017;70:1181–5.
11. Beidas OE, Gusenoff JA. Common complications and management after massive weight loss patient safety in plastic surgery. Clin Plast Surg 2019;46:115–22.
12. Almutairi K, Gusenoff JA, Rubin JP. Body contouring. Plast Reconstr Surg 2016;137:586e–602e.
13. Lockwood TE. Lower-body lift. Aesthetic Surg J 2001;21:355–69.
14. Srivastava U, Rubin JP, Gusenoff JA. Lower body lift after massive weight loss: autoaugmentation versus no augmentation. Plast Reconstr Surg 2015;135:762–72.
15. Friedman T, O'Brien Coon D, Michaels J, et al. Fleur-de-Lis abdominoplasty: a safe alternative to traditional abdominoplasty for the massive weight loss patient. Plast Reconstr Surg 2010;125:1525–35.
16. Acevedo E, Nadhan KS, Everett M, et al. Corset trunkplasty: recommended with abdominal skin laxity and open cholecystectomy scar. Plast Reconstr Surg 2018;141:60–9.
17. Rubin JP, Gusenoff JA, Coon D. Dermal suspension and parenchymal reshaping mastopexy after massive weight loss: statistical analysis with concomitant procedures from a prospective registry. Plast Reconstr Surg 2009;123:782–9.
18. Rubin JP. Mastopexy after massive weight loss: dermal suspension and total parenchymal reshaping. Aesthetic Surg J 2006;26:214–22.
19. Rubin JP, Khachi G. Mastopexy after massive weight loss: dermal suspension and selective auto-augmentation. Clin Plast Surg 2008;35:123–9.
20. Gusenoff JA, Coon D, Rubin JP. Brachioplasty and concomitant procedures after massive weight loss: a statistical analysis from a prospective registry. Plast Reconstr Surg 2008;122:595–603.
21. Bossert RP, Dreifuss S, Coon D, et al. Liposuction of the arm concurrent with brachioplasty in the massive weight loss patient: is it safe? Plast Reconstr Surg 2013;131:357–65.

Indications of Oblique Flankplasty

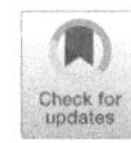

Peter Wirth, MD[a], Ahmed M. Afifi, MD[a,b,*]

KEYWORDS

• Flankplasty • Oblique flankplasty • Body contouring

KEY POINTS

- Oblique flankplasty is an adjunct to lipoabdominoplasty or an alternative to lower body lift in patients with prominent flanks.
- The oblique flankplasty provides the narrowest possible contour to the waistline when compared with other truncal body contouring procedures.
- Proper orientation of the excision can maximize the pull on surrounding tissues, including the lateral buttock and epigastrium.

BACKGROUND

Redundant skin and soft tissue of the lower back and flank are a challenging area for the plastic surgeon to address. An abdominoplasty or lower body lift in isolation does not provide a direct solution to the flank, and modifications to these procedures provide modest improvement to the patient with prominent flanks. Thus, in some patients, a more direct approach to the flank is needed. The oblique flankplasty as described by Hurwitz in 2019 allows for direct excision of flank deformity.[1] To understand the role of oblique flankplasty in body contouring, one must first review the relevant truncal body contouring procedures.

The primary goal of a traditional abdominoplasty is to address anterior abdominal laxity. In isolation, the traditional abdominoplasty provides no direct effect to the flank or back.[2–4] To circumvent this shortcoming, flank and lower back liposuction is commonly added to abdominoplasty, leading to the common practice of combining circumferential (commonly referred to as 360-degree) liposuction to many abdominoplasties. However, treatment of the flank and lower back area with liposuction alone does not address the excess skin in the area and can contribute to the appearance of a dog ear at the lateral aspect of the abdominoplasty incision.[5]

Many surgeons extend the incision to a circumferential or near-circumferential abdominoplasty to help provide more definition to the waist and flank. These circumferential abdominoplasties can have many variations and nomenclatures, including belt lipectomy and lower body lift (LBL).[6,7] The incision in a belt lipectomy is higher, with the goal of surgery being improvement in the waist and lower back. The incision in the lower body lift is lower, with the goal of surgery being primarily improvement of the buttocks and lateral thighs.[8,9] On the other hand, the extended or near-circumferential abdominoplasty is another common and effective technique that involves extending the abdominoplasty incision past the iliac crest to tighten the excess skin of the waist while avoiding the risks associated with the circumferential abdominoplasty.[5,10,11]

However, extending the incision posteriorly along the same horizontal line, even when combined with extensive liposuction, will still have limited effect on the flanks in patients with

[a] Division of Plastic and Reconstructive Surgery, University of Wisconsin School of Medicine and Public Health, University of Wisconsin, G5/352 Clinical Science Center, 600 Highland Avenue, Madison, WI 53792, USA; [b] Division of Plastic and Reconstructive Surgery, University of Wisconsin School of Medicine and Public Health, University of Wisconsin, G5/356 Clinical Science Center, 600 Highland Avenue, Madison, WI 53792, USA
* Corresponding author.
E-mail address: afifi@surgery.wisc.edu

Clin Plastic Surg 51 (2024) 111–117
https://doi.org/10.1016/j.cps.2023.06.004

significant flank rolls for multiple reasons. First, these rolls often extend cephalad further away from the LBL incision, making that incision less effective in eliminating the whole flank roll. Second, the excision in LBL or extended abdominoplasty is along the vertical plane, while often the excess skin is three-dimensional. Finally, the skin of the lower back can be quite thick and might not recoil sufficiently after liposuction.

The concept of an oblique flankplasty therefore becomes clear; a direct excision of the flank roll is the most effective and consistent technique to narrow the waistline. The obvious drawback is the scar location. However, the technique offers distinct advantages that will be discussed and can make it the better choice for many patients.

INDICATIONS

Effect on the Flank

A basic concept in skin lifting procedures is that the closer the incision is to the target area, the more effective the vector of pull. For example, in a brow lift, the ratio of brow elevation to width of skin excision decreases as the incision moves further cephalad (from above the eyebrow, to the midforehead, to the hairline, and finally to the scalp). Pascal stresses this concept in the LBL, stating that to have maximal effect on the infrabuttock crease, the incision needs to be lowered. He proposed the "16 cm rule," that the effect of the skin excision does not extend past 16 cm from the incision.[12] While the authors are not familiar with strong evidence for a specific distance beyond which an excision has no effect, and it likely varies among patients, they believe that this is an important concept that universally applies: the closer the incision is to the target area, the more effective the surgery will be. It therefore becomes clear why the oblique flankplasty is the most effective technique for addressing flank rolls and for narrowing the waist and lower back.

Oblique flankplasty is most appropriate for patients with Pittsburgh grade 2 (distinct rolls) and grade 3 (severe deformity consisting of laxity, ptotic, or oversized rolls) flanks (**Fig. 1**).[13,14] An important consideration of oblique flankplasty is understanding the oblique vector of pull that accurately and reproducibly narrows the waist by addressing horizontal and vertical laxity of the flank. This contrasts to the lower body lift, which consists of a vertical line of pull upwards. This vector provides no direct improvement to flank deformities. In fact, the lower body lift can accentuate the flank by providing a poorly contoured torso with circumferential band of recessed scar (**Fig. 2**).[1] This results in an area of relative fullness to the torso and a narrowed hip, which runs counter to the ideal waist-to-hip ratio and aesthetic.

Effect on the Buttock and Lower Body

Buttock sagging and deflation are common complaints among patients and are important considerations when deciding between oblique flankplasty and LBL, as each technique addresses buttock aesthetics differently. As a result, patients will need to prioritize their wishes and concerns. There are three important considerations with regards to the buttock when counseling patients on oblique flankplasty.

First, is the effect of oblique flankplasty and LBL on buttock ptosis. As explained previously, the closer the incision to the area of concern, the more effective the lifting will be. Therefore, the superiorly positioned incision of the flankplasty will have little effect on buttock ptosis or the infrabuttock crease. If this area is the patients' main concern, they should opt for an LBL.

Second, is the interplay between the waist and the buttock, or simply the waist-to-hip ratio. Research suggests that the most attractive waist-to-hip ratio is approximately 0.65, from a less curvy 0.7 several decades ago.[15] The oblique flankplasty allows for maximal narrowing of the waist and helps improve the definition of the buttock and the waist-to-hip ratio. Even without directly changing the buttock, the patient can appear to have a much more defined buttock by simply defining the waist (**Fig. 3**).

Finally, one must consider that buttock fat grafting has become extremely popular in the last decade and gives the surgeon significant latitude in shaping the buttock. The remote location of the incision in oblique flankplasty away from the buttock allows for more liberal buttock fat grafting when compared with lower body lift, where the proximity of fat grafting recipient areas to the incision makes contouring more challenging.

Healing and Scarring

The skin of the back is some of the thickest in the body. As a result, this skin is more durable, less attenuated, and better able to hold sutures. Additionally, the orientation of the scars along the lower back is favorable, as they naturally follow Langer's lines. The obliquity of the resection runs parallel with relaxed skin tension lines, like the latissimus dorsi flap as described by Hammond, in which marked improvement in scar quality was noted with this orientation.[16]

Furthermore, the incisions of the oblique flankplasty heal considerably faster and with fewer

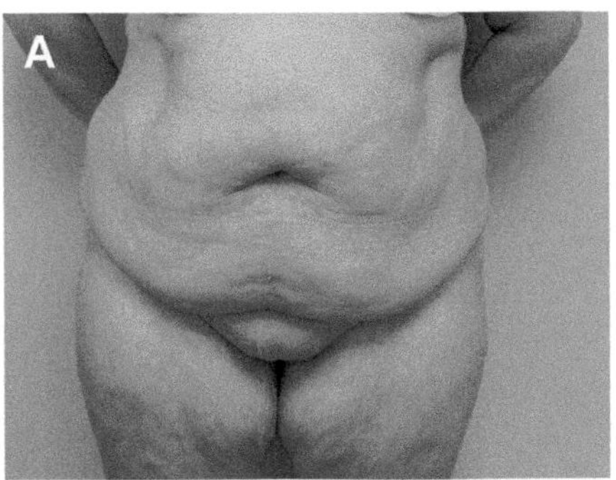

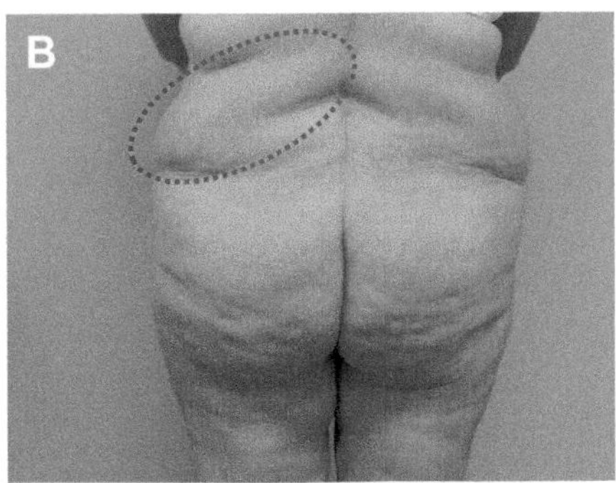

Fig. 1. 53-year-old woman presenting for body contouring following massive weight loss of 85 kg following sleeve gastrectomy. (*A*) Frontal view. (*B*) Posterior view, with flank roll identified (*red dotted oval*).

complications when compared with the lower body lift. In the original technique paper, only 2 patients developed delayed wound healing of less than 5 cm out of the first 30 patients (6.7%).[1] This compares to the rate of delayed wound healing in lower body lifting that exceeds 30%.[17–20] The difference is likely attributable to the relative lack of mechanical stress across the incision, as the motion of the lower back is relatively little when compared with the waist. Additionally, there is minimal to no undermining of the flank tissues. As mentioned previously, the dermis is this area is some of the thickest in the body, as opposed to the elastic and thin dermis that is along the LBL incision.

Despite favorable scar formation of the lower back, the location of the scars in the oblique flankplasty is not discreet. Other truncal body contouring procedures are designed to be well-concealed by clothing. In the case of a lower body lift or abdominoplasty, even relatively high scars can be concealed by certain garments. In an oblique flankplasty, 2-piece swimwear and standard undergarments will not cover the scars. Patients must understand this trade-off preoperatively. The authors recommend that this be carefully documented by the surgeon and strongly encourage the use of photos while counseling patients.

Unfortunately, these criticisms have been a major source of dismissal of the oblique flankplasty technique by plastic surgeons. The authors have been surprised in their practice that patients will often prioritize an improved waist over scar location. In fact, many patients are not bothered by the scar at all. Notably, the authors still recommend proactive scar management with silicone sheeting, kinesio taping, and early profractional laser for all patients.

Alternative to Fleur-de-lis Abdominoplasty

The fleur-de-lis (FDL) abdominoplasty is used to treat excess epigastric laxity in the horizontal and vertical axes and has become a mainstay in the massive weight loss population.[21,22] However, the long vertical scar in a visible location and the high complication rate are major drawbacks.[23,24]

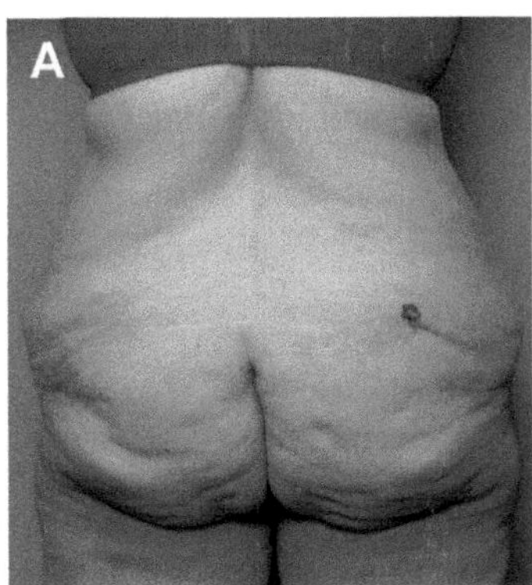

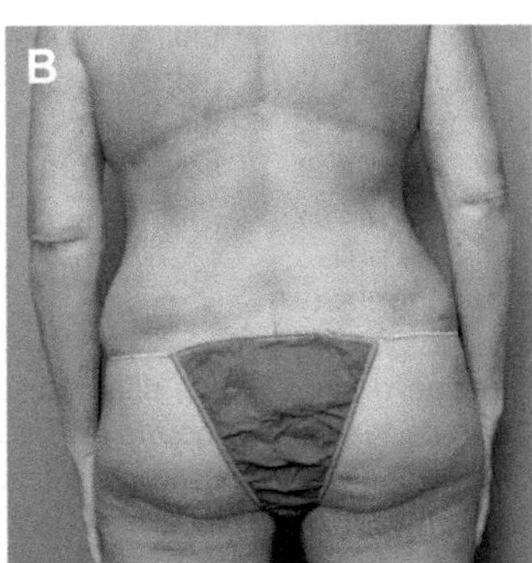

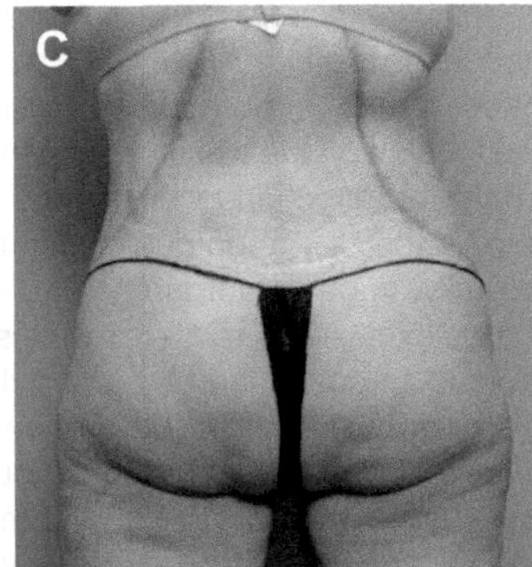

Fig. 2. 51-year-old woman who presented for body contouring following massive weight loss of 85 kg following gastric band. (*A*) Posterior view at time of consultation. (*B*) Posterior view following lower body lift and staged upper body lift with residual flank deformity. (*C*) Posterior view following oblique flankplasty.

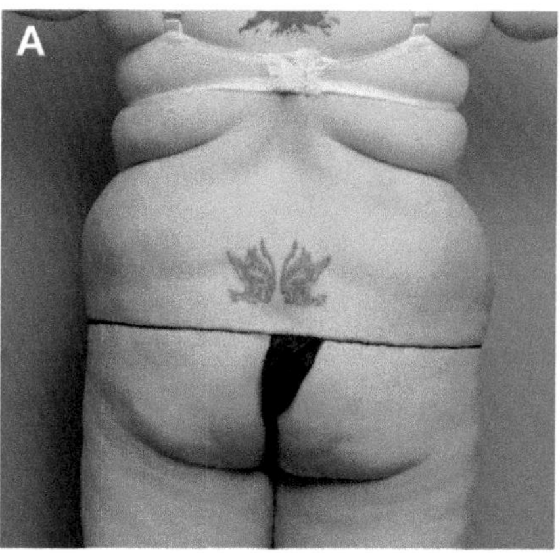

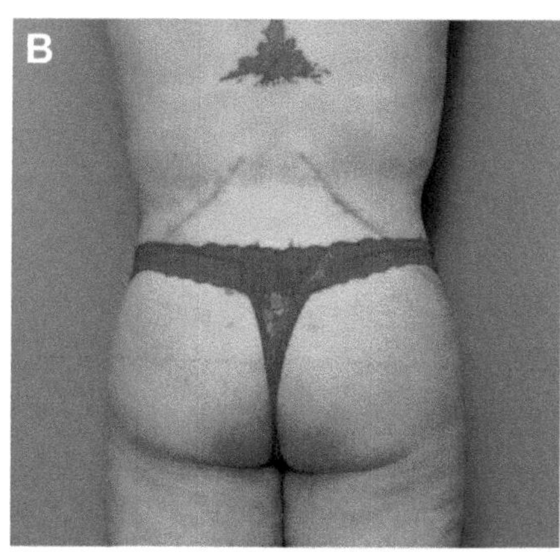

Fig. 3. 40-year-old woman treated with extended lipoabdominoplasty and oblique flankplasty. (*A*) Posterior view preoperatively. (*B*) Posterior view postoperatively with marked improvement in buttock aesthetics with well-defined infrabuttock crease.

The oblique flankplasty has been proposed to be an alternative to FDL, as the vertical direction of pull can improve epigastric horizontal skin laxity (**Fig. 4**). While this can be true in some patients, one must be wary of how much epigastric tightening will be achieved. As described previously, the proximity of the incision to the target area is directly related to how effective it will be. In many patients, the oblique flankplasty excision might be too far away to significantly improve the epigastrium. The authors strongly believe that oblique flankplasty will not eliminate the need for FDL in certain patients, particularly those with a high body mass index (BMI) or with significant epigastric skin laxity (**Fig. 5**). FDL is still the most effective option for correcting horizontal laxity in the epigastrium.

However, there is more to oblique flankplasty in correcting epigastric laxity than just the direction of the scar. To understand this, the reader should be familiar with the landmark article by Lockwood, in which he described the high lateral tension (HLT) abdominoplasty.[25] The HLT abdominoplasty is often misunderstood, as it is not about decreasing the tension on the closure in the midline, but rather about the direction of pull of the abdominoplasty flap. In the HLT abdominoplasty, the flap is pulled laterally. In other words, the HLT abdominoplasty is not exclusively related to incision design, but instead the direction of pull on the tissue during closure of the incision. This concept can be tested by pulling on one's shirt in an outward (laterally) and downward direction and comparing it to pulling inwards (medially) and downwards. Pulling laterally improves horizontal skin laxity in the epigastrium. HLT is therefore an excellent option for patients with moderate epigastric laxity that can improve this area and obviate the need for an FDL. The reader is referred to the article by Rosenfield published in a previous edition of this journal to learn more about HLT abdominoplasty.[26]

The importance of oblique flankplasty becomes clear when considering the need for an effective HLT abdominoplasty. To perform a HLT abdominoplasty, the lateral extent of the incision needs to be more oblique (less horizontal), and there is often a dog ear created that will necessitate extending the scar. Surgeons have traditionally pulled the abdominoplasty flap medially during closure to decrease the lateral dog ear, so the lateral direction of pull in an HLT will naturally make the dog ear more prominent. However, the location of the HLT scar and dog ear are precisely in line with the origin of the oblique flankplasty resection. The authors believe that an oblique flankplasty therefore allows for a more effective HLT abdominoplasty and can be thought of as a glorified dog ear excision of the HLT abdominoplasty. Albeit too simplistic, this explanation will help the learner grasp the location of the scar, the direction of pull, and the effect on the epigastrium.

TECHNICAL PEARLS

Determining Scar Location

As discussed previously, determination of scar location is based on achieving maximal waist narrowing. The incisions are placed alongside the skin roll, and curve upwards away from the midline. The bury test can be used while marking the patient to ensure adequate laxity for closure with minimal tension. This test is performed again intraoperatively before making incisions. Importantly, the

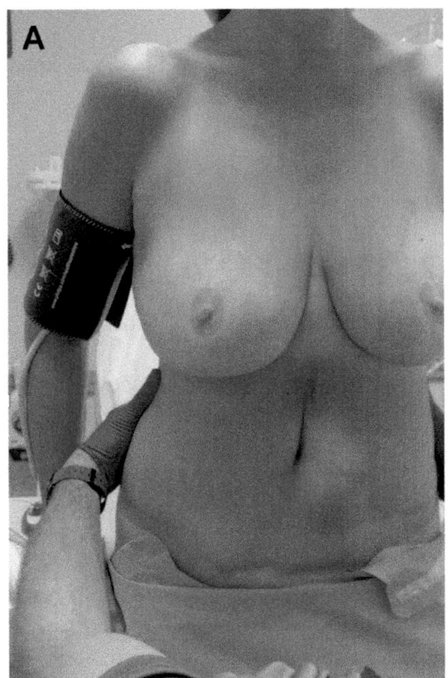
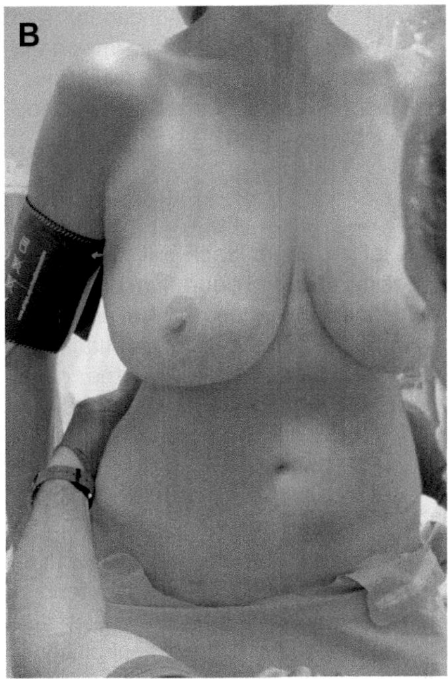

Fig. 4. 51-year-old woman (see Fig. 2), demonstrating effectiveness of the vector of pull in the oblique flankplasty on horizontal abdominal laxity. (*A*) At rest. (*B*) Posteriorly directed pull.

planned resection is dissected down to muscle fascia with minimal to no undermining. Poor planning may result in an overly tight closure requiring undermining, which places this area at increased risk of delayed wound healing. Closure should include the strong SFS in that area.[25,27]

Adjustments to incision placement can help address saddlebags and anterior upper abdominal laxity. If planned correctly, a posterior vector of pull along the upper incision closure in an oblique flankplasty can avoid the need for an FDL abdominoplasty in many cases, as this can be sufficient at addressing the horizontal laxity of the upper abdomen. Inferiorly positioned lower incisions will efface saddlebags and provide a lateral thigh and buttock lift.

Areas at Risk of Bleeding

Massive weight loss patients have many large vessels that traverse the subscarpa's fat. These vessels exist in a deflated tissue plane and can be difficult to identify before unintentional injury and subsequent bleeding occurs. In an oblique flankplasty, the deep fat immediately superior to the iliac crest has a particularly high density of these

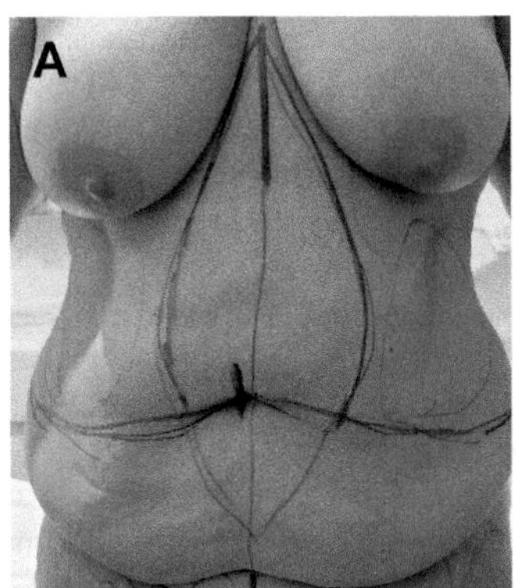
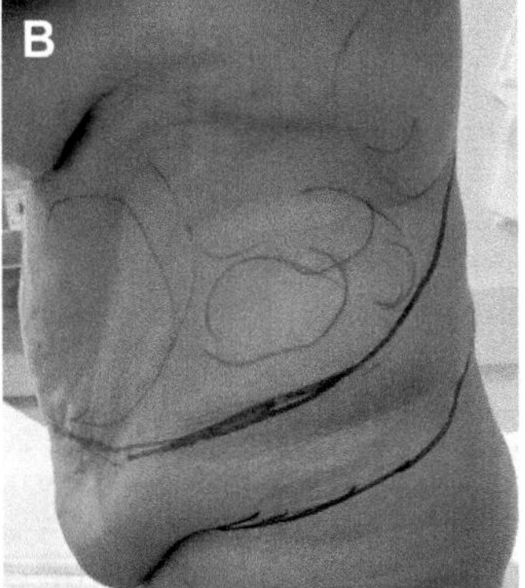
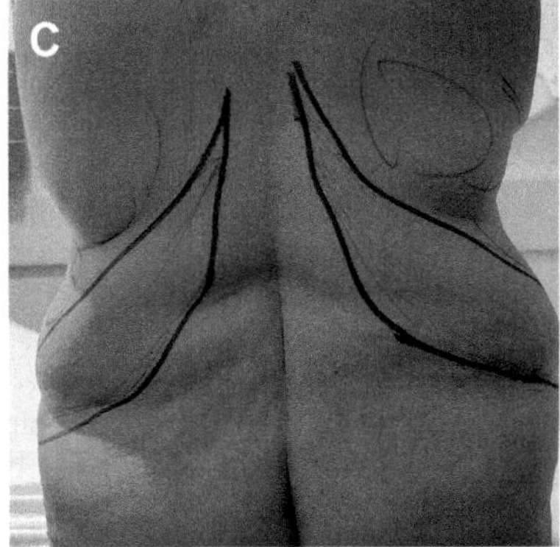

Fig. 5. 53-year-old woman (see Fig. 1) with preoperative markings prior to oblique flankplasty, fleur-de-lis abdominoplasty, and thigh liposuction. (*A*) Frontal view with fleur-de-lis markings. (*B*) Lateral view with posterior extension of fleur-de-lis markings, transitioning to oblique flankplasty. (*C*) Posterior view with oblique flankplasty markings.

vessels. Careful dissection, identification, and control of the vessels in this area is important. Careful hemostasis will pay dividends, with reduction of overall blood loss and decreased likelihood of postoperative bleeding.

Upper Back Roll

The presence of an upper back roll should not impact the design of the oblique flankplasty. No improvement should be expected for an upper back roll given the vector of pull for the flank and relatively adherent tissues overlying the chest wall. This area should instead be treated separately with upper back lift, if necessary.[28,29]

SUMMARY

As described previously, the oblique flankplasty is a natural progression of truncal body contouring procedures aimed at narrowing the waist and flank. The ideal patient for oblique flankplasty is one who is primarily interested in contouring of the trunk, achieving the narrowest possible waist, and has prominent flank rolls. Several secondary goals of the oblique flankplasty include better defining the upper border of the buttock and improvement in horizontal upper abdominal laxity. Finally, there are several important areas that are less impacted by the oblique flankplasty, including the medial thigh and buttock. While most dramatic improvement in the overall appearance of the flanks can be achieved, the tradeoff is high riding posterior incisions to create a natural, concave flank. Although the incisions are visible, they are away from the buttock, which helps maintain lower back aesthetics and allows for independent treatment of the buttock with fat grafting.

CLINICS CARE POINTS

- Oblique flankplasty can be combined with lipoabdominoplasty to treat patients with Pittsburgh grade 2 and 3 flank deformities.
- The combined vertical and horizontal vectors of pull improve the contour to the lateral buttock and thigh as well as epigastric horizontal laxity, which can obviate the need for fleur-de-lis abdominoplasty.
- Although scarring tends to be favorable in this area, patients must understand that the resulting scars will visible along the lower third of the back.

DISCLOSURE

P. Wirth: Nothing to disclose. A. Afifi: Nothing to disclose.

REFERENCES

1. Hurwitz DJ, Beidas O, Wright L. Reshaping the oversized waist through oblique flankplasty with lipoabdominoplasty. Plast Reconstr Surg 2019;143(5):960e–72e.
2. Matarasso A. Abdominolipoplasty: a system of classification and treatment for combined abdominoplasty and suction-assisted lipectomy. Aesthetic Plast Surg 1991;15(2):111–21.
3. Matarasso A, Matarasso DM, Matarasso EJ. Abdominoplasty: classic principles and technique. Clin Plast Surg 2014;41(4):655–72.
4. Matarasso A. Traditional abdominoplasty. Clin Plast Surg 2010;37(3):415–37.
5. Shestak KC. The extended abdominoplasty. Clin Plast Surg 2014;41(4):705–13.
6. Lockwood TE. Lower-body lift. Aesthetic Surg J 2001;21(4):355–69.
7. Lockwood T. The role of excisional lifting in body contour surgery. Clin Plast Surg 1996;23(4):695–712.
8. Lockwood TE. Transverse flank-thigh-buttock lift with superficial fascial suspension. Plast Reconstr Surg 1991;87(6).
9. Lockwood T. Lower body lift with superficial fascial system suspension. Plast Reconstr Surg 1993;92(6).
10. Swanson E. Near-circumferential lower body lift: a review of 40 outpatient procedures. Plast Reconstr Surg Glob Open 2019;7(12):E2548.
11. Sozer SO, Basaran K, Alim H. Abdominoplasty with circumferential liposuction: a review of 1000 consecutive cases. Plast Reconstr Surg 2018;142(4):891–901.
12. Pascal JF. Buttock lifting: the golden rules. Clin Plast Surg 2019;46(1):61–70.
13. Song AY, Jean RD, Hurwitz DJ, et al. A classification of contour deformities after bariatric weight loss: the Pittsburgh rating scale. Plast Reconstr Surg 2005;116(5):1535–44.
14. Song AY, O'Toole JP, Jean RD, et al. A classification of contour deformities after massive weight loss: application of the pittsburgh rating scale. Semin Plast Surg 2006;20(1):24.
15. Wong WW, Motakef S, Lin Y, et al. Redefining the ideal buttocks: a population analysis. Plast Reconstr Surg 2016;137(6):1739–47.
16. Hammond DC. Latissimus dorsi flap breast reconstruction. Plast Reconstr Surg 2009;124(4):1055–63.
17. Srivastava U, Rubin JP, Gusenoff JA. Lower body lift after massive weight loss: autoaugmentation versus

no augmentation. Plast Reconstr Surg 2015;135(3): 762–72.
18. Menardais B, Kerfant N, Chaput B, et al. Lower body lift in the massive weight loss patient: a new classification and algorithm for gluteal augmentation. Plast Reconstr Surg 2018;142(4):596E–8E.
19. Srivastava U, Rubin JP, Gusenoff JA. Lower body lift after massive weight loss. Plast Reconstr Surg 2013; 132:68.
20. Afifi A. Staging body contouring: how to handle the most complex patients, In: Plastic Surgery the Meeting; October 2022, 2022, Boston, MA.
21. Mitchell RTM, Rubin JP. The Fleur-de-Lis abdominoplasty. Clin Plast Surg 2014;41(4):673–80.
22. Castañares S, Goethel JA. Abdominal lipectomy: a modification in technique. Plast Reconstr Surg 1967;40(4):378–83.
23. Christopher AN, Morris MP, Patel V, et al. A comparative analysis of fleur-de-lis and traditional panniculectomy after bariatric surgery. Aesthetic Plast Surg 2021; 45(5):2208–19.
24. Derickson M, Phillips C, Barron M, et al. Panniculectomy after bariatric surgical weight loss: analysis of complications and modifiable risk factors. Am J Surg 2018;215(5):887–90.
25. Lockwood T. High-lateral-tension abdominoplasty with superficial fascial system suspension. Plast Reconstr Surg 1995;96(3):603–15.
26. Rosenfield LK. High tension abdominoplasty 2.0. Clin Plast Surg 2010;37(3):441–65.
27. Lockwood TE. Superficial fascial system (SFS) of the trunk and extremities: a new concept. Plast Reconstr Surg 1991;87(6):1009–18.
28. Shermak MA. Management of back rolls. Aesthetic Surg J 2008;28(3):348–56.
29. Soliman S, Rotemberg SC, Pace D, et al. Upper body lift. Clin Plast Surg 2008;35(1):107–14.

Spiral Flap Breast Reshaping with Transverse Upper Body Lift or J Torsoplasty

Dennis J. Hurwitz, MD[a,b,*], Dani Kruchevsky, MD[a]

KEYWORDS

- Upper body lift • Brachioplasty • Mastopexy • Breast reconstruction • Spiral flaps • J torsoplasty • Body contouring

KEY POINTS

- Spiral flaps are deepithelialized epigastric and lateral thoracic flaps from either a transverse UBL or J torsoplasty.
- Reverse abdominoplasty with a transverse back lift provides a UBL with scars along the bra line.
- J torsoplasty is an effective UBL with scars along the inframammary fold and lateral chest.
- J torsoplasty is performed in supine position.
- Seven esthetic subunits of the posterior torso assist aesthetic evaluation.

 **Video content accompanies this article at http://www.plasticsurgery.theclinics.com.**

INTRODUCTION/HISTORY/DEFINITIONS/BACKGROUND

From the mid-1990s, the senior author (DJH) applied body contouring and breast reshaping surgery to treat dozens of patients with skin laxity after massive weight loss (MWL), courtesy of University of Pittsburgh laparoscopic gastric bypass pioneer Phillip Schauer. The results were often esthetically disappointing, because the deformities were poorly understood, and the techniques inadequate with a high rate of wound healing complications. With the prevailing approach of independent operations for each region, intervening areas were inadequately treated with discard of potential donor sites for tissue sculpting.

With increasing understanding of psychological, nutritional, and metabolic deficiencies, our patients were better prepared for extensive lengthy surgery.[1–5] As the nature of the skin redundancy, laxity and deep adherences were being appreciated, improved skin resection patterns and combinations of procedures were being designed and better executed by experienced teams. Coordinated integration of each area in as few stages as possible led to upper and lower body circumferential transverse excisions, with at times harvest of flaps for breast and/or buttock augmentation and often with a fleur-de-lis (FDL) abdominoplasty, which the senior author (DJH) called total body lift (TBL) surgery.[6–8]

Concerned about TBL high complications and esthetic deficiencies, around 2010 DJH started oblique excision body lifts. The esthetic success of Boomerang pattern correction of gynecomastia, consisting of two sets of opposing oblique excisions of the anterior chest, spurred these modifications[9–11] (see Dennis J. Hurwitz and Dani Kruchevsky's article, "Maximizing the TULUA Abdominoplasty with Oblique Flankplasty," in this issue, Figure 3). The principle being that

[a] Pittsburgh Center for Plastic Surgery, 3109 Forbes Avenue #500, Pittsburgh, PA 15213, USA; [b] University of Pittsburgh
* Corresponding author.
E-mail address: drhurwitz@pghplasticsurgery.com

Clin Plastic Surg 51 (2024) 119–133
https://doi.org/10.1016/j.cps.2023.09.002

vertical and horizontal excess needs to be treated by either a combination of transverse and vertical excisions ("T" shaped) or simply elliptical.

With confirmation of the superiority of large elliptical excision techniques, contemporary TBL usually starts with oblique flankplasty with lipoabdominoplasty (OFLA)[9,12] and is then followed some months later with J torsoplasty,[13] spiral flap reshaping of the breasts,[14] and L brachioplasty[15,16] and modified L thighplasty.[17]

Before fully describing the evolution of transverse upper body lift (UBL) to J torsoplasty, we define posterior torso deformities and esthetic goals with the aid of observing seven esthetic subunits in Case 1 single-stage oblique excisions TBL and Case 2 multistage TBL with transverse UBL.

CASE 1: SINGLE-STAGE OBLIQUE EXCISIONS CONTEMPORARY TOTAL BODY LIFT

A 29-year-old woman, BMI 24, after 100-pound weight loss, is treated for moderate to severe lipodystrophy with skin laxity of her arms, torso, breasts, and thighs with two oblique lifts, lipoabdominoplasty, and Wise pattern mastopexy with spiral flap reshaping by three operative teams in less than 5 hours. Vertical medical thighplasty was performed 7 months later (**Figs. 1–3**).

Fig. 3, right, of Case 1 introduces the correctable posterior torso seven *esthetic subunits*. Lateral to the breast (1) *Chest* may have rolls extending around the back that flatten to reveal muscles. (2) *Scapula* may have distinct rolls in the mid-back that flatten to even reveal bone. (3) *Flank* may have bulges which may include the hip that surgery creates obliquely oriented depressions smoothly transitioning between scapula and hip. (4) *Hip* may have descending bulges stopped by the lateral gluteal unit that are transformed to small prominences distinct from the flank and lateral gluteal unit. (5) *Lateral gluteal* may have skin wrinkling and depressions that smooth to flat or rounded in females and flat to depressed in males. (6) *Buttock* may have descending bulges to join the lateral thigh saddlebag deformity, which are diminished and raised to be the fullest width along the inferior buttocks. (7) *Lateral thigh* may expand with buttock descent for saddlebag deformity that reduced and firmly tapered from the buttocks to the lateral thigh.

Case 1 generalized esthetic improvement is as follows:

1. Asymmetrical deformity becomes symmetric result.
2. Pale, symmetric, and well-positioned, non-constricting scars.
3. Rolls and bulges are esthetically reduced and appropriately contoured.
4. Abdominal skin is form-fitting, symmetrically tight, and accentuates muscularity.
5. Oversized upper body is reduced, smooth and shapely tapered, but larger than the mid body.
6. Upper arms and axillae are smaller and contoured with shorter descend of posterior axillary folds.

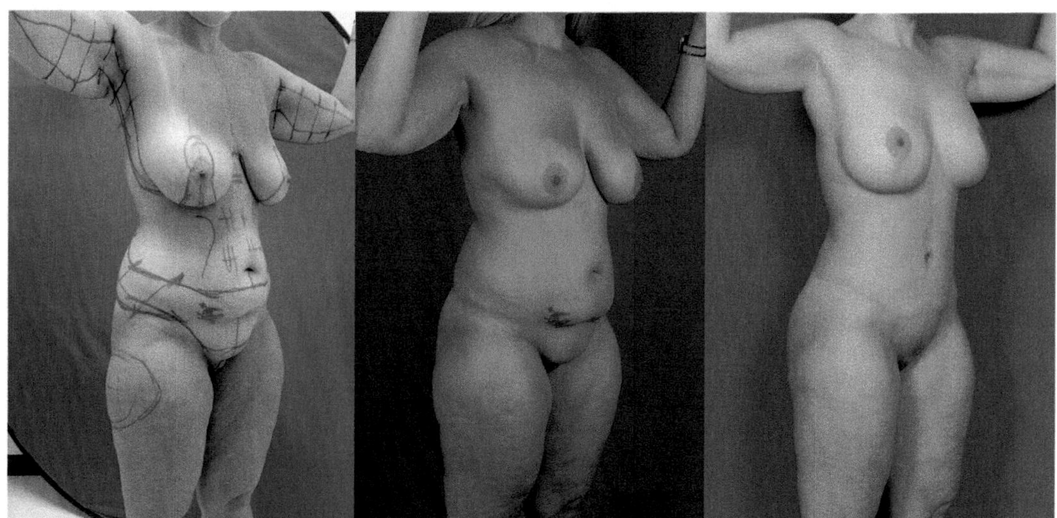

Fig. 1. Case 1. Before and after right anterior oblique patient views: *Left* with deformity and markings for VASERlipo (pluses), OFLA, J torsoplasty, spiral flap/Wise breast reshaping, and L brachioplasty, and *middle* before with Pittsburgh Grade 3 hanging bulges of lateral chest, back, flanks, hips, abdomen, and medial thighs and breast ptosis, and *right* 1 year after TBL with no deformity.

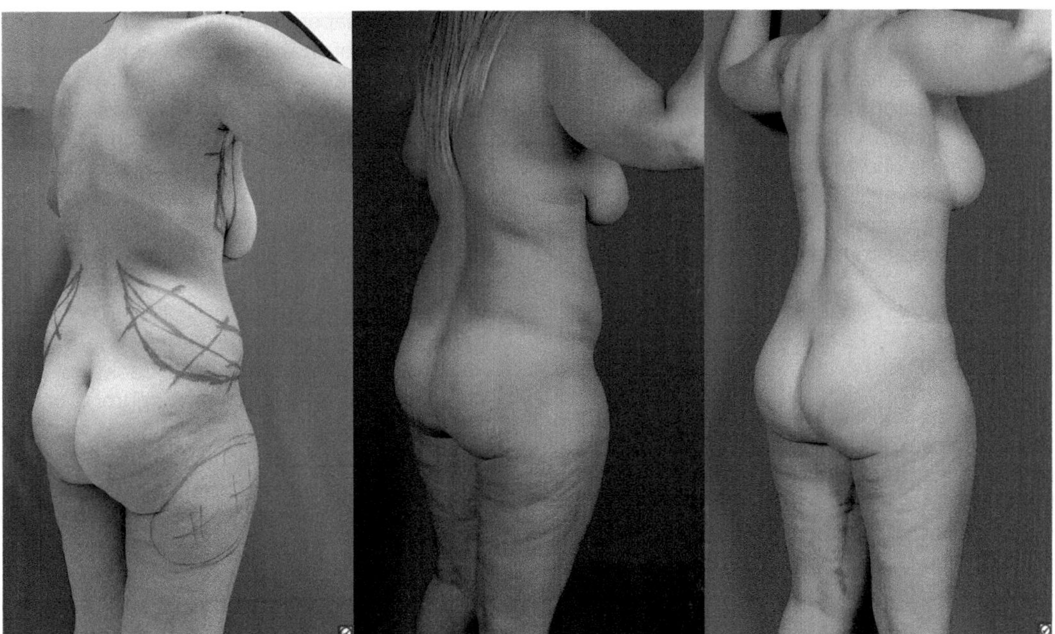

Fig. 2. Case 1. Before and after right posterior oblique patient views: *Left* before with deformity and markings, *middle* before with deformity, and *right* 1 year after TBL with no deformity.

7. Attractively enlarged breasts are the greatest width of the upper body with correction of ptosis and deflated upper pole.
8. Slightly raised breasts expose the inframammary fold (IMF) for a longer and tighter upper abdomen.
9. The mons pubis is slightly round and smoothly transitions.

Case 1 esthetic subunits demonstrates as follows:

1. Removal of the lateral *chest* rolls helps define the lateral breasts and lateral pectoral and latissimus borders.
2. Oversized combined flank/hip roles transform to deeply recessed *flanks* smoothly transitioned

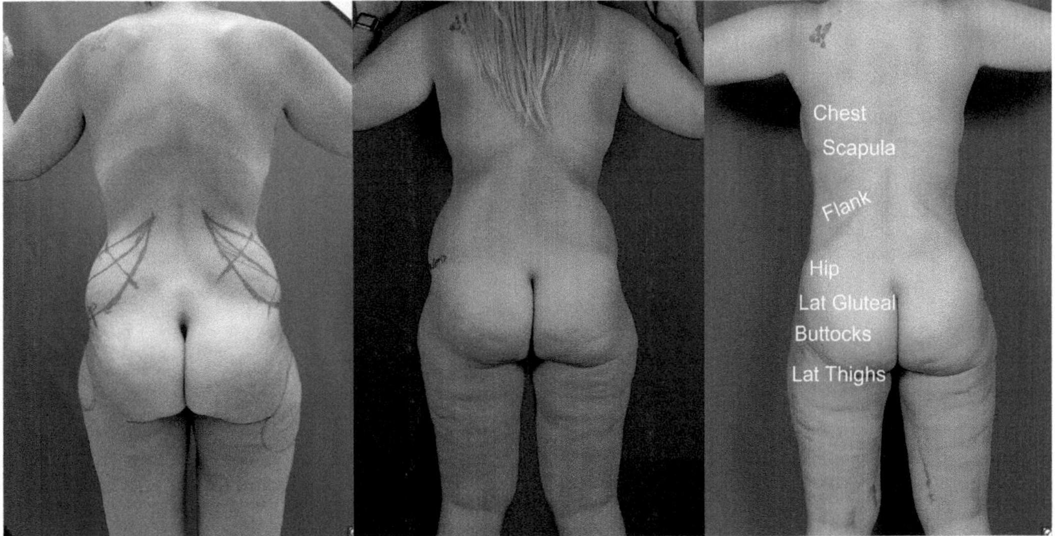

Fig. 3. Case 1. Before and after posterior patient views: *Left* before with deformity and markings, *middle* before with deformity, and *right* 1 year after TBL without deformity. Each of the seven marked *esthetic subunits* exhibit improvement.

from a flat *scapula* area to small defined curved *hips*.
3. The buttocks have smoothly round projections centrally flatted into the lower back, full in *lateral gluteal* areas, widest of the torso along the *buttock* line and well defined from the posterior thigh.
4. Cylindrically contoured thighs without loose skin or saddlebags at the *lateral thighs*.

CASE 2: TRANSVERSE UPPER BODY LIFT AFTER OBLIQUE FLANKPLASTY WITH LIPOABDOMINOPLASTY

With severe back skin folds approaching the posterior midline, Case 2 represents the contemporary use of a transverse UBL after an OFLA. .A transverse UBL is better than J torsoplasty for severe mid-back redundancy, especially when the scapula folds approach the posterior midline (**Figs. 4–6**).

EVOLUTION TO CONTEMPORARY TOTAL BODY LIFT

Returning to the origins of TBL surgery and its evolution to oblique excision surgery, the senior author (DJH) early on approached the upper body, breasts, and arms as a unit. Ptotic flat breasts need the nipple areola complexes (NACs) reduced and lifted and the parenchyma esthetically shaped. Surrounded by circumferential skin rolls of the chest and back, the breasts usually descend several interspaces. Wise pattern mastopexy improves NACs and breast shape, but leaves a low-lying small and poorly projecting breast, surrounded by rolls of skin. The senior author (DJH) and others conceived a reverse abdominoplasty along the IMF continuing transversely posterior to the spine to raise the IMF and the breast footprint and to circumferentially reduce mid-torso skin laxity.[18,19]

Although planned to be hidden under a wide brassiere strap, the transverse back scars may widen, hypertrophy, depress, and/or constrict. Even when the scar is fine, there is a discordance of a fuller upper torso across the scar to a narrower mid-torso, because after removal of the transverse strip two different body widths are approximated. To further accentuate this discrepancy, the circumferential scar may constrict like a barrel stave. To eliminate the mid-back transverse scar and body width discrepancies, we originated the J torsoplasty UBL, which is limited to the posterolateral chest. The inspiration was limited but unsuccessful experience with lateral thoracoabdominoplasty, which failed to treat scapula or flank rolls.[20,21]

Nevertheless, there remain indications for transverse lifts and FDL abdominoplasty. A transverse lower body lift (LBL) best treats oversize, sagging

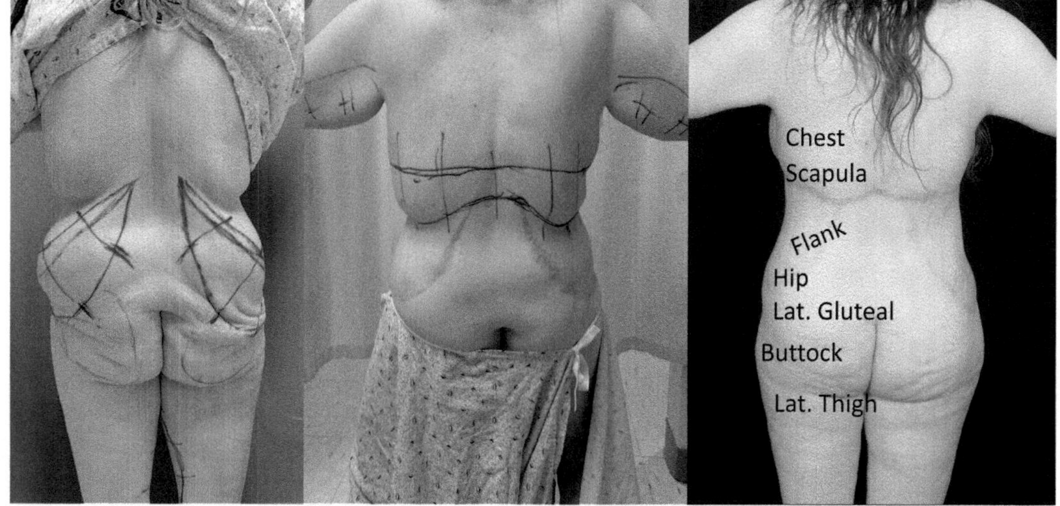

Fig. 4. Case 2. Posterior views of 31-year-old woman after 110-pound weight loss with severe posterior mid-torso skin laxity for two-stage TBL 2021/2022. *Left*: lipodystrophy with chest/scapula and flank/hip rolls with wrinkled lax lateral gluteal unit with markings for oblique flankplasty, vertical thighplasty, and lipoaugmentation of buttocks. *Middle*: improved flanks, hips, and buttocks. Severe chest and medially oriented scapula rolls is marked for transverse UBL, and L brachioplasty. *Right*: nearly 2 years after second stage shows faint flankplasty scars within smoothly depressed flanks. The arms, upper, and midback bag are smaller with correction of chest/scapula rolls so that the lateral breasts are seen. The transverse bra line scar is slightly widened. All *seven esthetic subunits* are improved.

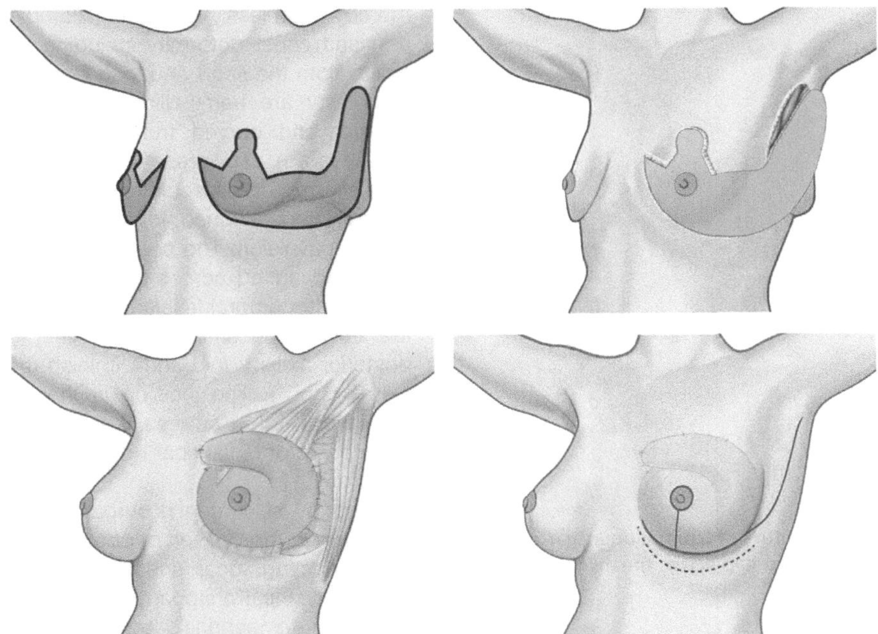

Fig. 5. J torsoplasty UBL with spiral flap reshaping of the breasts. *Upper left*: the J torsoplasty includes inferior and a lateral extension of a Wise pattern mastopexy. *Upper right*: after deepithelialization, the perimeter is incised. *Lower left*: the lateral flap spirals superiorly to the second cartilage, and the epigastric flap is flipped up over the inferior pole and secured to the fourth cartilage. *Lower right*: through transparent skin, flaps position at completion.

hips and lateral gluteal region in the absence of enlarged flanks. A transverse UBL is better than J torsoplasty for severe mid-back redundancy, especially if it approaches the posterior midline as in Case 2, or if greater tissue volume is needed for the spiral flap than is available along the lateral chest. FDL is reserved for transverse epigastric laxity associated with a long midline scar, or refusal of oblique flankplasty.

Fig. 6. Completed L brachioplasty markings with truncated hemi ellipses along the medial arm and lateral chest.

As mastopexies after MWL usually bottom out, with or without gel implant augmentation, we searched for nearby soft tissue augmentation. Considerable excess soft tissue surrounds the breasts with abundant vascularity for potential flaps. Despite prior abdominoplasty, excess superior epigastric skin is usually available. Leaving this soft tissue attached to the lower pole of the breast, a broad-based deepithelialized flap is flipped up to augment the lower pole (see **Fig. 5**). Likewise, instead of harvesting the skin roll lateral to the breast and transversely across the back, a short C-shaped posterior extension heading vertically to the axilla is deepithelialized and advanced under the superior breast pole. Suture suspension of these flaps to the second and fifth costochondral cartilages securely centralizes and suspends the flap augmented breast.

The blood supply of the epigastric flap is from the descending branches of the fifth and sixth intercostals. The lateral flap blood supply is serratus perforators along the anterior axillary line. The spiral course of these two flaps lends the appellation.

The vertical limb of the J torsoplasty continues cephalad into the short limb of the L brachioplasty,

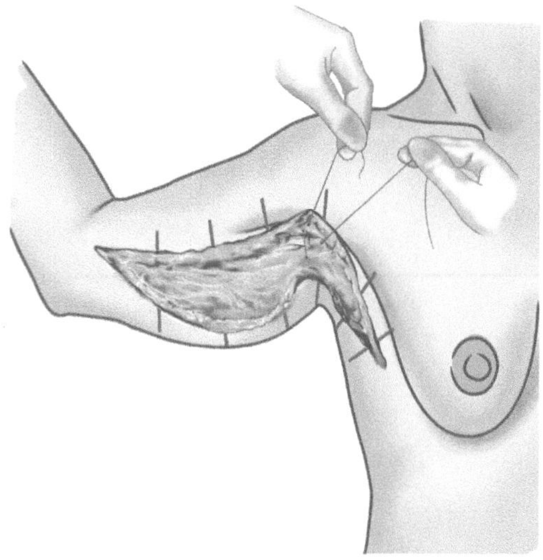

Fig. 7. Anchoring suture of L brachioplasty from proximal posteriorly based flap across the axilla to the deltopectoral fascia.

thereby seamlessly correcting complex proximal arm and chest deformity including an oversized axilla. Both the short and long limbs of the L brachioplasty are hemi ellipses with straight lines anterior and curved truncated limbs posterior (see **Fig. 6**). To preserve delicate underlying medial arm neurovasculature, the excision site is radically liposuctioned, followed by scalpel assisted skin avulsion. The posteriorly based proximal flap is advanced across the axilla and anchored to the deltopectoral fascia to tense and straighten the curved posterior incision line, elevate the posterior axillary fold and diminish the oversized axilla (**Fig. 7**). The incision is then closed with two-layer barbed sutures, leaving an inconspicuous posteromedial scar on a slightly bowed upper arm.

Currently, all surgery is outpatient except for the medically compromised or obese. The routine use of long-acting local anesthetic Exparel (Pacira Bioscience Inc, Parsippany, NJ) and effective infusion of epinephrine, tranexamic acid, with

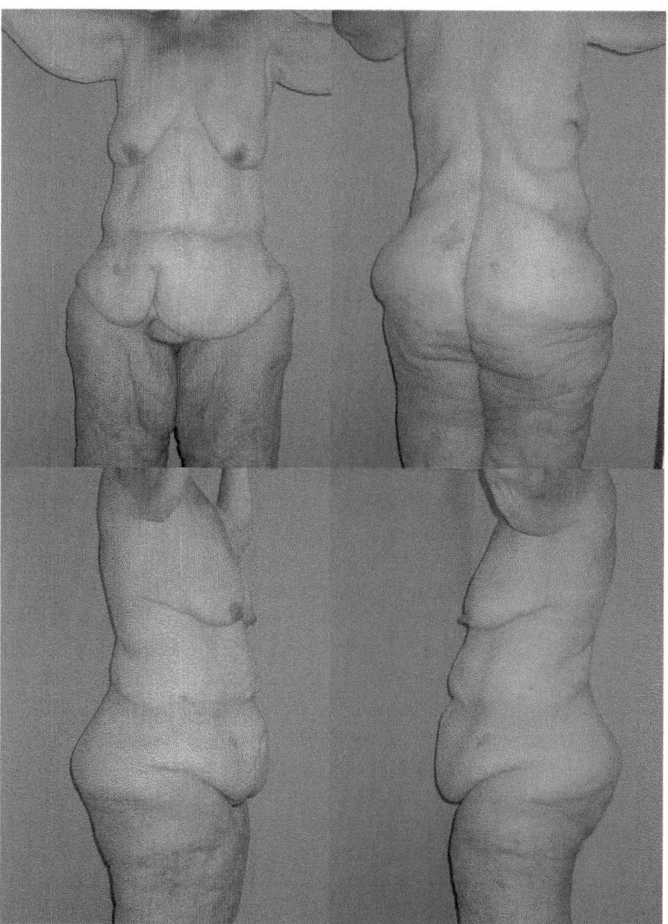

Fig. 8. Case 2. After nearly 200-pound weight loss, a 45-year-old woman, BMI 30 presents with severe hanging skin and lipodystrophy with deflated, hanging breasts. She requests TBL. *Upper left*: anterior. *Upper right:* left posterior. *Lower left*: right lateral. *Lower right*: left lateral.

continuous hemostasis, has virtually eliminated unplanned hospital admission. Anticoagulant prophylaxis is reserved for patients with a history of deep vein thrombosis, pulmonary embolism, or factor V deficiency. With the use of rechargeable battery-powered sequential compression stockings, there have been no symptomatic deep vein thrombosis (DVT) or pulmonary embolism (PE).

EVALUATION/APPROACH

With adequate upper body soft tissue excess, the pivotal physical variables in deciding spiral flap for breast reshaping is breast volume and position. When the breast is oversized, a reduction is performed, which may be suture or mesh suspended. When the ptotic breast is adequate in volume, and the IMF and breast footplate have not descended, a dermal suspension mastopexy is favored.[22] In patients who do not wish to accept the risk of flap augmentation or have inadequate neighboring tissue, silicone implants are placed subpectoral before a Wise pattern mastopexy.

After pushing and gathering skin, conservative preoperative incision lines are marked for moderate tension and for harvesting quality flaps. If preliminary approximation of the excision site proves the width inadequate, subsequent rims of tissue are removed.

SURGICAL ORDER

Markings start with Wise pattern mastopexy and reverse abdominoplasty. Then, the L brachioplasty is drawn from elbow to mid-lateral chest. Finally, the UBL is drawn as a transverse extension of the lateral Wise pattern or a J shape excision connecting the lateral Wise pattern to the short limb of the L brachioplasty.

The transverse UBL starts prone with harvest of two laterally based flaps, with an excision wide enough on closure to efface mid-back skin rolls. After a turn supine, the L brachioplasty usually precedes the mastopexy with flaps, which is followed by the reverse abdominoplasty. With the J torsoplasty, the entire operation is supine. After the breast mound is

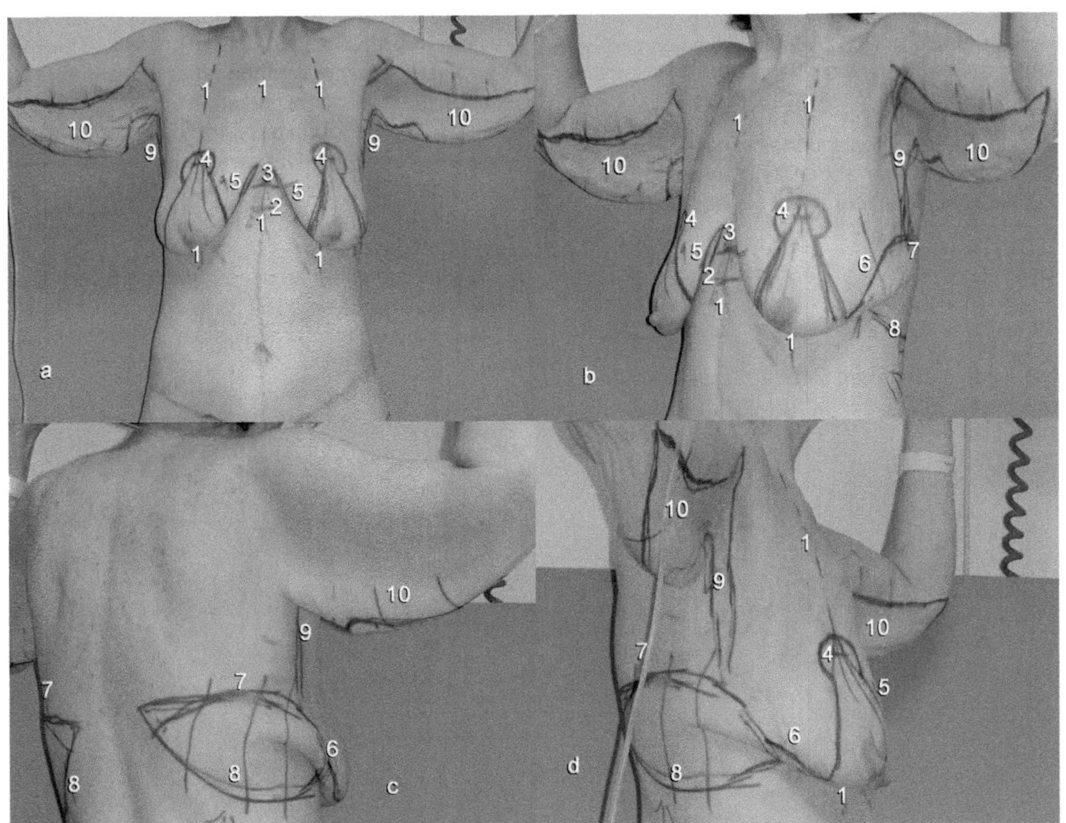

Fig. 9. Case 3. Second-stage TBL. One year after her FDL abdominoplasty, transverse LBL, vertical medial thighplasty, she is marked for L brachioplasty, Wise pattern mastopexy, transverse bra line UBL, with overlay sequential numbering. *Upper left*: anterior view. *Upper right:* left anterior oblique view *Lower left*: right posterolateral view. *Lower left*: right lateral view.

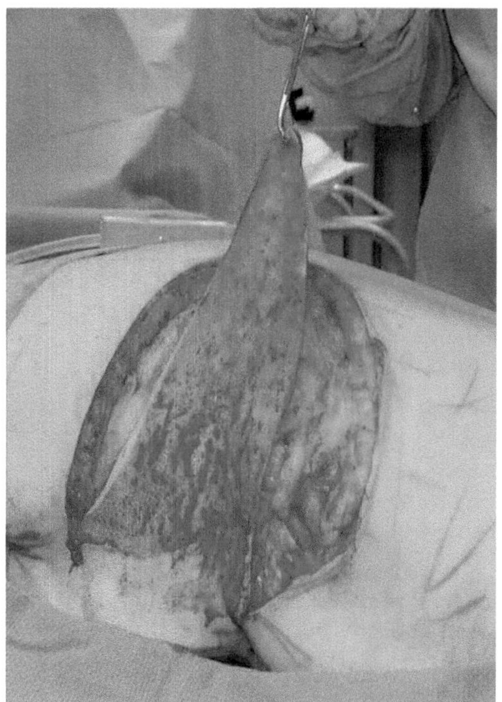

Fig. 10. Case 3. Intraoperative prone showing left back with head to left. Deepithelialization and isolation of the transverse back flap, raised from latissimus dorsi fascia.

shaped with the flaps and the reduced NAC is positioned, the reverse abdominoplasty and J lateral torso advancement complete the operation.

CASE 3: TRANSVERSE UPPER BODY LIFT, SPIRAL FLAP BREAST RESHAPING, AND L-BRACHIOPLASTY

A 46-year-old woman, 5′ 6″, 202-pounds (BMI 33), previously 427 pounds (BMI 69) before open

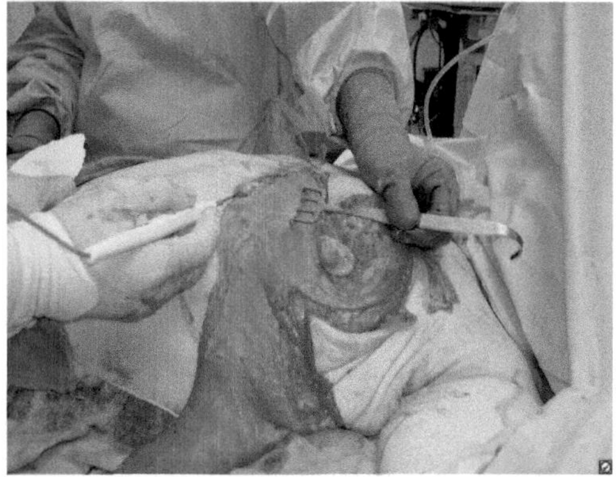

Fig. 11. Case 3. Intraoperative supine showing left chest as IMF incision is being made with electrosurgery. Entire Wise pattern is deepithelialized and perimeter elevated.

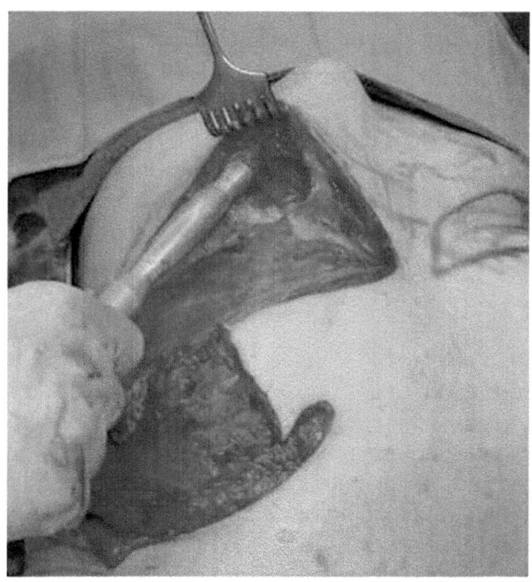

Fig. 12. Case 3. Using a blunt-tapered dissector, discontinuous inferior chest flap undermining to beyond the costal margin.

bypass surgery, requests TBL surgery. She has generalized skin excess, lipodystrophy especially along the hips, and deflated breasts. There are long vertical anterior abdominal midline and right lower adherent scars and severely ptotic mons pubis (Fig. 8). Although operated on before the J torsoplasty or OFLA was available, she is a better candidate for transverse UBL harvest due to inadequate lateral chest volume and FDL due to midline scar.

Six months after an uncomplicated FDL abdominoplasty, transverse LBL, and vertical thighplasty, she is marked for L brachioplasty, transverse UBL,

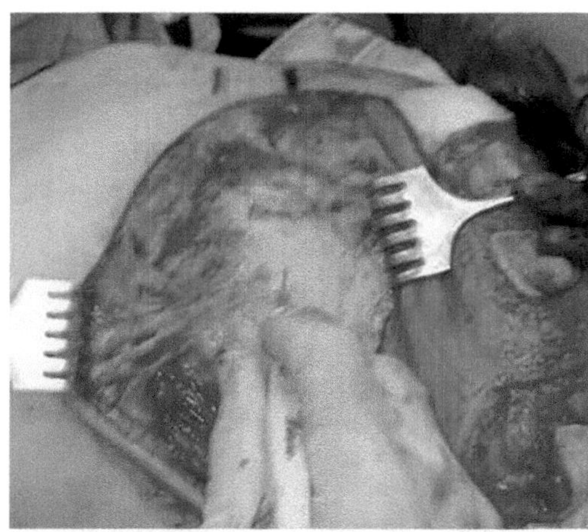

Fig. 13. Case 3. Direct electrosurgical undermining of the epigastric flap extension of the breast to the presternal marked new IMF location.

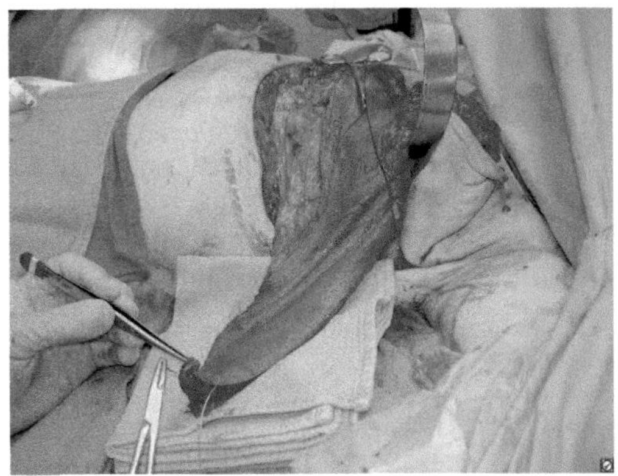

Fig. 14. Case 3. After checking for adequate blood supply, a pull through suture is placed into medial tip of flap to aid entrance through lateral pectoral window exposed with a retractor.

reverse abdominoplasty, and Wise pattern mastopexies with spiral flap reshaping (Fig. 9). Vertical chest midline [1] and nipple meridians [1] are drawn. IMFs [2] are registered on the chest midline. The desired superior breast location is found by pushing the breast and excess epigastric skin up and sighting the raised IMF and registering it [3] some centimeters above the current IMF [2]. The entire breast is superiorly positioned and cradled, searching for the optimal nipple location. The keyhole pattern [4] hangs from the desired new NAC with 10 cm vertical limbs. This long and narrow pattern accommodates the added breast volume. A line [5] is drawn from the medial vertical to the parasternal base of the breast to meet parallel the new IMF. From [6] line extends a level transverse upper pattern line [7] above the bra (IMF) line to a posterior paramedian point. By pinch gathering of the inferior skin, the proper width of back skin resection is determined for a line [8] drawn to form the parallel excision lines, ending at the posterior midline.

The short limbs [9] of the L brachioplasty descend from the axilla. The long arm limbs [10] of the L brachioplasty are marked from axilla to elbow.

Transverse UBL starts prone with simultaneous harvest of flaps. After deepithelialization, the perimeter is incised (Fig. 10). After elevation of laterally based flaps from over the latissimus dorsi muscle, the donor sites are closed with two-layered barbed suture.

Turning supine, the breast foot plate will be superiorly positioned by suturing attached inferior and lateral spiral flaps to the sixth and second costal cartilages, respectfully. To avoid distorting the breast, the lateral chest and epigastric skin will be suture advanced to chest musculoskeleton. The surgical steps are as follows:

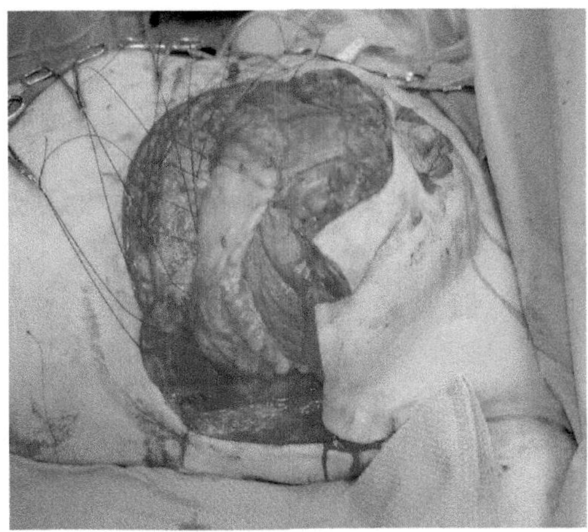

Fig. 15. Case 3. Braided sutures are placed from the leading edge of the reverse abdominoplasty flap along the sixth rib and lateral chest. As the epigastric flap is pushed into position, these sutures are serially tied and then cut. The keyhole closure has started over the shaped breast mount created by flip up of the contiguous epigastric flap and suprapectoral spiraled advancement of the lateral thoracic flap to the second intercostal cartilage.

- Deepithelialize Wise pattern and spiral flaps, followed by incision and undermining of surrounding skin (Fig. 11).
- Discontinuous undermine reverse abdominoplasty to costal margin (Fig. 12).
- Undermine epigastric flap extension of inferior pole of the breast (Fig. 13) and then the superior breast over the pectoralis, leaving central and transverse pedicles to breast.
- Through a lateral suprapectoral window tunnel the back flap over pectoralis muscle to the second costal cartilage (Fig. 14).
- After the centralized breast mount is augmented and suture shape by the spiral flaps. The reverse abdominoplasty flap is

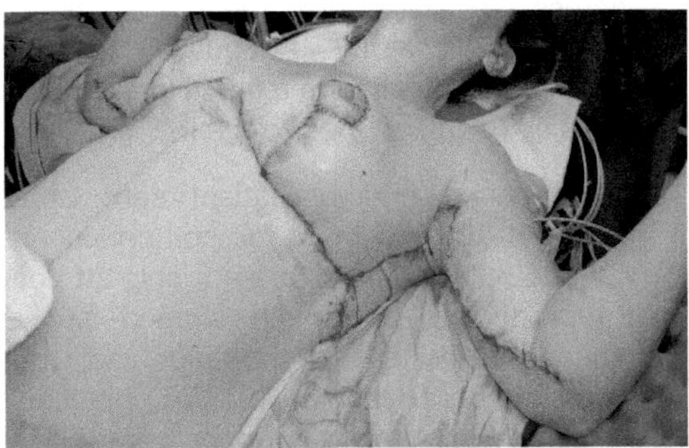

Fig. 16. Case 3. Immediate postoperative result shows well-shaped symmetric breasts surrounded by tightly sutured well-contoured reduced chest and arms.

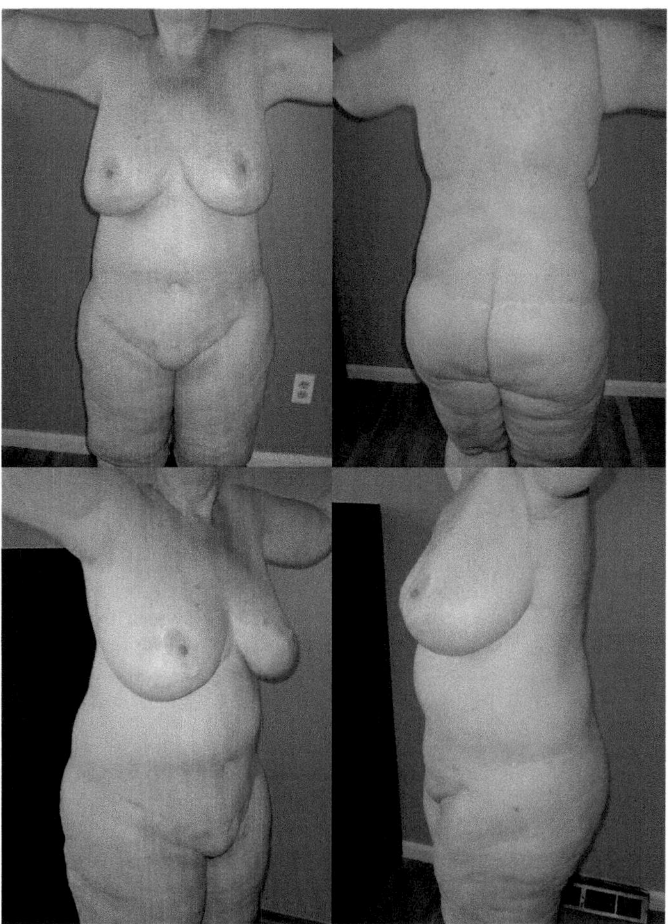

Fig. 17. Case 3. Comparing to **Figs. 8** and **11**, improved body, breast and arm appearance after 30 pound weight gain and 7 years post-op. *Upper left*: anterior. *Upper right:* posterior. *Lower left*: right anterior oblique. *Lower right*: left lateral.

suture raised to the sixth rib IMF and the lateral chest skin along the musculoskeletal anterior axillary line (**Fig. 15**).

- Liposuction is followed by resection of the medial arm skin. Key suture proximal advancement of the posterior triangular flap to deltopectoral fascia is followed by two-layer barbed suture closure from elbow across the axilla down the lateral chest to the transverse UBL. Adequately mobilized Wise pattern flaps form a tight closure around NAC and vertical limbs to the IMF (**Fig. 16**).

The 30-pound heavier patient sent photos 7 years post-op (**Fig. 17**), for comparison see **Figs. 8** and **9**. The breasts are not only attractive and appropriately sized and shaped but are harmonious with the neighboring and much improved torso and arms. The NAC position is well maintained. Adequate upper pole fullness and high breast position persists. There are tapering tails of the breasts with full lateral breasts that stop abruptly at the mid-lateral chest and not marred by lateral folds. Her numerous scars are inconspicuous. The UBL and IMF have not descended while the posterior LBL only a little. Although there are no back rolls, there is also no defined waist or depressed flanks. She has been transformed from a bizarre habitus to a well-shaped full-bodied woman.

CASE 4: J TORSOPLASTY, SPIRAL FLAP BREAST RESHAPING, AND L-BRACHIOPLASTY

A 38-year-old, 5′, 7″ and 200-pound female requests a TBL after losing 156 pounds (**Fig. 18**). Her ptotic small breasts are surrounded by rolls of skin. Mid-torso rolls and lower abdominal rolls are huge. Three months after FDL abdominoplasty and transverse LBL with adipose fascial flap buttock augmentation, she returns for her L brachioplasty, Wise pattern mastopexy with spiral flaps harvested from a reverse abdominoplasty, and J torsoplasty.

Her breast and arm markings are like the previous case, except for the J-shaped lateral

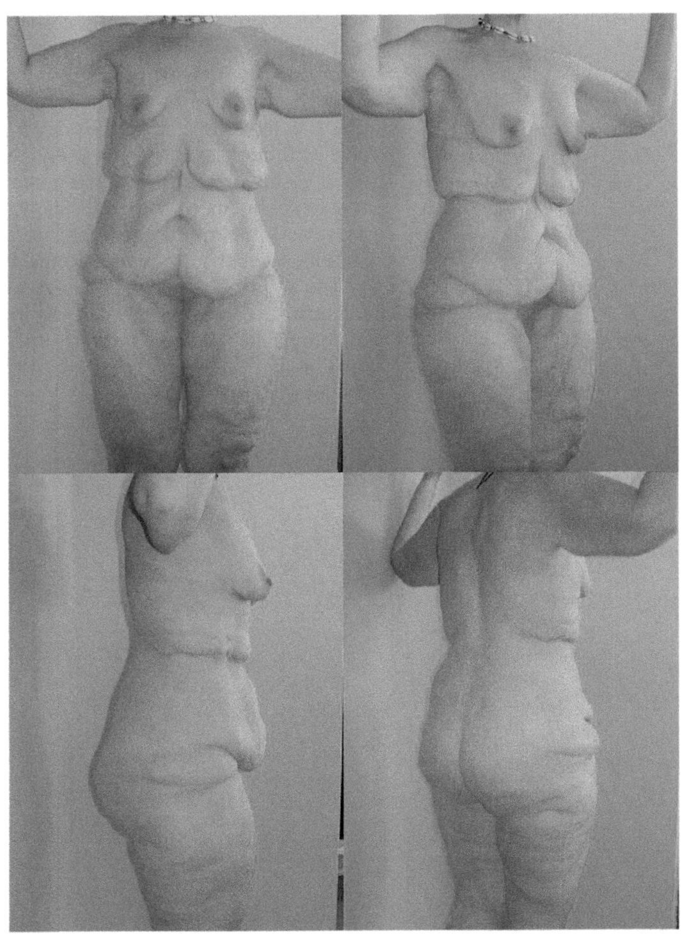

Fig. 18. Case 4. A 42-year-old woman, who lost 190 pounds, seeks TBL for lipodystrophy with severe anterolateral mid-body (Scapula) rolls, hip excess, and breast hypoplasia with ptosis. *Upper left*: anterior. *Upper right:* right anterior oblique. *Lower left*: right lateral. *Lower left*: right lateral. *Lower right*: right posterior oblique.

connection (**Fig. 19**, Video 1). With the excess back skin pushed firmly anterior at the level of the third rib, a vertical line is drawn from the inferior axilla along the mid-lateral chest. Before reaching the level of the IMF, the back skin from the lumbar region is also pushed obliquely superior and anterior. While still holding the skin up, this line is continued to the previously marked reverse abdominoplasty line. When the skin is dropped, the resulting line from the axilla to the IMF resembles a J on the left and a reverse J on the right. To estimate the width of the vertical resection, the lateral chest excess is pinched to the lateral pectoral border. Here, a more medial line is drawn parallel to the outer J line. Between the two lines is the width of resection for the back lift. Because the lateral thoracic and epigastric flaps are deepithelialized and harvested contiguous to the central breast mound, their dimensions are predetermined with minimal intraoperative adjustments.

After the left brachioplasty is completed, the breast with its lateral chest and inferior epigastric flap extensions are isolated (**Fig. 20**, *upper right*). After mobilization, the flaps are flipped and spiraled into position to both augment and suspend (see **Fig. 20**, *lower left*). The J torsoplasty reverse abdominoplasty is discontinuously undermined, and sutures are in place to frame the breast to the advance IMF and lateral chest wall (see **Fig. 20**, *lower right)*. The second stage surgery took 4 hours with no blood transfusion.

One year later and 15 pounds heavier, she is better shaped (**Fig. 21**). The enlarged breasts are symmetric high, round, and supported. Reduced arms and thighs have relatively inconspicuous inner longitudinal scars. Esthetic feminine contours are created without bra line scars.

DISCUSSION

After two decades, we confirm that spiral flap breast reshaping and suspension succeeds with either transverse back or J torsoplasty UBLs. For moderate to severe back laxity, our preference is

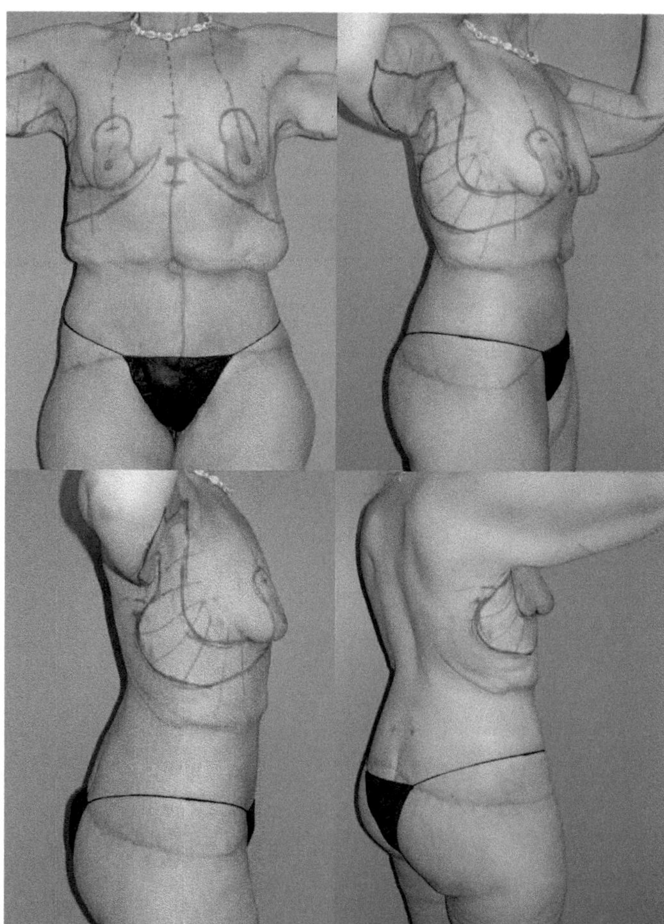

Fig. 19. Case 4. Contiguous surgical markings for L brachioplasty through J torsoplasty to Wise pattern mastopexy 3 months after FDL abdominoplasty with transverse lower body lift and L thighplasty in same views as **Figs. 11** and **18**. The FDL has pulled the scapula mid-torso roll slightly anterior. To obliterate the large lateral scapula role, the C-shaped extension of the J torsoplasty needs to extend far posterior, causing difficult closure aligning much longer outer to inner incision lines. Lower body and thigh shapes are excellent.

for the less conspicuous scar J torsoplasty. As the J torsoplasty closure runs parallel to the oblique flankplasty, these techniques synergistically reduce all torso skin laxity. However, a wide J pattern demands tedious suture approximation of the shorter inner incision to the longer outer, sometimes causing difficult to treat radiating folds to the back.

Some lateralization of the breast mound may occur. With a bulky base to the lateral flap, preservation of the trans-anterior serratus perforators may leave too much lateral fullness that may need to be reduced later. If the lateral chest advancement flap is not adequately secured to the musculoskeleton, the breast will be pulled toward the back. Favoring a slight medial positioning of the raised NAC may anticipate that adverse dynamic.

The broad-based epigastric flap is reliable to augment the lower pole of the breasts and is especially useful for correcting constriction. As the narrow-based lateral flap advances and rotates over the pectoralis major muscle to the second costochondral junction, it may turn ischemic, which is not discovered until palpably firm. On a few occasions, flap necrosis has led to suppuration, requiring drainage, multiple debridements with months of wound care. Surgical revision, fat, or silicone implant augmentation may be needed. While unusual, patients need to be prepared for flap necrosis and its prolonged care. Initiates to these techniques should select candidates with generous skin laxity and blood supply.

We respect that some experienced plastic surgeons reject complex upper body surgery. They do not accept simultaneous interwoven operations on the breast, upper torso, and arms. As these surgeons wish to focus on one area at a time, their patients require more operative sessions. They do not trust surgeon assistants to perform part of the operation, whereas they are preoccupied on another area. These reluctant surgeons understand that intertwined operations make intraoperative adjustments to one procedure difficult. For wary surgeons, the use of large pedicle flaps

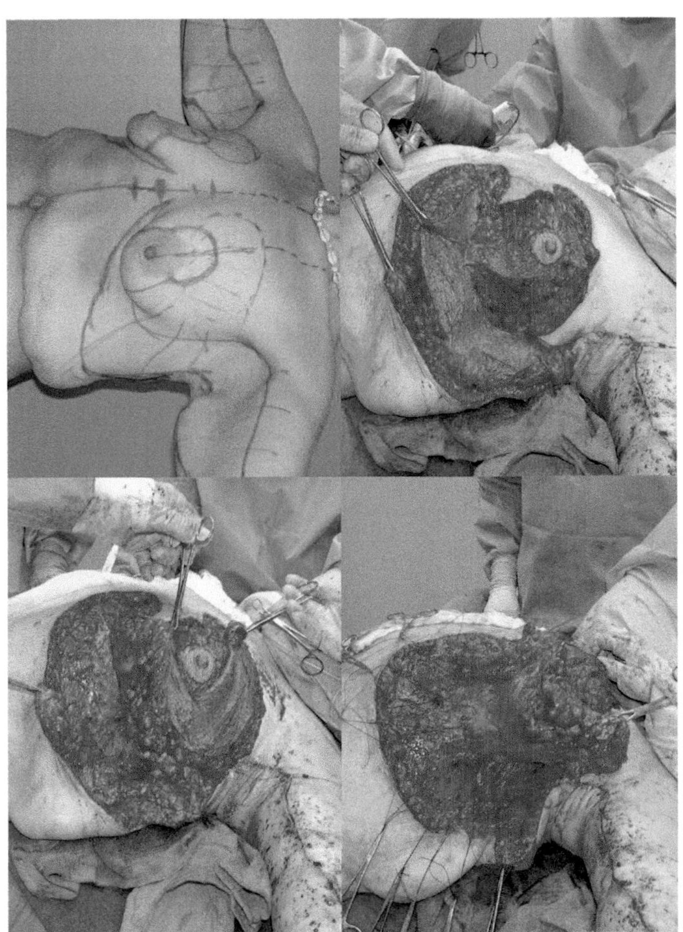

Fig. 20. Case 4. Intraoperative views of J torsoplasty, Wise pattern mastopexy, and spiral flap reshaping, and L brachioplasty. *Upper left*: left upper body, breast, and arm markings as would appear on the operating room table. *Upper right:* after the long limb of the L brachioplasty is closed, the deepithelialized chest and breast flaps are isolated. *Lower left*: the flaps are positioned in a spiral to augment and suspend breast. *Lower right*: as the breast and surrounding flaps are pulled superior, sutures are placed to advance the J torsoplasty UBL to raise the footprint of the breast.

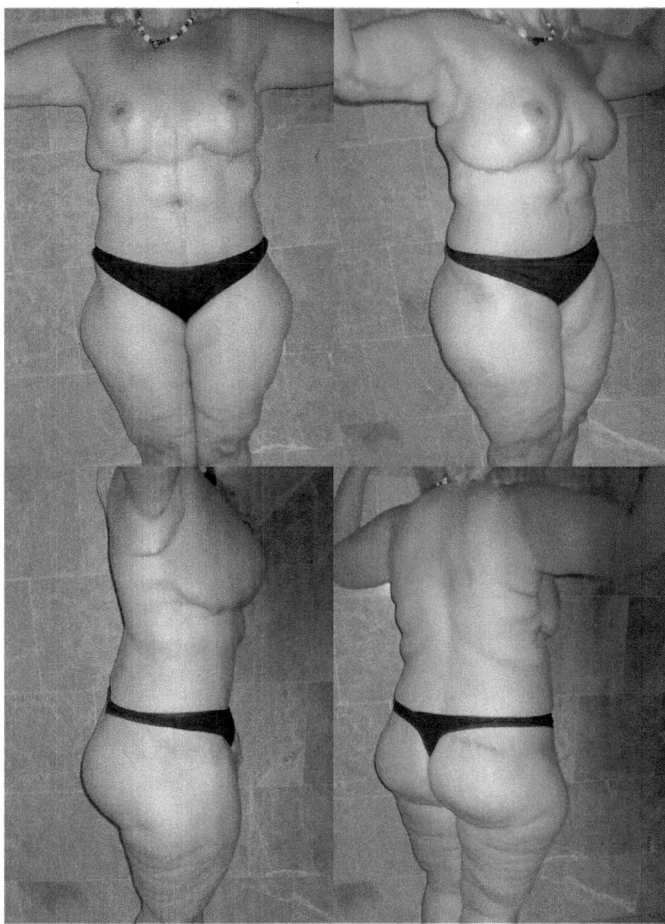

Fig. 21. Case 4. One year later and 20 pounds heavier, the patient sends photos which are arranged to compare to **Fig. 18**. The lipodystrophy was mostly corrected. The arms, body, and breast have improved shape and position with small upper abdominal residual skin rolls and posterior radiating lateral chest folds. These were reduced by minor revision several years later.

with even slight uncertainty of vitality has no place in cosmetic surgery.

With this complex interplay of three operations and deepithelialization of buried tissue, most all incisions are set at the onset. Having all the moving parts from several teams come together symmetrically is a foreboding challenge that is incredibly satisfying. Thoughtful experience is presented in this article to present strengths and weaknesses of using spiral flaps reshaping of the breast with either transverse or J torsoplasty UBL as well as the integration with OFLA into the contemporary TBL.

CLINICS CARE POINTS

- Spiral flap reshaping mastopexy esthetically repositions, shapes, and suspends the deflated, sagging and mispositioned breast with surrounding skin flaps.
- Deepithelialized epigastric and lateral thoracic flaps reshape the breast from either a traditional transverse upper body lift (UBL) or J torsoplasty.
- In moderate cases of upper torso skin and adipose redundancy, J torsoplasty effectively provides an effective UBL with scars along the inframammary fold and lateral chest.
- In severe cases of upper torso skin and adipose redundancy, a reverse abdominoplasty with a transverse back lift provides a more effective UBL with scars along the inframammary fold to across the central back.
- J torsoplasty may extent across the axilla through the L brachioplasty for optimal skin and adipose reduction, recontouring and scarring.
- With the J torsoplasty being performed entirely supine, simultaneous team surgery on the arms and also upper body/breasts safely expedites the operations.
- Distal necrosis of the lateral flap is an uncommon but serious complication.
- Care must be taken to avoid lateralization of the breasts.
- Use esthetic subunits to evaluate posterior torso results.

DISCLOSURE

Nothing to disclose.

SUPPLEMENTARY DATA

Supplementary data related to this article can be found online at https://doi.org/10.1016/j.cps.2023.09.002.

REFERENCES

1. Taylor J, Shermak M. Body contouring following massive weight loss. Obes Surg 2004;14(8):1080–5.
2. Sanger C, David LR. Impact of significant weight loss on outcome of body-contouring surgery. Ann Plast Surg 2006;56(1):9–13.
3. Agha-Mohammadi S, Hurwitz DJ. Potential impacts of nutritional deficiency of postbariatric patients on body contouring surgery. Plast Reconstr Surg 2008;122(6):1901–14.
4. Gusenoff J, Rubin J. Plastic surgery after weight loss: current concepts in massive weight loss surgery. Aesthetic Surg J 2008;28(4):452–5.
5. Colwell A, Borud L. Optimization of patient safety in postbariatric body contouring: a current review. Aesthetic Surg J 2008;28(4):437–42.
6. Hurwitz D, Aghamohammadi S, Ota K, et al. A clinical review of total body lift surgery. Aesthetic Surg J 2008;28(3):294–303.
7. Hurwitz D. Total body lift, reshaping the breasts, chest, arms, thighs. Hips, back, waist, abdomen and knees after weight loss, Aging, and pregnancies. MD Publish; 2005.
8. Hurwitz DJ. Single-staged total body lift after massive weight loss. Ann Plast Surg 2004;52(5):435–41.
9. Hurwitz DJ. Aesthetic refinements in body contouring in the massive weight loss patient. Plast Reconstr Surg 2014;134(6):1185–95.
10. Hurwitz DJ. Boomerang pattern correction of gynecomastia. Plast Reconstr Surg 2015;135(2):433–6.
11. Hurwitz D. Enhancing masculine features after massive weight loss. Aesthetic Plast Surg 2016;40(2):245–55.
12. Hurwitz DJ, Beidas O, Wright L. Reshaping the oversized waist through oblique flankplasty with lipoabdominoplasty. Plast Reconstr Surg 2019;143(5):960e–72e.
13. Clavijo-Alvarez JA, Hurwitz DJ. J Torsoplasty. Plast Reconstr Surg 2012;130(2):382e–3e.
14. Hurwitz DJ, Agha-Mohammadi S. Postbariatric surgery breast reshaping. Ann Plast Surg 2006;56(5):481–6.
15. Hurwitz DJ, Jerrod K, L-Brachioplasty. An adaptable technique for moderate to severe excess skin and fat of the arms. Aesthetic Surg J 2010;30(4):620–9.
16. Hurwitz DJ, Holland SW. The L brachioplasty: an innovative approach to correct excess tissue of the upper arm, axilla, and lateral chest. Plast Reconstr Surg 2006;117(2):403–11.
17. HURWITZ D. Medial thighplasty. Aesthetic Surg J 2005;25(2):180–91.
18. Hunstad JP, Repta R. Bra-line back lift. Plast Reconstr Surg 2008;122(4):1225–8.
19. Agha-Mohammadi S, Hurwitz DJ. Management of upper abdominal laxity after massive weight loss: reverse abdominoplasty and inframammary fold reconstruction. Aesthetic Plast Surg 2010;34(2):226–31.
20. RAHBAN S, GROSS J. A new approach to correction of truncal redundancy after massive weight loss—the lateral thoracoabdominoplasty. Aesthetic Surg J 2007;27(5):518–23.
21. Hurwitz D. Comprehensive body contouring: theory and practice. Springer Verlag; 2016. p. 117–41.
22. Rubin JP, Khachi G. Mastopexy after massive weight loss: dermal suspension and selective autoaugmentation. Clin Plast Surg 2008;35(1):123–9.

Interplay of Oblique Flankplasty with Vertical Medial Thighplasty

Dennis J. Hurwitz, MD[a,b,*], Dani Kruchevsky, MD[a]

KEYWORDS

• Oblique flankplasty • Thighplasty • Thigh lift • Lower body lift • Massive weight loss

KEY POINTS

- Oblique flankplasty with lipoabdominoplasty (OFLA) has major advantages over traditional circumferential lower body lift in both improved esthetics of the flanks, hips, buttocks, and upper lateral thighs, and lower complication rates.
- Medial thighplasty by L-shape excision, facilitated by preliminary excision site liposuction allowing scalpel assisted skin avulsion, is preferred due to effective reduction, relatively inconspicuous scar, and low rate of complications.
- Short, horizontal limb vertical extensions of the medial thighplasty complete a three-sided picture frame rounded and smoothly transitioned pubic monsplasty
- Through proximal anterolateral thigh secure suspension, OFLA, either immediately or as a first stage, complements medial thighplasty for optimal circumferential esthetic result.

 **Video content accompanies this article at http://www.plasticsurgery.theclinics.com.**

INTRODUCTION

Massive weight loss (MWL) patients request treatment of excess skin and adipose of both torso and proximal extremities. As the keystone of total body lift (TBL) surgery,[1] circumferential lower body lift usually proceeds and has considerable impact on upper body lift and medial thighplasty.

Over the past decade, we replaced traditional transverse posterior lower body lift and abdominoplasty with oblique flankplasty and lipoabdominoplasty (OFLA).[2,3] OFLA provides long-lasting improvement of shape and skin tightness of the central and lower torso. By avoiding suture adherences of the skin flap to abdominal muscular fascia, our lipoabdominoplasty transfers all upward tension to elevate sagging mons pubis and proximal anterior thigh. Through the secure broad rotation advancement of the oblique flankplasty inferior flap, the lateral buttocks and thighs are optimally suspended. With liposuction, saddlebags are corrected. For severe lateral buttock thigh adiposity, we introduce the posterior wedge resection modification.

Either a T- or L-shaped thighplasty provides the remaining and dominant thigh reduction and shaping. Both cosmetic and radical excision site liposuction (ESL) are routinely used.[4] If the patient requests a shorter vertical scar ending at the mid-medial thigh, extensive bipolar radiofrequency energy provides distal thigh skin contraction.

This report reflects our past 6 years of over 50 cases of OFLA with either T- or L-shaped thighplasty with liposuction and occasional radiofrequency skin tightening. Through Case 1, OFLA operative technique is described followed by a more detailed exposition of limited L-shaped thighplasty with radiofrequency skin tightening,

[a] Hurwitz Center for Plastic Surgery, 3109 Forbes Avenue, Suite 500, Pittsburgh, PA 15213, USA; [b] University of Pittsburgh
* Corresponding author. Hurwitz Center for Plastic Surgery, 3109 Forbes Avenue, Suite 500, Pittsburgh, PA 15213.
E-mail address: DrHurwitz@Hurwitzcenter.com

Clin Plastic Surg 51 (2024) 135–146
https://doi.org/10.1016/j.cps.2023.06.013

including videos of the markings and the operation. Three brief instructive cases follow.

COMPLEX SURGERY OF BODY AND THIGHS

Our customary outpatient treatment of oversized and loose skinned thighs is in two stages, starting with OFLA, followed some months later by vertical medial thighplasty. The goal is gender-specific sculpture of the body and thighs, through skin and adipose excision, liposuction and at times lipoaugmentation. After removal of excess tissue, we drape the patient's skin with appropriately thick subcutaneous tissue esthetically about the musculoskeletal system. By correcting the thigh circumferentially, an aesthetic tapered cone extends from the torso to the knee. Unfortunately, after MWL and aging, there is unmeasurable dermal and subcutaneous tissue structural deterioration that may result in postoperative tissue laxity.

Case 1 is a 48-year-old, 5′, 4″ and 185-pound, BMI 32, woman requesting improvement of the appearance of her torso and thighs. She desires a curvaceous tight-skinned torso and tapering tight-skinned thighs without a long scar. Stage 1 is OFLA. Stage 2 is limited L-shaped thighplasty with VASERlipo and radiofrequency skin tightening.

Planning Oblique Flankplasty and Lipoabdominoplasty

Surgical markings to treat skin excess and skin laxity, and adiposity and adipose atrophy, are drawn standing (**Fig. 1**). The orientation and degree of skin excision follow a preconceived pattern adjusted by skin gathering techniques. With limited to no direct undermining of the closing flaps, strategic liposuction of bulging adipose and vertical etching of the abdomen and back is drawn.[2]

After an orienting vertical line dropped from the xyphoid to the genital labial commissure, encircle the umbilicus. Lateralized umbilicus will be later centralized. Places within encircled adiposity indicate magnitude of liposuction. Leaning over, epigastric skin redundancy is estimated. If possible, the superior transverse incision is drawn across the abdomen through the umbilicus. The inferior incision just superior to the mons pubis is drawn horizontal about 7 cm to either side of the vertical midline. From each end, symmetric lines are drawn that rise just inferior and past the anterior superior iliac spine.

The upper abdominoplasty horizontal line ends inferior to the mid-lateral pelvic crest. Superior to this incision, the skin is firmly adherent to the lateral torso. The lower abdominoplasty horizontal incision line is adjusted laterally while vigorously pushing superiorly on the lax lateral thigh and buttocks to meet the upper incision line along the midlateral torso. The width between these transverse lines varies from 5 to 25 cm. Liposuction of trochanteric bulges (saddlebags) increase lateral thigh skin laxity. The flankplasty lines of excision meet these terminating transverse incisions.

Oblique orientation of the flank excisions follows the natural course of the redundant rolls of skin and fat from the mid-back paraspinous region to the hips. A guideline is drawn along the crest of the flank bulge. Near the middle of this line, the redundant tissue is gathered equally on either side and marked. From these marks, tapered excisions extend superomedial to paraspinous regions. Inferior extensions of the mid-flank marks run roughly parallel to end at the previously drawn lateral termination of the abdominoplasty. Areas for liposuction are encircled and quantified by pluses, including the flank excision site if harvested fat is needed.

From paraspinous location to the abdomen, the superior marked line of the flank excision is roughly 25% shorter than the longer inferior line (along the buttocks). As the superior line of the flankplasty continues as the superior line of the abdominoplasty a reverse line discrepancy occurs across the abdomen, which is also roughly 25% longer than the inferior incision of the abdominoplasty. Guided by 10-cm interval hash marks of both flankplasty incisions, the superior flap in rotated and advanced posteriorly, which distributes the inferiorly advanced epigastric flap also posteriorly, thereby reducing transverse laxity and obviating a midline abdominal vertical excision as in a fleur-de-lys. Following these hatch marks provide a smooth symmetric posterior advance of the epigastric flap to the inferior closure along the sacral region and lateral buttocks. Later, when the abdominoplasty is closed, the incision lines are equal in length, instead of the excessively long superior line in the usual abdominoplasty.

Flankplasty

The patient is rolled prone onto large gel rolls placed under the costal margins and upper thighs, thereby suspending the loose-skinned abdomen for unimpeded posterior advancement of the mid-torso skin.

Because the buttock and thigh tissues are superiorly mobile, the initial incision is along the inferior marked line through skin and multilayer Scarpa's fascia and then to a variable extent through globular buttock fat to lumbodorsal fascia about the

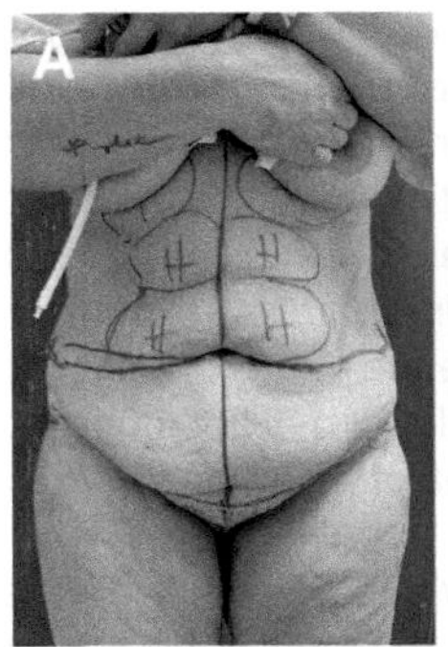
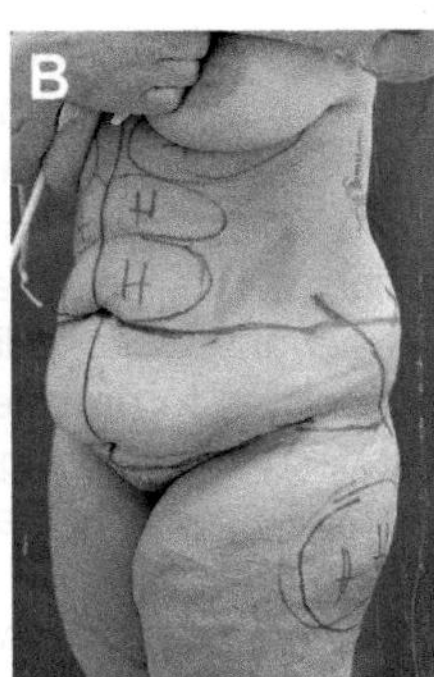
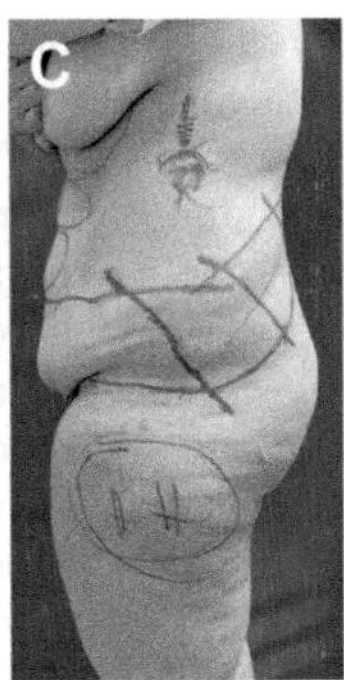
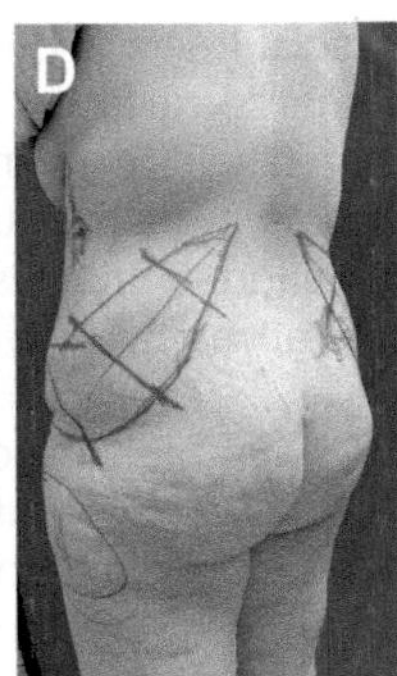
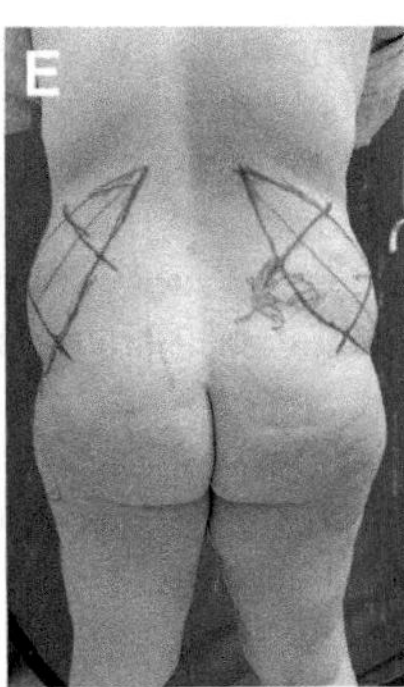

Fig. 1. Case 1. OFLA markings. (*A*) Frontal (*B*) Left Anterior Oblique (*C*) Left Lateral (*D*) Left Posterior Oblique (*E*) Posterior. Instead of tapering the incision lines to each other, they were extended directly lateral and wide enough to remove excess skin between the lateral buttocks and thighs. The flank excisions ascend over the greatest projection of the flank rolls.

level of the palpable posterior superior iliac spine. The incision is completed to the upper lateral thigh. Oversized upper lateral thighs are liposuctioned flat, which aids in superior advancement of the lateral thigh.

Once the inferior incision is completed, the buttock skin edge is grabbed with towel clamps and pulled up to the anticipated superior incision. After confirming the width of the resection, the superior incision is made to latissimus dorsi muscle and lumbodorsal fascia. Starting medially, the tissue between the two incisions is electrosurgically excised, leaving a thin layer of areolar tissue over the muscular fascia. About 2 cc's of liposomal bupivacaine (Exparel; Pacira Pharmaceuticals, USA) is injected for 11 and 12 intercostal nerve blocks along the easily palpable ribs for near painless recovery of OFLA.

The superficial subcutaneous fascia system of the buttocks and lower back is approximated using #2 USP polydioxanone (PDO; Quill, Surgical Specialties, Inc, Wyomissing, PA), including a bite to the underlying muscular fascia. Intradermal running 2 to 0 Quill Monoderm (Surgical Specialties, Inc, Wyomissing, PA), and skin glue completes the closure except for the lateral openings that lead to the abdominoplasty, which are temporarily stapled. The patient is then turned supine for lipoabdominoplasty.

Lipoabdominoplasty

After superwet infusion of saline with xylocaine and epinephrine, VASERLipo (Solta Medical–Bausch Health Companies, Inc, Bothell, WA) with five ring probes ii 80% pulsed mode is applied, followed by VenTx 3.5 mm diameter cannula aspiration. Thorough abdominal deep liposuction proceeds until reaching the desired epigastric flap thickness.

After isolation of the umbilicus, the superior transverse incision is made perpendicular to muscle fascia. A narrow midline tunnel elevates the epigastric flap to the xiphoid. Indirect undermining is through spreading the LaRoe Dissector (ASSI, 300 Shames Drive, Westbury, NY). The mobilized superior flap is pulled toward the planned inferior incision, which is adjusted as necessary. This approach leaves the lower abdomen covered as long as possible, which keeps exposure to a minimum, reducing hypothermia and contamination.

The lower transverse incision is made across the groins to the level of Scarpa's fascia with preservation of about 6 cm of sub-Scarpa's lymphatics and superior to the mons pubis to the level of the rectus muscle anterior sheath. This now isolated hypogastric skin is rapidly excised over supramuscular areolar tissue from side to side. With significant diastasis recti, a vertical ellipse is drawn to include the medial rectus muscle for expeditious #2 PDO Quill suture plication. In some, lower abdominal protrusion may be flattened with a transverse plication of the lower rectus muscle fascia.

The umbilicoplasty creates both an anesthetic structure along with high central tension by suture advancing small deepithelialized epigastric flaps to the rectus muscle fascia at the base of the umbilicus. The superior tension accentuates the epigastric linea alba depression and reduces tension on the relatively ischemic suprapubic closure.[5]

For Case 1, the tissue resection weight of the flanks was 2400 g, and the abdominal resection was 1881 g. The volume of aspirated fat from the back was 400 cc's, from lateral thighs 300 cc's and from the abdomen 325 mL.

Suction drainage is through high pressure Interi (IC Surgical, Grand Rapids, MI, USA). Although minimal undermining is performed, liposuction opens subcutaneous fascial tracts and leaves residual fluids within traumatized tissues. Four thin channels are placed in multiple locations to exit as a single drain through a mons pubis stab wound. Weeks of well-fitted compression garments and early postoperative massage aid rapid recovery.

The lower abdominal wound is closed with #2 PDO barbed suture (Surgical Specialties, Inc, Wyomissing, PA, USA) through Scarpa's fascia and 3 to 0 Quill Monoderm (Surgical Specialties, Inc, Wyomissing, PA, USA) intradermal. Superficial judicious liposuction can now define the rectus abdominis muscles. Skin glue and then Primapore bandages cover the closures.

Most operations were performed in an outpatient surgical center. Within a week, the umbilical sutures are removed, and lymphatic massage started. The patient wears elastic garments continuously for 4 weeks. Three months after uncomplicated healing, Case 1 proceeded with an L-shaped limited vertical medial thighplasty with VASERlipo and BodyTite.

Planning Medial Thighplasty

While standing, thighs, mons pubis, and buttocks are observed for symmetry. For ease of execution, markings are then made supine and then confirmed standing.

When the proximal posterior thigh bordering the buttocks has objectionable rolls of skin, a T-shaped excision is designed with the horizontal limb crossing the entire inferior gluteal fold and then spiraling up between the labia majora and the thighs lateral to the mons pubis. A crossing vertical excision extends the entire length of the thigh to the knees and if necessary, beyond to the calf.[4] With mild to moderate proximal posterior thigh skin redundancy, the T-shaped excision is replaced by an L.

Case 1 4 month pleasing result from her OFLA and markings for her L-shaped limited medial vertical thighplasty is captured (**Fig. 2**). She was planned for an L-Shaped thighplasty with the short limb along the labia majora thigh junction and the long limb at a right angle continuing down the medial thigh.[6] The L-shaped medial vertical thighplasty horizontal component extends posteriorly to the medial buttock thigh crease to include skin redundancy at the ischial tuberosity. The vertical component of the excision continues at a right angle from labia majora toward the medial knee and if needed beyond to the calf. A limited vertical thighplasty with its shorter vertical scar is possible when the distal thigh skin redundancy is minimal with the excision ending just beyond mid-thigh and supplemented with distal BodyTite bipolar radiofrequency energy and cosmetic VASERlipo.

While frog-legged, markings start with a line along the labial thigh junction (Video 1). With thigh adduction, the tissues inferior to this line are gathered superiorly along a line parallel to the labial crease incision to provide the width of horizontal resection. The right angle turn from horizontal to vertical incision is near the palpable ischial tuberosity.

In addition to proper width of excision, positioning the excision along the medial thigh is critical. Medial thigh closures should be hidden between the legs and not seen unless one leg is advanced. This location is achieved by gently pushing the anteromedial thigh skin posteriorly to a point several centimeters posterior to the medial midline, which marks the anterior incision of the vertical excision. Once the anterior vertical incision is marked, the width of skin excision is determined by gathering at the mid-thigh and then tapered distally to meet at the knee.

After reinking the vertical incision, the two legs are pushed together to imprint the first markings on to the other thigh. The adequacy of excision is checked and adjusted (**Fig. 3**A).

The areas for VASERlipo of excess adiposity of the anterior thigh are drawn from + to +++ for magnitude of fat removal. In addition, radical ESL is performed along the vertical limb to allow for skin only resection for preservation of medial thigh neurovasculature. As Case 1 requests a shorter vertical excision, bipolar radiofrequency skin tightening is planned for the mid and distal thighs. The patient then stands for adjustments.

Medial Vertical Thighplasty

Under general anesthesia, frog-legged and after superwet saline infusion, radical liposuction is performed along the vertical limb (Video 2). Esthetic VASERlipo and radiofrequency skin tightening with BodyTite (InMode, Tel Aviv, Israel) proceeds elsewhere and continues during the excision surgery, leaving a pristine margin along the closure. VASER and power-assisted lipoplasty was followed by BodyTite (**Fig. 3B**, C). The aspirate volume was 2000 cc, and the BodyTite energy was 170 KJ. First the posterior and then the anterior vertical incisions are made through the skin and superficial fascial system after verification of the markings (**Fig. 3**D). Through scalpel-assisted avulsion, the skin is dissected off the defatted superficial subcutaneous system (SFS) (**Fig. 3**E). The vertical wound is closed using #1 PDO barbed suture (Surgical Specialties, Inc, Wyomissing, PA, USA) for the fascia and 3 to 0 Quill Monoderm

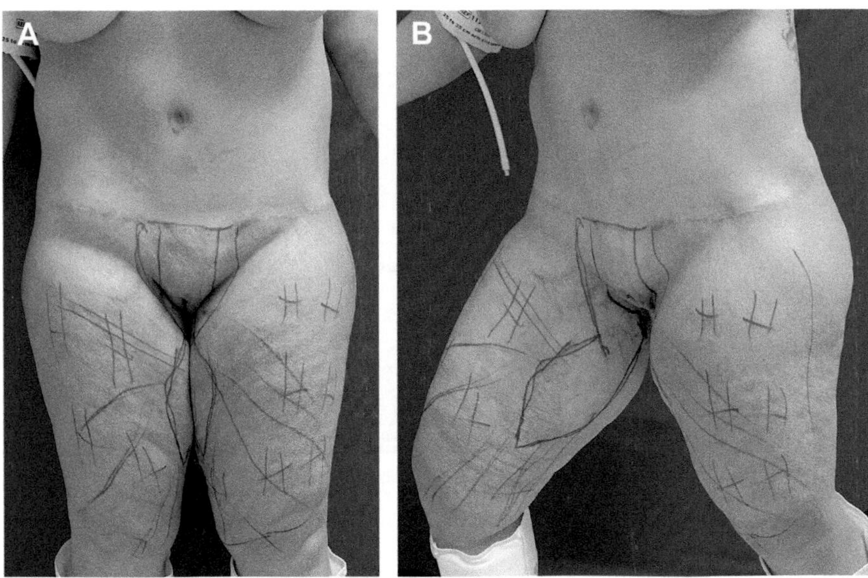

Fig. 2. Case 1: (*A*) Frontal (*B*) Left anterior Oblique. L-shaped limited medial thighplasty markings supplemented with BodyTite bipolar radiofrequency energy and VASERlipo.

(Surgical Specialties, Inc, Wyomissing, PA, USA) for the dermis. The mid-portion of the horizontal limb is suture suspended in the fascia of the adductor magnus tendon and pubis with 2/0 Vicryl (Ethicon, Inc, Somerville, NJ) sutures. This wound is also closed with barbed sutures (**Fig. 3**F–H). Topical skin glue is followed by Primapore Telfa dressing (Smith & Nephew; Sydney, Australia).

The result 5 months after her OFLA and 2 months post-thighplasty meets patient expectations and can be compared with her preoperative images (**Fig. 4**).

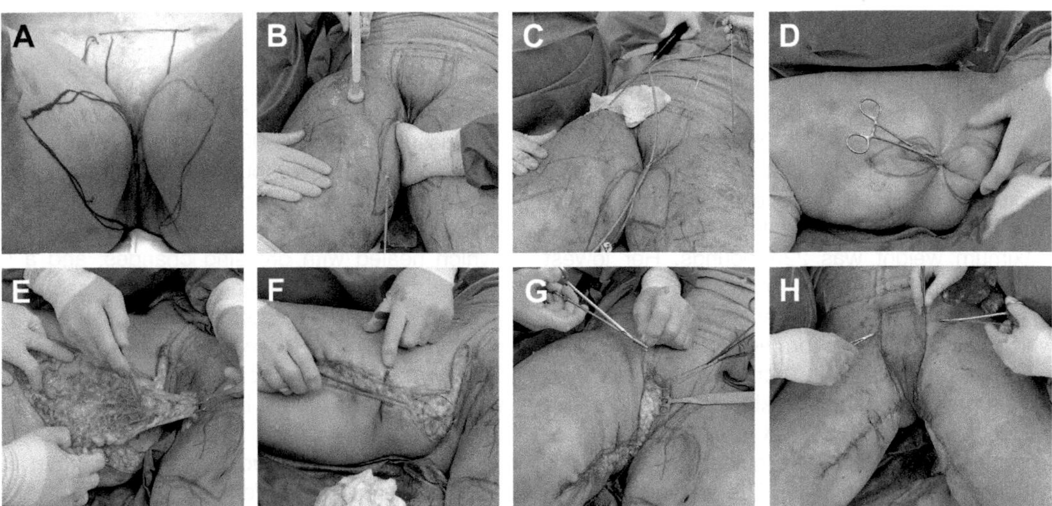

Fig. 3. Case 1: (*A*) After reinking the vertical incision markings, the two legs are pushed together to imprint the first markings on to the other thigh, afterward verified standing. (*B*) Superwet saline infusion to the operated area. Followed by BodyTite, VASERlipo (*C*) and power-assisted lipoplasty. (*D*) Following radical excision site liposuction, the markings are verified for appropriate tension. (*E*) Excision of the marked skin through scalpel assisted avulsion. For preserved neurovasculature, (*F*) #1 polydioxanone (PDO) barbed suture closes the SFS. (*G*) The mid-portion of the horizontal limb is suture suspended in the fascia of the adductor magnus tendon and pubis with 2/0 Vicryl suture. (*H*) Dermal closure is achieved 3 to 0 Quill Monoderm.

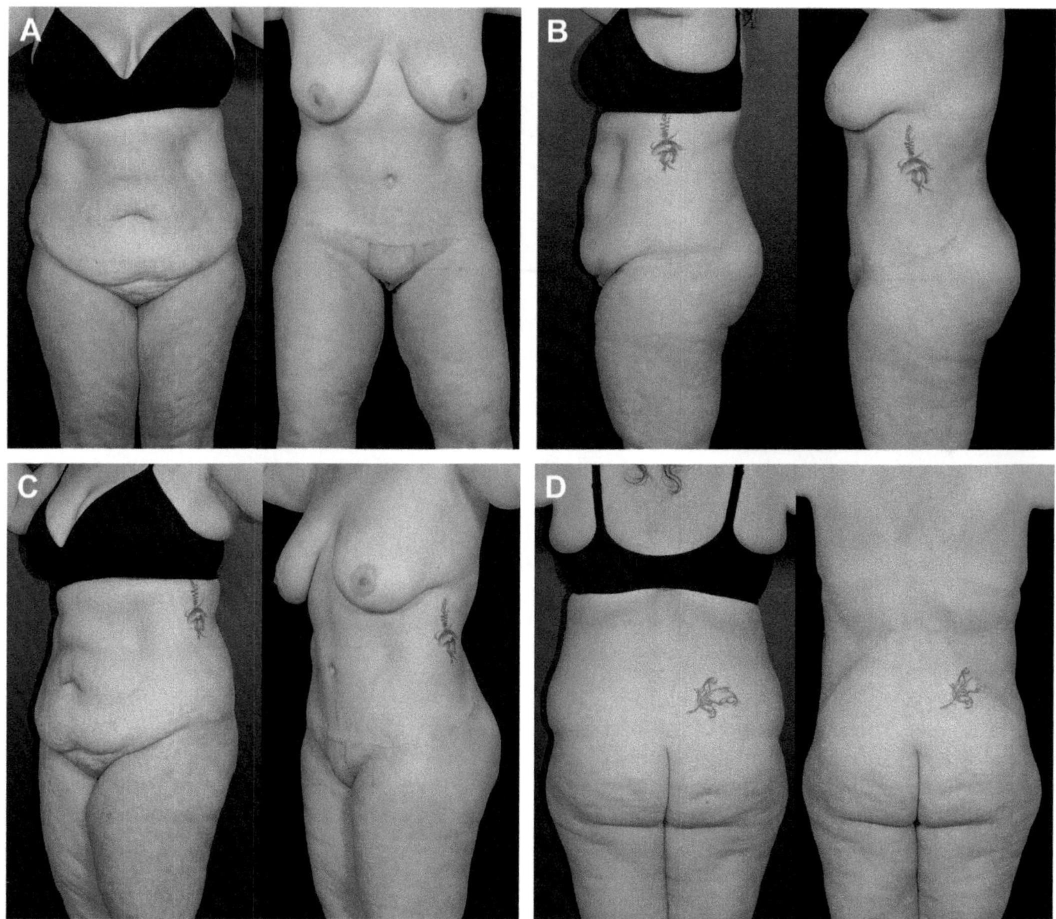

Fig. 4. Case 1: The result 5 months after OFLA and 2 months thighplasty (*right*) can be compared with her preoperative images (*left*). (*A*) Frontal (*B*) Left Lateral (*C*) Left Anterior Oblique (*D*) Posterior.

single-stage total body lift, followed by L-shaped vertical medial thighplasty

A 36-year-old, BMI 28, healthy woman requests a single-stage TBL to improve appearance of her arms, breasts, torso, and legs after MWL. Her maximum weight was 225 pounds. Her lowest weight through lifestyle change was 125 pounds, which slowly increased to her current 158 pounds, which has been stable for over 6 months.

Clinical photos showing her post-weight loss lipodystrophy with sagging skin, and preoperative markings for OFLA, L-brachioplasty, J-torsoplasty, and spiral flap reshaping with Wise-pattern mastopexy (**Fig. 5**). The method of upper body markings is found in Chapter 11.

On May 2022, her TBL starts prone with oblique flankplasty yielding 1020 g. After a two-layer closure, she was turned supine with separate operative teams for the arms, abdomen, and chest/breasts. The volume of fat aspirated from lateral hips was 800 cc on the left and 200 cc from the epigastrium. The excised lower abdominal tissue weighed 2100 g. After her 5 hours surgery and a two-hour recovery, she was discharged home. Her postoperative course was uneventful except for a 3-cm left axillary wound, which healed with dressing changes, and a left elbow seroma eliminated by a single aspiration. Her TBL surgery replaced trunk, breast, and arm lipodystrophy with loose skin for a feminized tight 360° wrap with fading scars. Her arms are reduced with natural curvatures. Her breasts are raised and better shaped.

With the lateral buttocks and thighs firmer and well-shaped, an L-Vertical Thighplasty with VASERlipo of the thighs and legs was performed 6 months later (**Fig. 6**). At the beginning of the procedure, the fat was disrupted using five-ring cannulas at 70% setting. The fat aspirate was 500 cc's, not including the excision site. Three areas of delayed healing on the left thigh responded to removal of dermal sutures. Six

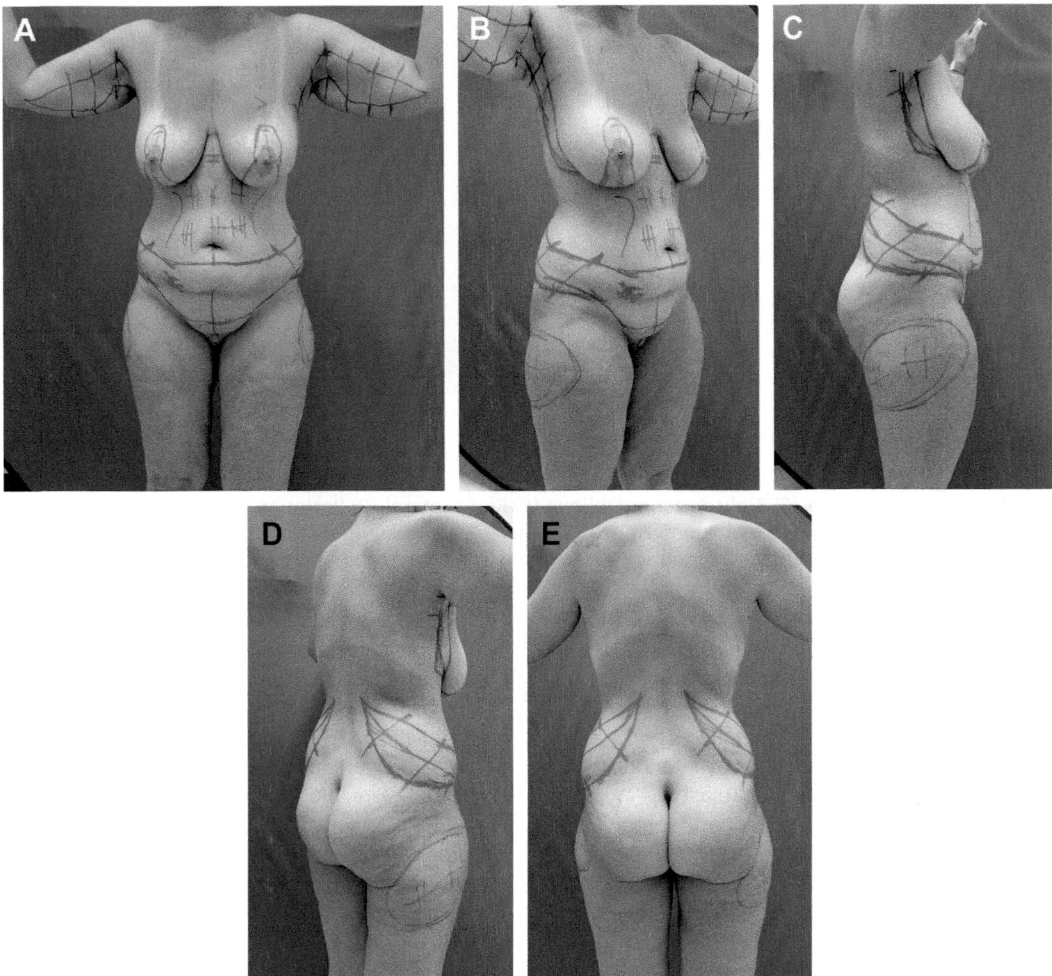

Fig. 5. Case 2: A 36-year-old patient has body and arm weight loss deformity with presurgical markings for single-stage TBL with L-brachioplasty. (*A*) Anterior (*B*) Right Anterior Oblique (*C*) Right Lateral (*D*) Right Posterior Oblique (*E*) Posterior.

months later, the patient was pleased with the feminine contours and skin tightening from her TBL and subsequent vertical thighplasty and VASERlipo (**Fig. 7**).

Case 3 is an example of combining flankplasty with a T-shaped vertical thighplasty at the same stage following failed lower body lift and liposuction debulking of the thighs.

This 58-year-old 5′8″ 180# woman has maintained her 100-pound weight loss after gastric bypass surgery 15 years ago. She requests surgical improvement 12 years after her lower body lift and ultrasonic assisted lipoplasty (UAL) debulking of her thighs performed by the senior author. She suffers from post lower body lift deformity of bulging flanks, sagging, flat hips, lateral gluteal depressions, sagging buttock saddle bags, and elongation of her posterior gluteal crease. Her thighs are oversized, loose, and irregularly contoured with infragluteal-transverse rolls of skin (**Fig. 8**). Bilateral oblique flankplasty (**Fig. 9**) revised her posterior lower body lift with lifting and shaping of the lateral gluteal region and thigh. T-shaped vertical thighplasty reduced, tightened, and smoothed her thighs, leaving a natural medial gap, as seen 1 year later (see **Fig. 8**). The posterior transverse extension of the customary L-thighplasty by running the entire length of the infragluteal fold has smoothed the posterior superior thigh, leaving better defined infragluteal folds. Her buttocks are better shaped and firm with a shorter intergluteal crease.

This case demonstrates revision of a failed lower body lift (LBL) with oblique flankplasty, and successful intraoperative combination with T-shaped vertical thighplasty. The L-thighplasty needs to be converted to the T shape when the posterior thigh, infragluteal areas have rolls of skin. Although

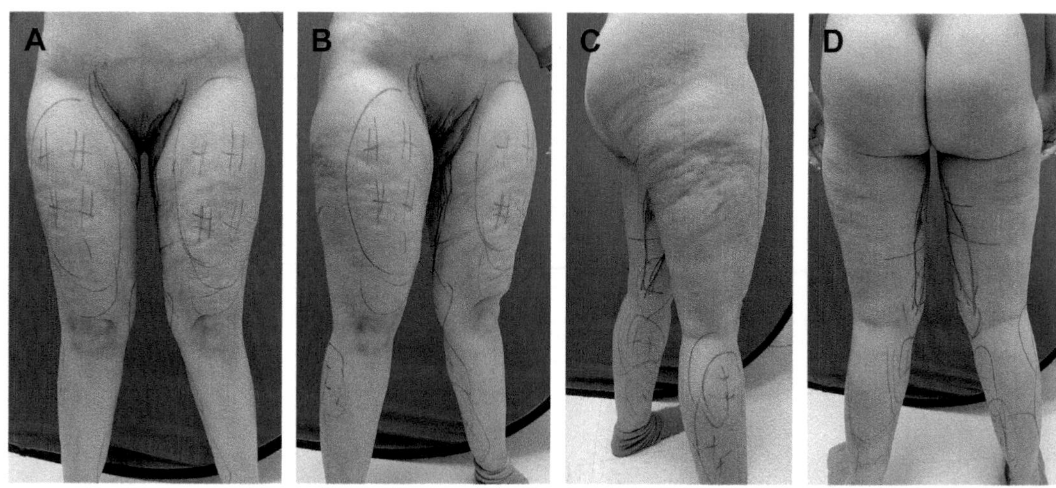

Fig. 6. Case 2: (*A*) Anterior (*B*) Right Anterior Oblique (*C*) Right Lateral (*D*) Posterior. Immediately before stage 2, she shows moderate adiposity of the anterior thighs, medial knees, and lower legs with mild to moderate skin laxity of the anteromedial thighs marked for VASERlipo and L vertical thighplasty.

breakdown at the T junction is common, this did not occur in this case. While pleased, she is considering further liposuction and radiofrequency skin tightening of her distal thighs and legs.

Case 4 is an example of correcting severe lateral buttock and thigh lipodystrophy by inferior incision wedge excision of oblique flankplasty.

A 57-year-old, 5′ 8″, 150-pound woman complains of progressive bulging of her buttocks and lateral thighs. Twenty years earlier she was pleased with her lipoabdominoplasty and liposuction of the flanks, performed by the senior author. As she gained 15 pounds over several years, she noticed disproportionate severe fatty enlargement of her buttocks and upper thighs (**Fig. 10**). The lateral buttock and thighs were slightly sagging with anticipation that there would be looser skin after debulking liposuction, so bilateral oblique flankplasty was planned. After liposuction of 1200 cc's from each buttock and medial thigh, more skin excess than anticipated prompted intraoperative posterior wedge resections of superior buttock skin along the inferior incision line. VASERlipo was also performed through her abdomen and upper medial thighs. For balance, each inferior buttock was lipografted 150 cc's. Two years later, her waist is narrower, the hips defined, and the buttocks and upper thighs are well shaped and proportional (see **Fig. 10**).

This inferior incision line wedge resection has been successfully performed in several other cases of lateral buttock and thigh lipodystrophy,

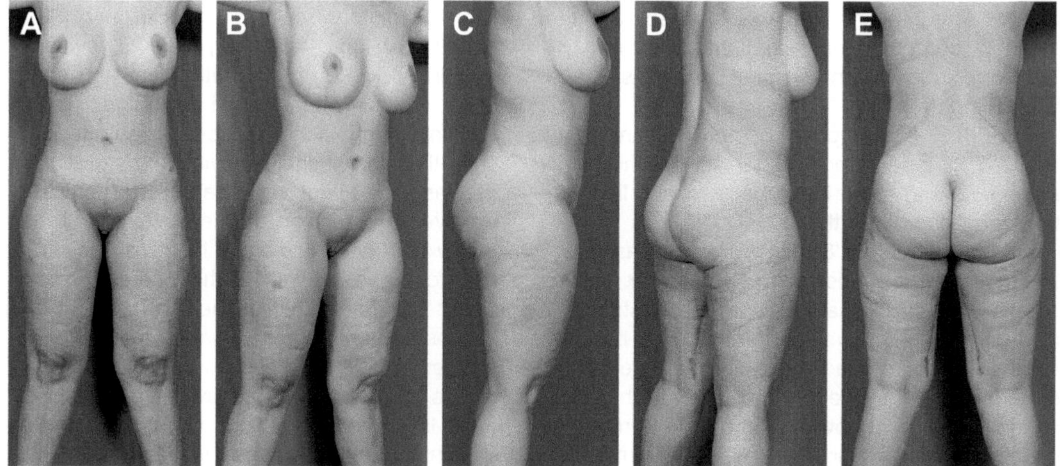

Fig. 7. Case 2: One year following her TBL and 6 months following her thighplasty with lower extremity VASER-Lipo, she shows maintenance of her dramatic contour changes, except for some minor breast ptosis. (*A*) Anterior (*B*) Right anterior oblique (*C*) Right Lateral (*D*) Right Posterior Oblique (*E*) Posterior.

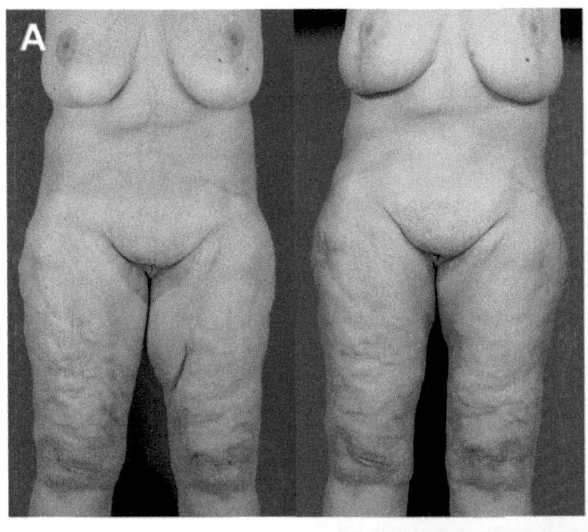

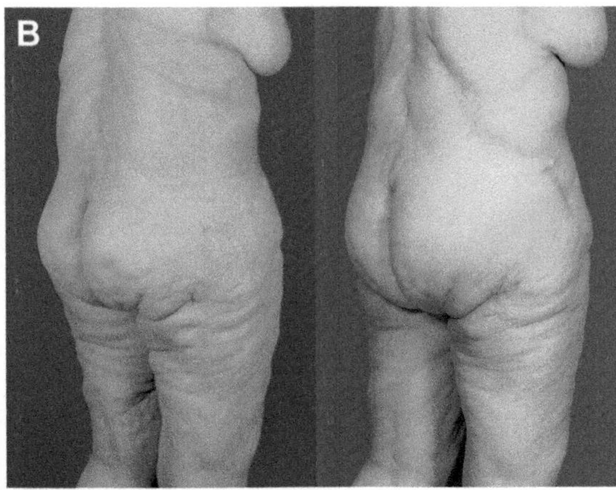

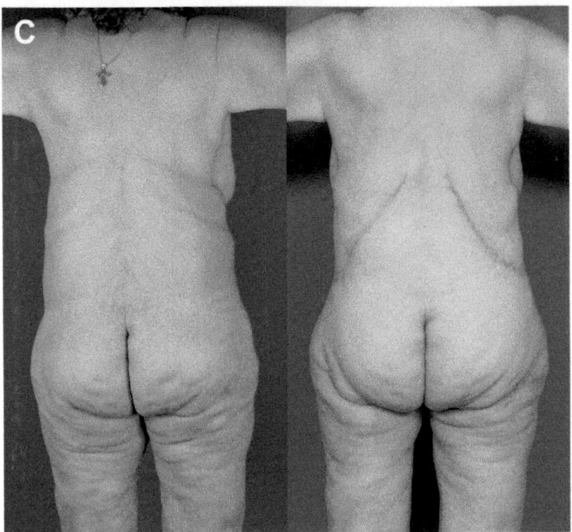

Fig. 8. Case 3: (*A*) Anterior (*B*) Right Lateral (*C*) Right Posterior Oblique C. Posterior. Pre-op (left) and post-op (right) demonstrate how the single-stage surgery transitioned the oversized, loose, and irregularly contoured thighs with infragluteal-transverse rolls of skin to tighter and smoother thighs, leaving a natural medial gap, as well as improving the lower body lift deformity to achieve deeper flanks and shaping of the lateral gluteal region and thigh.

leading to recommendation of modified oblique flankplasty for severe lateral buttock and thigh lipodystrophy. Unlike the prevalent midlateral skin wedge resection for severe lateral thigh lipodystrophy,[7] this modified operation has no visible lateral scar or flattening of the desirable mid-lateral rounded contour. Whatever dog ear there is flows into the natural buttock prominence.

DISCUSSION

After a decade and over 100 cases, we confirm that OFLA not only shapes a smoothly deep waist but also preserves hip prominence while raising the buttocks and lateral thighs.

Despite the back scars above underwear, OFLA is our posterior lower body lift procedure of choice. The scars fade and are not seen in the mirror frontal view. LBL ignores and may even accentuate flank deformity. LBL wound healing complication rate approaches 40%,[8] probably due to pressure on the closures over boney prominence. Whereas flankplasty has a minor delayed wound healing less than 10%, LBL primarily reduces vertical skin excess and thereby raises but also flattens the buttocks and hips. Commonly, the lateral gluteal area is depressed, elongates the gluteal crease, and indents along the circumferential scar.[9]

Owing to poor lateral tissue anchoring, by 6 months LBL often sags along the hip, buttocks, and upper thighs. On the other hand, the long-term stability of the OFLA lateral buttock and hip rotation advancement is attributable to dense

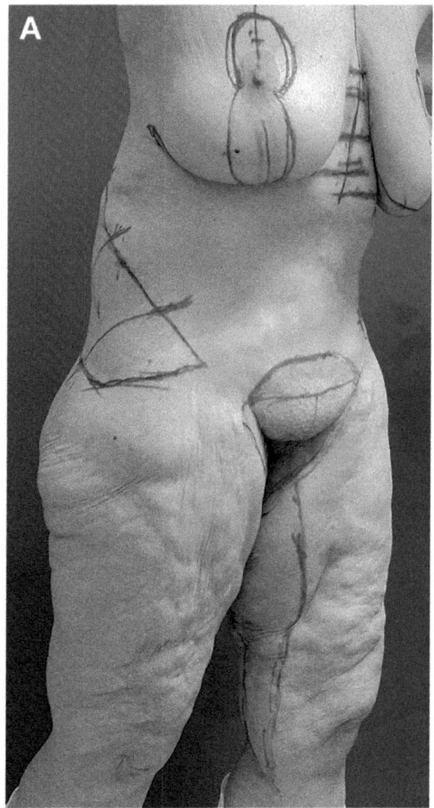

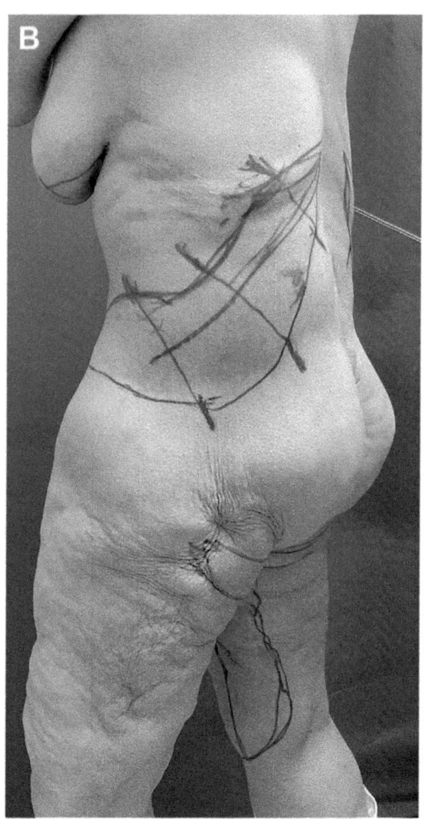

Fig. 9. Case 3: Marking of oblique flankplasty and T-shaped vertical thighplasty, running the posterior limb to entire length of the infragluteal fold. (*A*) Right Anterior Oblique. (*B*) Left Posterior Oblique.

adherence to lumbodorsal fascia.[10] Primary healing along the entire flankplasty is consistent due to minimal undermining, excellent blood supply, and closure within body recess devoid of prominences and shear forces.[2] Through a stable OFLA, medial thighplasty whether performed at the same time or more commonly later yields a tapered, smaller, cylindrical, and firm thigh with the least conspicuous medial vertical scar.

Medial thighplasty has the highest complication rate of body contouring surgery, up to 70%,[11,12] including wound dehiscence, seroma, wound infection, scar migration, hypertrophic scarring, lymphocele, skin necrosis, and suture granulomas. To reduce complications, we embrace ESL for expeditious scalpel-assisted skin avulsion, which preserves underlying neurovasculature. We are pleased that Schmidt and colleagues[13] subsequently confirmed our observations.

Another strategy to reduce complication is avoiding T-shape excision whenever possible because of the potential for delayed healing at the three-point closure. The L-shape excision with the right angle as far posterior as technically possible is preferred. The infragluteal extension, which is the source of the T shape, is added only in cases of significant posterior thigh and lower buttock skin laxity (Case 3).

For severe lateral buttock thigh adiposity, we introduced the posterior wedge resection that results in a more concealed scar and avoids flattening of the desirable mid-lateral rounded contour (case 4).

To tighten proximal thigh skin and better define the labia majora while fixing the horizontal scar to the labial crease, we favor anchoring sutures from the upper medial thigh horizontal excision to fascia overlying the pubis and adductor magnus tendon. We find this anchor with 2/0 Maxon (Ethicon, Inc, Somerville, NJ) sutures reliable, reproducible, while avoiding the potential complications of permanent sutures. We have found anchoring to Colles fascia unreliable[14] and have not found the need to create dermal flaps.[15]

Some[15] suggest that concomitant liposuction of the anterior and posterior thigh injures the neurovascular, leading to higher rates of complications. We have found that esthetic liposuction, optimally using VASER, and radiofrequency skin tightening are safe and the flaps are not undermined.

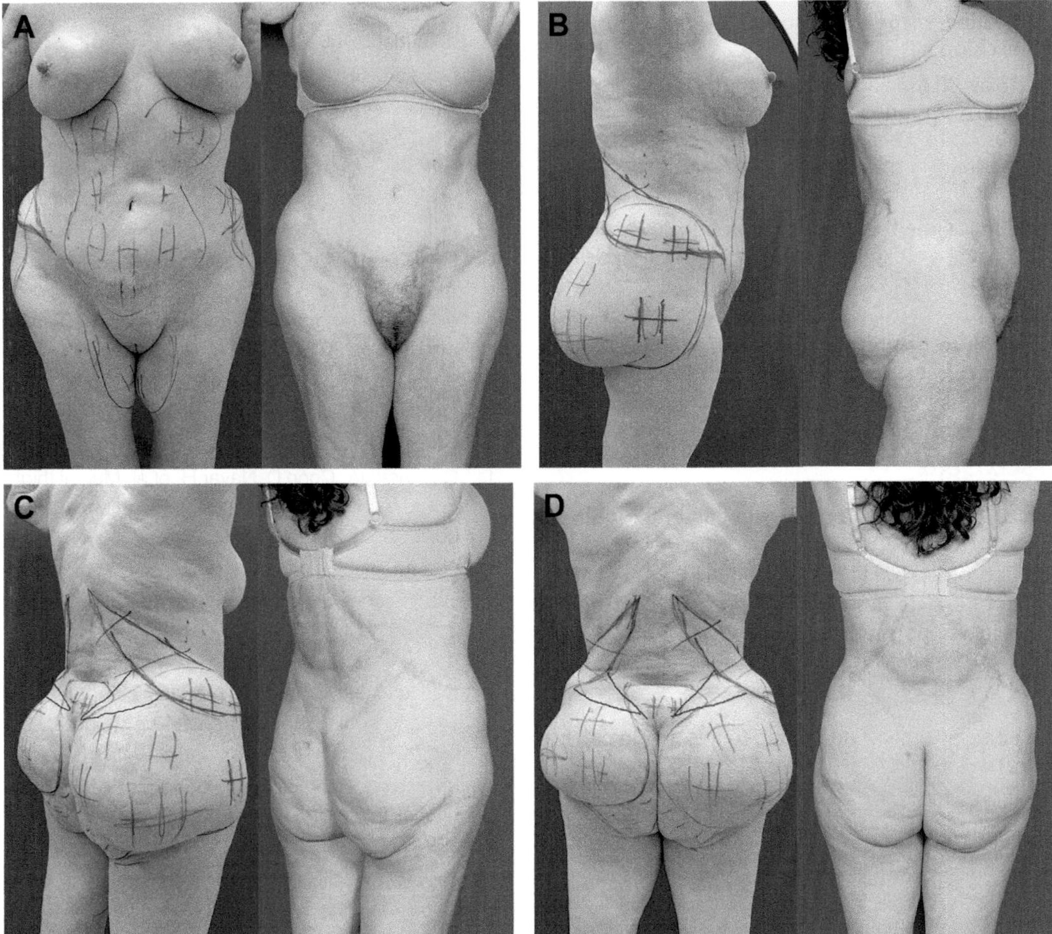

Fig. 10. Case 4: (*Left*) Severe lipodystrophy of buttocks and upper thighs treated by modified by wedge resection oblique flankplasty, Liposuction of marked areas and lipografting of inferior buttock were planned. (*Right*) Two years following the surgery her waist is narrower, the hips defined, and the buttocks and upper thighs are well shaped and proportional. (*A*) Anterior (*B*) Right Lateral (*C*) Right Posterior Oblique (*D*) Posterior.

Liposuction facilitates tissue advancement through indirect undermining.

The challenging closure of wound edges swollen with residual injected saline with xylocaine and epinephrine is met by running #1 Quill PDO with relief of damaging tension as one proceeds.[16]

Owing to the lack of undermining and reliability of garment compression, we avoid thigh drains. Moreover, negative pressure may open partially injured lymphatic channels. Since ESL, there have been no seromas or prolonged leg edema. A few lymphoceles have resolved with aspiration.

To reduce swelling and risk for deep vein thrombosis (DVT), our patients wear compression garments,[17] and are provided lymphatic massage.[18] Deep venous thrombosis chemoprophylaxis is prescribed only to high-risk patients..[19]

CLINICS CARE POINTS

- Circumferential lower body lift including abdominoplasty, either immediately or as a first stage, proceeds upper body lift, brachioplasty, and medial thighplasty.
- Oblique flankplasty not only shapes smooth deep flanks, but has a substantial and long-lasting effect on raising the buttocks and lateral thighs, leaving defined hip prominences
- Preliminary ESL allows expeditious scalpel assisted skin avulsion, which preserves underlying neurovasculature and reduces the risk of complications.
- Medial thighplasty with L-shape excision is preferred to reduce the risk of delayed

healing at the three-point closure of T-shape excision.

- To avoid drifting of the horizontal scar and/or lateralization of the genitalia, we favor absorbable anchoring sutures from the upper medial thigh horizontal excision to fascia near the pubis and adductor tendon fascia.
- Concomitant esthetic liposuction and radiofrequency skin tightening of non-excised areas is safe.
- In most patients, optimal circumferential thigh reshaping with tight skin combines oblique flankplasty with lipoabdominoplasty with L thighplasty.

DISCLOSURE

Dr D.J. Hurwitz was a paid investigator for InMode from 2010 to 2013 and has purchased stock through options. He has accepted $5000 in fees for lectures. He has received no editing or direct financial support for this article.

SUPPLEMENTARY DATA

Supplementary data related to this article can be found online at https://doi.org/10.1016/j.cps.2023.06.013

REFERENCES

1. Hurwitz DJ. Single-staged Total body lift after massive weight loss. Ann Plast Surg 2004;52(5):435–41.
2. Hurwitz DJ, Beidas O, Wright L. Reshaping the oversized waist through Oblique flankplasty with lipoabdominoplasty. Plast Reconstr Surg 2019;143(5):960e–72e.
3. Hurwitz DJ. Aesthetic refinements in body contouring in the massive weight loss patient. Plast Reconstr Surg 2014;134(6):1185–95.
4. Hurwitz D. Medial thigh lift. In: Hoschander A, Salgado C, Kassira W, et al, editors. Operative procedures in plastic, aesthetic and reconstructive surgery. CRC Press, Taylor and Francis Group; 2015.
5. Hurwitz DJ. Invited discussion on: simplified technique for creating an umbilicus with scarless caudal aspect and superior hooding. Aesthetic Plast Surg 2022;46(3):1290–2.
6. HURWITZ D. Medial thighplasty. Aesthetic Surg J 2005;25(2):180–91.
7. Davison SP, Clemens MW, Chang S. Modified circumferential Torsoplasty for the massive-weight-loss patient. Ann Plast Surg 2007;59(4):453–8.
8. Carloni R, De Runz A, Chaput B, et al. Circumferential contouring of the lower trunk: indications, operative techniques, and outcomes—a systematic review. Aesthetic Plast Surg 2016;40(5):652–68.
9. Afrooz PN, Shakir S, James IB, et al. Dynamics of gluteal cleft morphology in lower body lift. Plast Reconstr Surg 2015;136(6):1167–73.
10. Taylor DA. Zones of adhesion of the abdomen: implications for abdominoplasty. Aesthetic Surg J 2017;37(2):190–9.
11. Gusenoff JA, Coon D, Nayar H, et al. Medial thigh lift in the massive weight loss population. Plast Reconstr Surg 2015;135(1):98–106.
12. Fischer JP, Wes AM, Serletti JM, et al. Complications in body contouring procedures. Plast Reconstr Surg 2013;132(6):1411–20.
13. Schmidt M, Pollhammer MS, Januszyk M, et al. Concomitant liposuction reduces complications of vertical medial thigh lift in massive weight loss patients. Plast Reconstr Surg 2016;137(6):1748–57.
14. Lockwood TE. Fascial anchoring technique in medial thigh lifts. Plast Reconstr Surg 1988;82(2):299–304.
15. Özkaya Ö, Yasak T. Vertical medial thigh lift with the 'anchor L liposculpture' technique in massive weight loss patients: preliminary results. Aesthetic Plast Surg 2022;46(1):276–86.
16. Matarasso A, Hurwitz DJ, Reuben B. Quill barbed sutures in body contouring surgery: a 6-year comparison with running absorbable braided sutures. Aesthetic Surg J 2013;33(3_Supplement):44S–56S.
17. Agu O, Hamilton G, Baker D. Graduated compression stockings in the prevention of venous thromboembolism. Br J Surg 2002;86(8):992–1004.
18. Marxen T, Shauly O, Goel P, et al. The utility of lymphatic massage in cosmetic procedures. Aesthet Surg J Open Forum 2023;5. https://doi.org/10.1093/asjof/ojad023.
19. Griffin M, Akhavani MA, Muirhead N, et al. Risk of thromboembolism following body-contouring surgery after massive weight loss. Eplasty 2015;15:e17.

The Role of Noninvasive and Minimally Invasive Techniques in Open Surgical Interventions for the Purpose of Body Contouring

Evgeni Vanyov Sharkov, MD

KEYWORDS

• Radiofrequency • BodyTite • Ultrasound • VASER • Abdominoplasty • Thigh lift • Brachioplasty

KEY POINTS

- How and when to combine minimal invasive and noninvasive procedures with excisional techniques in body contouring surgery.
- What types of minimal invasive procedures to combine with excisional techniques in one stage surgery for altering the results and avoid possible side effects.
- What types of minimal invasive procedures to combine when choosing to stay away from excisional techniques.

INTRODUCTION

Using noninvasive and minimally invasive techniques in open body contouring surgery optimizes aesthetic results. Because of skin tightening, bipolar radiofrequency procedures (BodyTite, FaceTite, and AccuTite) can be alternatives to excisional techniques. Those technologies are also applicable as secondary procedures after excisional surgery and can treat neighboring areas.

Radiofrequency microneedling procedures like Morpheus 8 and Morpheus 8 Body tighten and improve skin quality. They are used in combination with ultrasound lipoplasty (Vaserlipo) and/or excisional procedures, providing optimal long-lasting results.

Ultrasonic-assisted lipoplasty (Vaserlipo) allows contour definition with vessel sparing that could be applied to excisional procedure. Vaserlipo combined with vibration-assisted liposuction defines contours during low tension closure of excisional body contouring surgery.

CLINICAL POINTS

Lower torso

- Bipolar radiofrequency in open surgery limits the size of the excision and scar length.
- Bipolar radiofrequency can be an alternative to excisional procedures. BodyTite and Morpheus 8 Body are alternatives of reverse abdominoplasty (**Fig. 1**). Mini-abdominoplasty with BodyTite and Morpheus 8 Body of the epigastrium is an alternative to mini-abdominoplasty with reverse abdominoplasty.
- Vaserlipo in combination with abdominoplasty provides optimal aesthetics.

Thighs

- BodyTite tightens skin and destroys fat. The procedure is an alternative to medial thigh lift. The aim is 50% to 70% improvement in aesthetics without excisional surgery.
- Vaserlipo provides optimal definition and minimizes contour irregularities. With good inner thigh skin elasticity, it is used as an isolated technique.

VDerm Clinic Private Practice, Str Oborishte 10, 1000 Sofia, Bulgaria
E-mail address: evgenisharcov@gmail.com

Clin Plastic Surg 51 (2024) 147–159
https://doi.org/10.1016/j.cps.2023.06.005

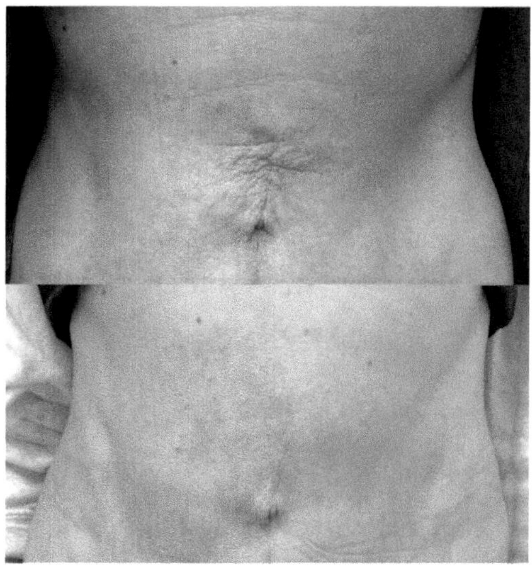

Fig. 1. BodyTite in combination with Morpheus 8 Body–before and 6 months after. BodyTite 1-sensor cannula, 20J were done on the skin above the umbilicus with parameters as follows – 40 energy; 40 °C external cut-off for tightening the skin. Morpheus 8 Body–burst mode – 7-5-3 mm/30 energy/3 stacks per place/25% to 30% of overlapping.

- Vibration-assisted lipoaspiration in combination with excisional technique and radiofrequency microneedling (Morpheus 8 Body) provides optimal contouring and skin tone with poor elasticity of the outer thigh and knee.

Upper limb

- BodyTite tightens the skin and destroys fat as an alternative to brachioplasty. The aim is to achieve 50% to 70% aesthetic improvement without excisional surgery.
- FaceTite and AccuTite in axilla and elbows with brachioplasty improve aesthetics.
- Morpheus 8 and Morpheus 8 Body with brachioplasty further tighten skin.
- Vaserlipo provides optimal definition in patients with preserved skin elasticity.
- Vibration-assisted lipoaspiration with excisional technique and bipolar radiofrequency (Morpheus8 Body, FaceTite, and AccuTite) optimizes contouring and elasticity
- Vaserlipo combines with Morpheus 8 Body in patients with poor skin elasticity, who refuse brachioplasty scar.

MINIMALLY INVASIVE AND NONINVASIVE TECHNIQUES WITH ABDOMINOPLASTY

Intraoperatively

Radiofrequency procedures

Minimally invasive radiofrequency treatment cranial to skin excision is not recommended, because of coagulation of vessels risking wound necrosis. It is safe to apply radiofrequency in adjacent areas like the flanks, with the ultimate goal of achieving 360° lower torso definition. This type of combination, together with vibration-assisted liposuction is 3-dimensional abdominoplasty. BodyTite causes fat destruction and collagen contraction, providing lasting results with significant skin shrinkage.[1]

At the end of the operation, radiofrequency microneedling (Morpheus8 Body) could be applied to improve skin elasticity. Parameters are 7-5-3 mm Burst Mode depth with 30 kJ, 3 stacks per place, which can be repeated on the 45th and 90th postoperative days.

Ultrasound procedures

Ultrasound lipoplasty is possible in the area cranial to the excision and the flanks. As VASERlipo spares subdermal vasculature, it does not significantly compromise healing.[2] Vaserlipo and the subsequent vibration-assisted liposuction may precede or follow skin excision. The excision precedes superficial ultrasound lipoplasty, allowing more precise definition. When VASERlipo is performed with vibration-assisted aspiration on the back, it should precede excision because of increased risk of excess compression of the epigastric flap. This combination is 4-dimensional abdominoplasty, with the desired effect of excision of excess subcutaneous skin with muscular definition.

Vibration-assisted liposuction

Vibration-assisted liposuction is used as part of 3-dimensional abdominoplasty, after BodyTite in the flanks. Vibration-assisted liposuction is performed on the same area plus or minus vibration-assisted liposuction cranial to the abdominal excision.

It is also used as part of 4-dimensional abdominoplasty, in which ultrasound treatment is performed, followed by aspiration and definition of the flanks, after which excess of skin and subcutaneous fat the abdomen is excised, followed by superficial VASERlipo of the flap and flanks.[3]

SECONDARY PROCEDURE

Radiofrequency Procedures

BodyTite, FaceTite, and AccuTite correct residual contour irregularities and skin laxity. Use the specified tip depending on the area of the surgical defect. For large deformity, use the BodyTite cannula, and for small deformity, use the FaceTite and AccuTite cannulas. The goal is 70°C internal probe for destruction of subcutaneous fat with sublethal damage to the connective tissue and 40°C external probe for additional safe tightening of

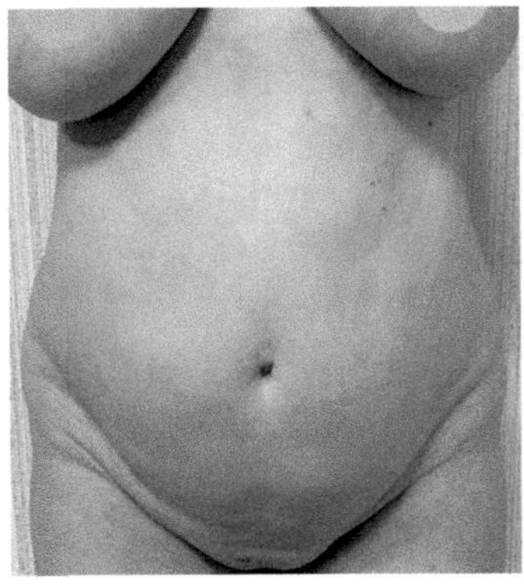
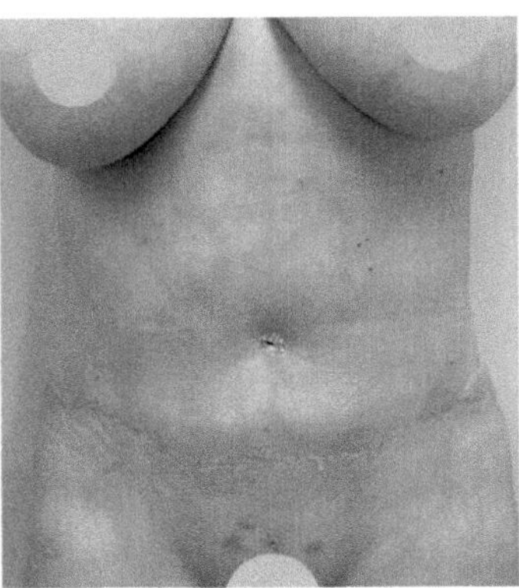
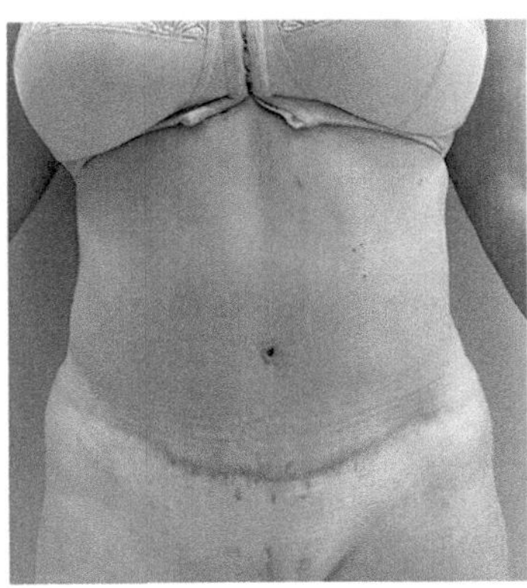

Fig. 2. Before, 3 months, and 1 year after 3-dimensional abdominoplasty–abdominoplasty with muscle plication + BodyTite radiofrequency lipolysis of the flanks and vibration-assisted liposuction of the flanks and abdomen (cranially from the navel, the liposuction is sparing with N4 long curved cannula of Mercedes type).

the skin. Usually deposit 8 to 10 kJ of energy per 10 cm^2.[4–6] After 6 months, the procedure is for contour irregularities from 3-dimensional and 4-dimensional abdominoplasty, overjumping scar to subcutaneous excess, skin excess cranial to umbilicus and in dog-ears.

For Morpheus8 Body, the parameters are 7-5-3 mm Burst Mode depth with 30 kJ, at 3 stacks. The procedure is performed 45, and possibly 90 days postoperatively, mainly in the epigastrium.

EVOLVE X is a noninvasive technique with radiofrequency energy that provides skin tightening, fat melting, and stimulation of the underlying musculature.[7] The procedure requires several sessions. Start after the 45th postoperative day, after open surgery.

Myostimulation–trueSculptfleX relies on electrical muscle stimulation for toning and tightening of the muscles in up to 8 areas. Electrostimulation of individual muscle groups is recommended after the fourth to sixth postoperative month, because of the need for complete resorption of postsurgical edema. After several sessions, muscle definition is improved 10% to 15%.

3-DIMENSIONAL ABDOMINOPLASTY

3-dimensional abdominoplasty further improves aesthetics. BodyTite and vibration liposuction of the abdomen and flanks are added to classic, extended, or high lateral tension abdominoplasty[8–20] (**Figs. 2–5**). Best candidates for 3-dimensional abdominoplasty are patients with subcutaneous excess in the abdomen and flanks with poor skin elasticity. These patient are older.

Position Prone

Infiltrate Klein solution. In the lower back and flanks, use bipolar radiofrequency lipolysis of subcutaneous fat at a depth of 3 to 6 cm, depending on pinch test. The purpose is to achieve 70°C heating (even reaching a destruction of 50% of

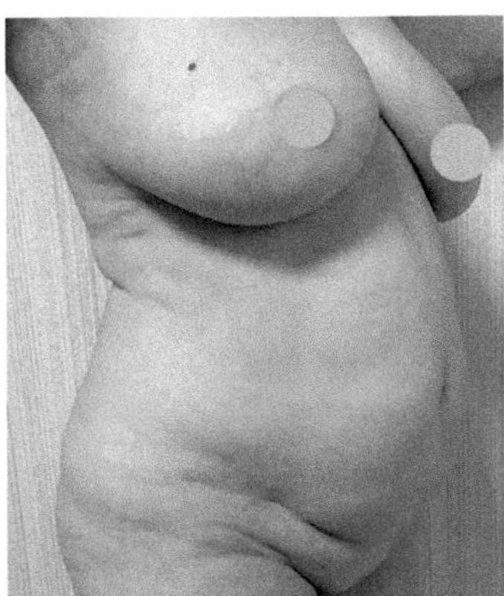
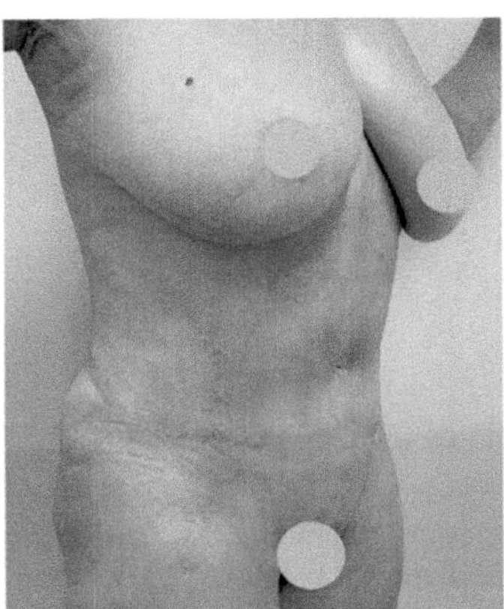
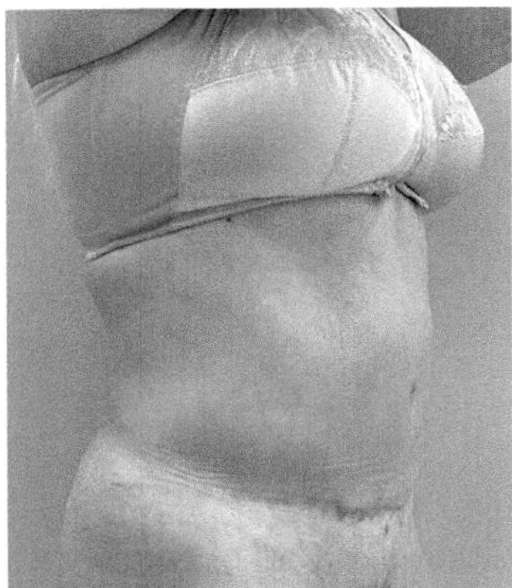

Fig. 3. Before, 3 months, and 1 year after 3-dimensional abdominoplasty–abdominoplasty with muscle plication + BodyTite radiofrequency lipolysis of the flanks and vibration-assisted liposuction of the flanks and abdomen (cranially from the navel, the liposuction is sparing with N4 long curved cannula of Mercedes type).

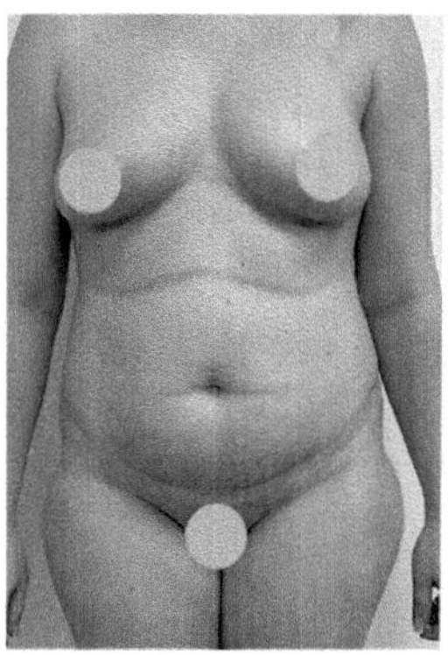
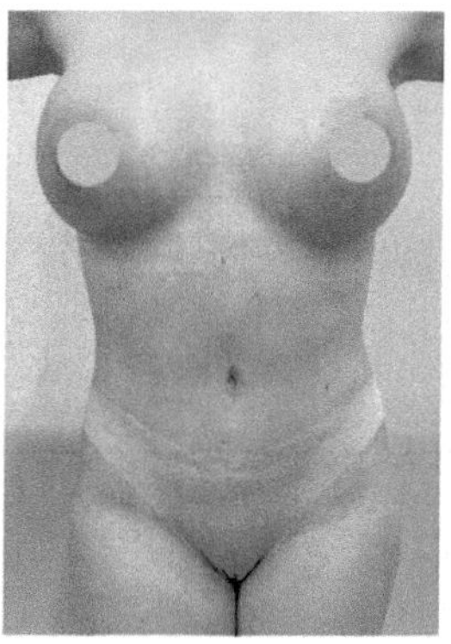
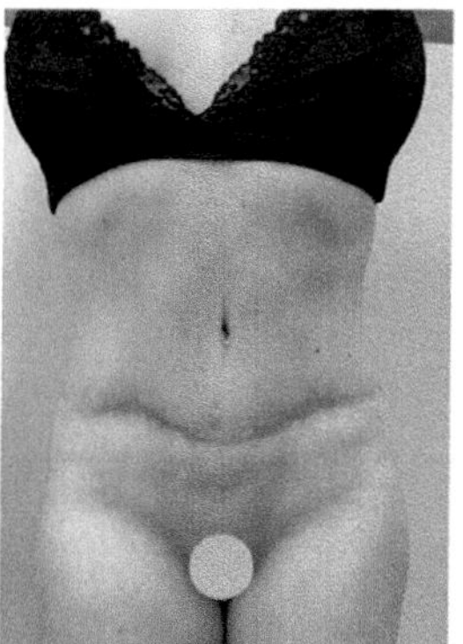
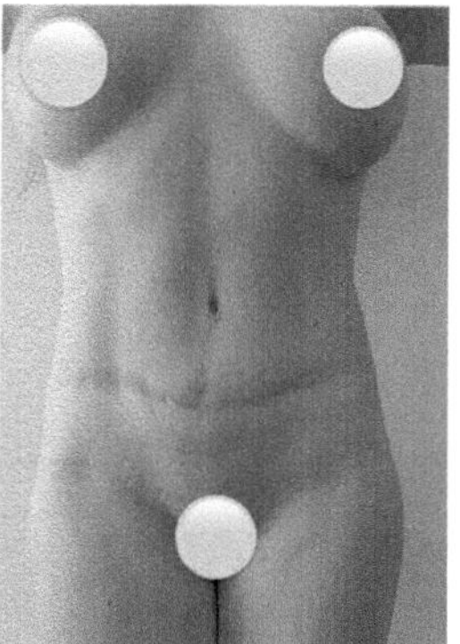

Fig. 4. Before, 3 months and 1 year after 3-dimensional abdominoplasty–abdominoplasty with muscle plication + BodyTite radiofrequency lipolysis of the flanks and vibration-assisted liposuction of the flanks and abdomen (cranially from the navel, the liposuction is sparing with N4 long curved cannula of Mercedes type). 1-stage augmentation mammoplasty was performed with BodyTite radiofrequency lipolysis and vibration-assisted liposuction of the hips with N3 and N4 long curved cannula of Mercedes type.

the fat cells will enable 50% less fat deposits in the area). Apply superficial bipolar radiofrequency at 1 to 2 cm for skin contraction. Optimal energy is 8 to 10 kJ per 10 cm. After the radiofrequency, proceed to vibration-assisted liposuction with 3 and 4 mm Mercedes type of cannulas.

Position Supine

Infiltrate Klein solution. Aspirate with vibration-assisted liposuction with N4 straight and curved cannula in the flanks and epigastrium. Skin incision is according to the preoperative markings. Centrally elevate epigastric flap with preservation of lateral rectus perforating vessels and umbilicus. If necessary, plicate diastasis of rectus abdominis, obliqus abdominis, and lower abdomen transversely. Excise excessive lower abdominal skin and subcutaneous fat. Perform pull-through umbilicoplasty. Apply Baroudi plication sutures. Close surgical incision under appropriate tension with drains.

4-DIMENSIONAL ABDOMINOPLASTY

High-definition Vaserliposculpting in the abdomen with/without the flanks area is added (**Figs. 6–8**).

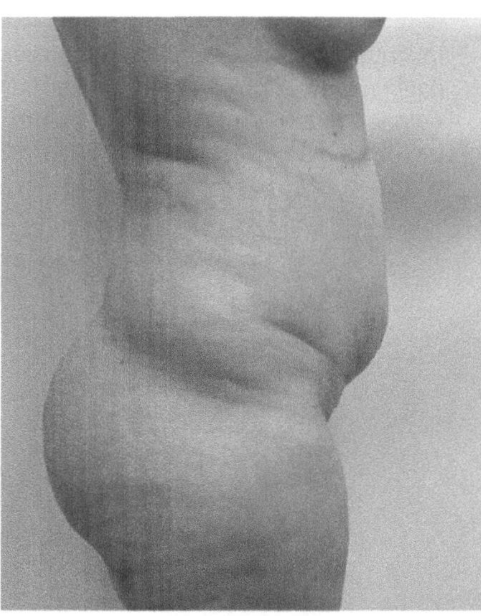
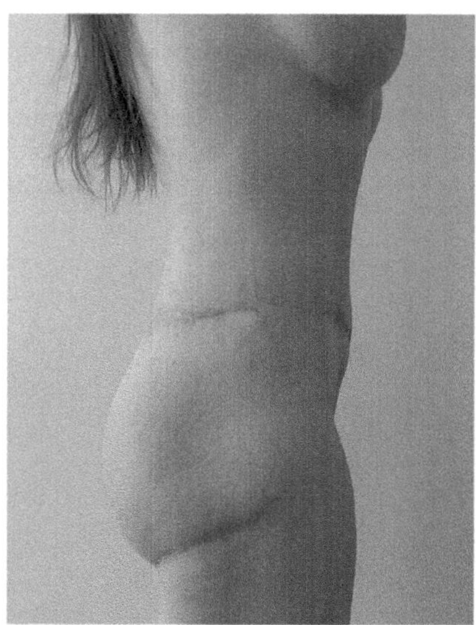

Fig. 5. Before and 1 year after 3-dimensional Abdominoplasty–abdominoplasty with muscle plication + BodyTite radiofrequency lipolysis of the flanks and vibration-assisted liposuction of the flanks and abdomen. One-stage augmentation mammoplasty was performed with BodyTite radiofrequency lipolysis and vibration-assisted liposuction of the hips with N3 and N4 long curved cannula of Mercedes type. Postoperative scars in the lower back and buttock area from gluteoplasty procedure done 6 moths after the combination of procedures from above.

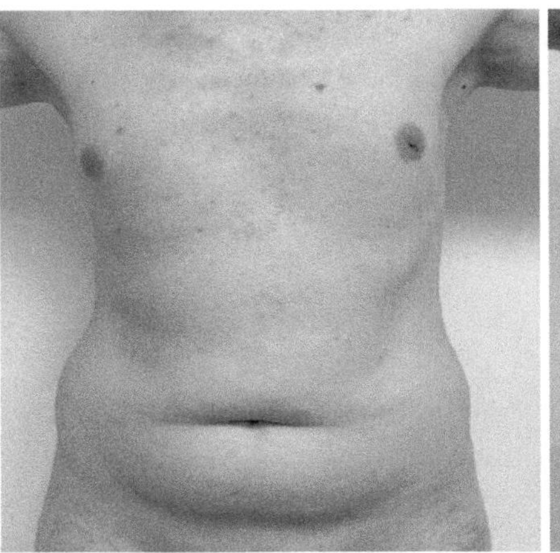
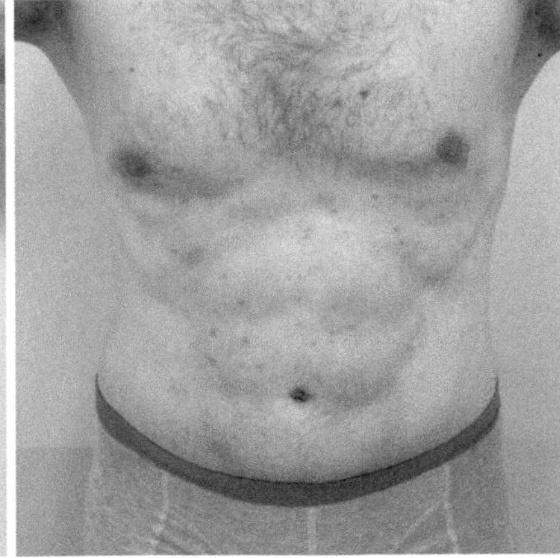

Fig. 6. Before and 6 months after ultrasound liposuction with abdominoplasty – 4-dimensional abdominoplasty.

Best candidates for 4-dimensional abdominoplasty have subcutaneous excess in the abdomen and flanks and preserved skin elasticity and desire definition. These most often include healthy young patients.

Start prone for VASERlipo of back and flanks.

- Vaser with 2 ring cannula at 80% pulse mode for superficial treatment, at 1 minute per 100 mL of infiltrated solution and until overcoming resistance; switched to 80% continuous mode in deep subcutaneous fat[21–25]
- Vibration-assisted liposuction for definition and lipoaspiration, with straight, curved and angled 3 and 4 mm cannulas of Mercedes type

Turn supine.

- Incise along marking, depending on habitus, preference of underwear
- Elevate flap with preservation of umbilicus to the costal margin and 4 to 5 cm wide midline tunnel to the xyphoid
- If necessary, plicate diastasis of rectus abdominis, obliqus abdominis, low transverse fascia
- Excise excess skin and subcutaneous fat
- Suture pull through umbilicoplasty
- Infiltrate of Klein solution; VASERlipo analogous to the flanks, but defining muscle
- Place Baroudi sutures
- Close incision with redistribution of tension and drains

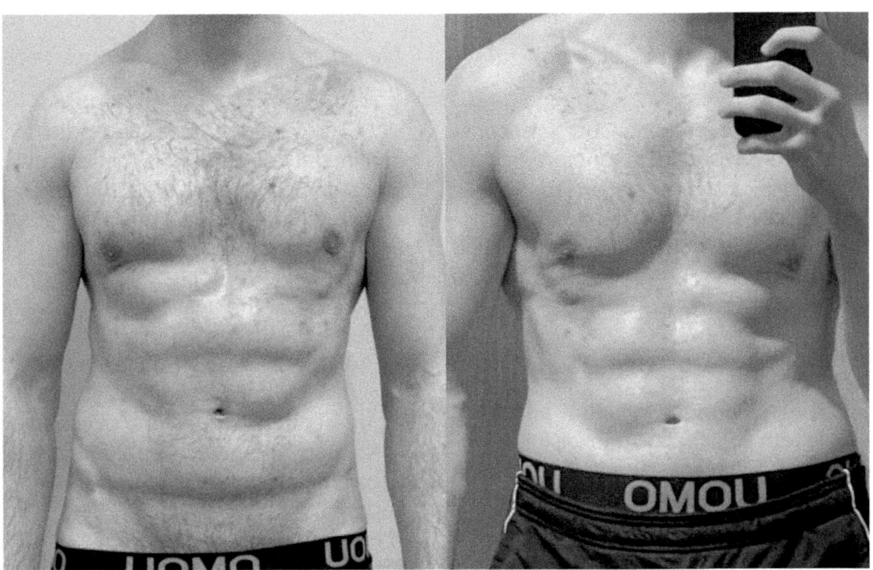

Fig. 7. 1 year after ultrasound liposuction with abdominoplasty–4D Abdominoplasty.

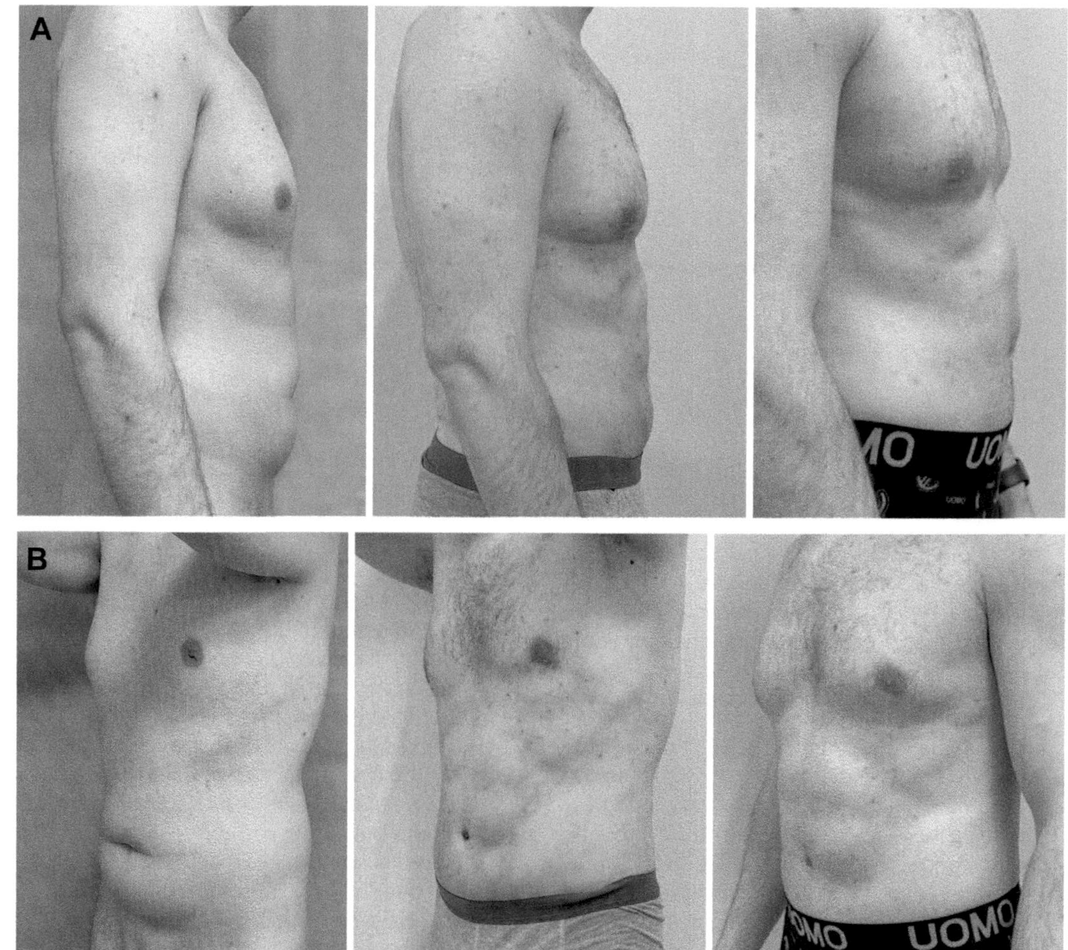

Fig. 8. (*A*, *B*) Before, 6 months after, and 1 year after ultrasound liposuction with abdominoplasty–4-dimensional abdominoplasty.

Thigh Lift Combined with Minimal and Noninvasive Procedures

Assess skin laxity. The presence of cutaneous-subcutaneous excess suggests postpregnancy, massive weight loss, and/or aging, which requires excisional techniques with or without liposuction.[26–28] With an accompanying adiposity and preserved skin elasticity, the procedures can be non- and/or minimally invasive.

With adiposity and compromised skin elasticity, options are:

- VASERlipo with radiofrequency intra- and postoperatively with anticipation of excisional procedure later because of insufficient skin retraction
- VASERlipo with excisional technique; VASERlipo with excisional technique and then Morpheus 8 Body to improve skin quality

Minimally Invasive Techniques with Medial Thighplasty

VASERlipo should be used with 2 ring probe continuous mode at 60% for inner and outer thigh areas, the banana roll area, the knees (and distant areas), followed by vibration-assisted liposuction using Mercedes type cannulas N3 и N4 long, short and curved (**Fig. 9**).

Excision of the available skin excess should be performed with medial thighplasty.

Using Morpheus8 Body, stay at least 1.5 cm away from the incision side; 7-5-3 mm Burst Mode depth with 30 kJ, no overlapping.

No BodyTite should be used in the inner thigh because of risk of compromising the blood supply.

For young patients with loose skin with potential for definition combinations for treating inner thighs are:

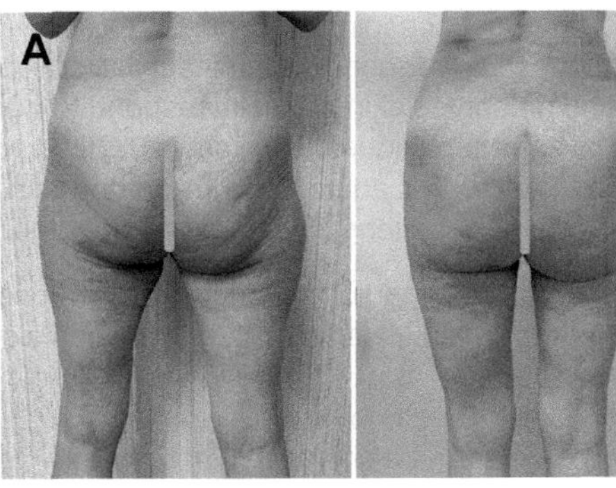

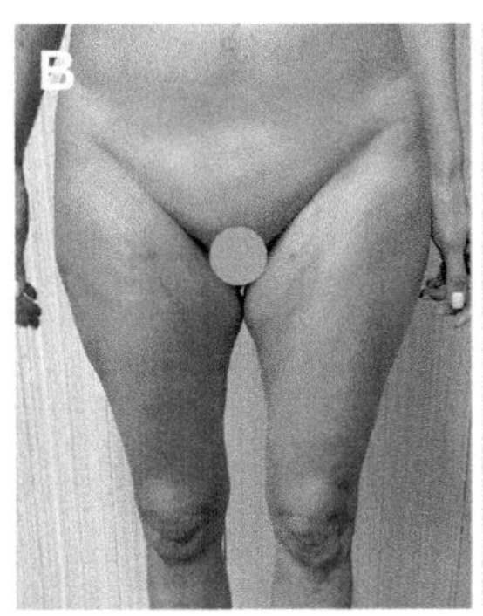

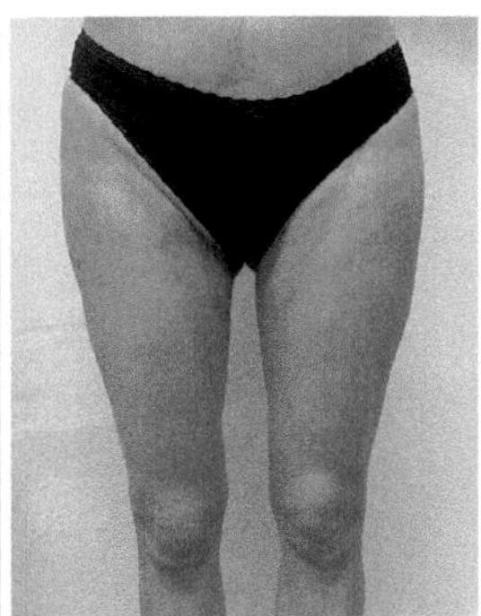

Fig. 9. (*A*, *B*) 1 year after vibration-assisted liposuction and 1-time excision (medial thigh lift) in the area of the inner thighs + vibration-assisted liposuction and BodyTite of the outer thighs.

VASERlipo (for definition) + Vibration-assisted liposuction (for lipoaspiration) + Excision (for removal of skin excess) + Morpheus 8 Body (for additional skin tightening caudal to the level of excision) – provides contouring and definition of the area + removal of the skin excess and tightening of the residual skin.

For thin and poor skin elasticity combinations for treating inner thighs are:

Vibration-assisted liposuction (for lipoaspiration) + Excision (for removal of skin excess) ± Morpheus 8 Body (for additional skin tightening caudal to the level of excision) – provides contouring and definition of the area + removal of the skin excess and tightening of the residual skin. This option is a more tissue-friendly option, and less risky.

Combined minimally invasive techniques include

- VASERlipo with 2 ring probe (continuous mode on 60% for deep) or inner and outer thigh areas, the banana roll area, the knees (and any distant area), followed by vibration-assisted liposuction using Mercedes type cannulas N3 и N4 long, short and curved
- To tighten skin–BodyTite 20W cannula with 1 sensor/20 power/40 external cut-off/8-10 kJ energy per 10 cm^2 of treated area then 7-5-3 mm burst mode depth Morpheus8 Body with 30 kJ, 3 stacks per place
- Additional tightening of the banana roll, with a FaceTite cannula can also be used for more suitable parameters
- Treat inner thigh with VASERlipo and Morpheus8 Body because of the thinness of the skin and adipose

Combination option for inner thighs includes

- *1* VASERlipo (for possible definition) + vibration-assisted liposuction (for lipoaspiration) + Morpheus8 Body – provides contouring and definition of the area and tightening of the skin
- *2* vibration-assisted liposuction (for lipoaspiration) + BodyTite + Morpheus8 Body – provides contouring of the area, tightening of the skin, long-lasting results regarding the reduction in fat deposits (**Fig. 10**)
- 3–BodyTite + Morpheus8 Body–provides optimal tightening of the skin and is a possible surgical excision in moderately loose skin (**Fig. 11**)

Secondary surgery

Radiofrequency procedures include

- BodyTite, FaceTite, AccuTite, used after 9 months to correct contour irregularities and/or additionally tighten the skin
- Morpheus8 Body: 7-5-3 mm burst mode depth with 30 kJ, 3 stacks, 30% to 40% overlap; EVOLVE X: for noninvasive contouring EvolveX requires several sessions with 15% to 20% improvement; the interventions start after the tenth postoperative day; the procedure contributes not only to the faster recovery, but also tightens underlying muscles and skin, with additional fat resorption

Brachioplasty Combined with Minimally Invasive Procedures

Brachioplasty excises cutaneous-subcutaneous excess plus or minus the lateral surface of the chest with/without accompanying liposuction.[29–32] Radiofrequency and VASERlipo are added for additional definition and/or the contouring of neighboring areas.

The magnitude of excess is essential. Cutaneous-subcutaneous excess with predominant skin laxity suggests massive weight loss and/or aging, and requires excisional techniques

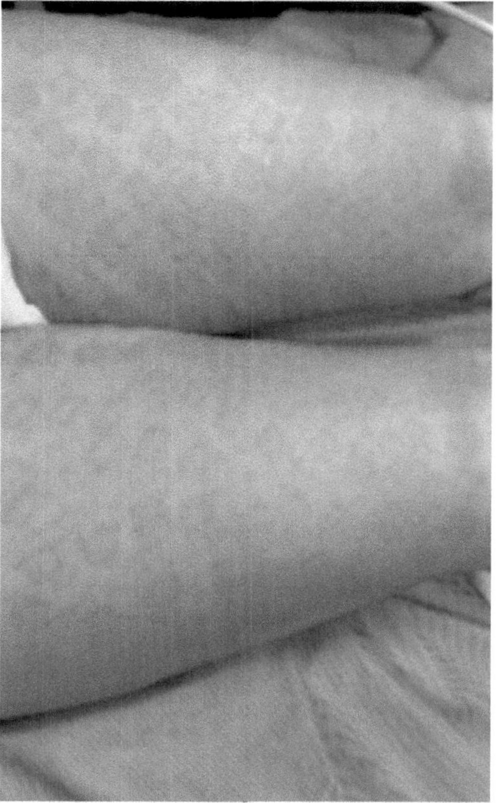

Fig. 10. Intraoperatively –vibration-assisted liposuction with BodyTite of the inner thighs in combination with Morpheus8 Body of the thighs and knees–40W cannula/70 internal cut-off/40 external cut-off/: the purpose is to achieve 8-10 kJ energy per 10 cm^2 of treated area, as–depending on the preoperative pinch test–it is worked at 2 or 3 cm ± 7-5-3 mm burst mode, 3 stacks per place, with 30 kJ, 30% to 40% overlapping.

with or without lipoaspiration procedures and with or without radiofrequency. Dominant fat component and preserved skin elasticity respond to minimally invasive techniques, such as VASERlipo and radiofrequency. For adiposity with compromised skin elasticity, 3 options exist in terms of surgery:

1. VASERlipo with radiofrequency intra and postoperatively with later excision for insufficient skin retraction
2. Lipoaspiration combined with excision
3. Lipoaspiration combined with excision and radiofrequency–Morpheus 8 Body and Morpheus 8 to improve skin quality.

Operation

There are several radiofrequency procedures:

- BodyTite: ± in combination with Vibration-assisted liposuction of the upper arms and in neighboring areas; the parameters are 20W cannula/70 internal cut-off/40 external cut-off/for 8-10 kJ energy per 10 cm^2 and a depth of 2 or 3 cm; the techniques are respectively stamping (melting the fat cells by reaching 70°C internal cut-off) and lining (tightening the skin by reaching 40°C external cut-off (**Fig. 12**)
- To further tighten: 20W cannula with 1 sensor/40 power/40 external cut-off to achieve 8-10 kJ energy per 10 cm^2 of treated area, working at a depth of 1-2 cm (**Fig. 13**); Do not use BodyTite for the upper arms in cases of excisional and/or combined lipoaspiration-excisional techniques, because of risk of compromising blood supply
- FaceTite: use in neighboring area (axilla) for overall aesthetics of the upper limb; use in combination with all options of brachioplasty; FaceTite handpiece set at 70 internal cut-off/40 external cut-off for 6-8 kJ energy. The

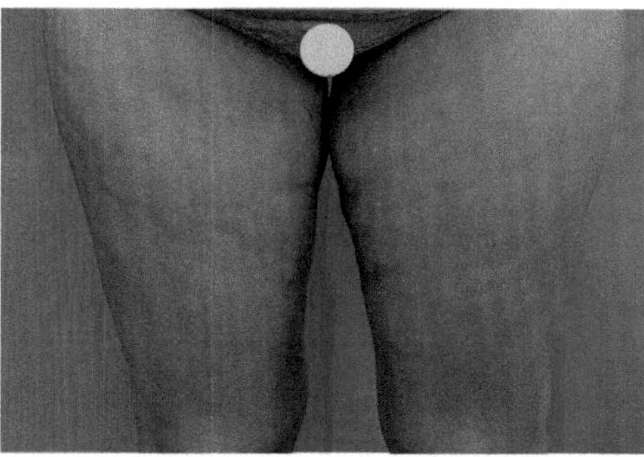

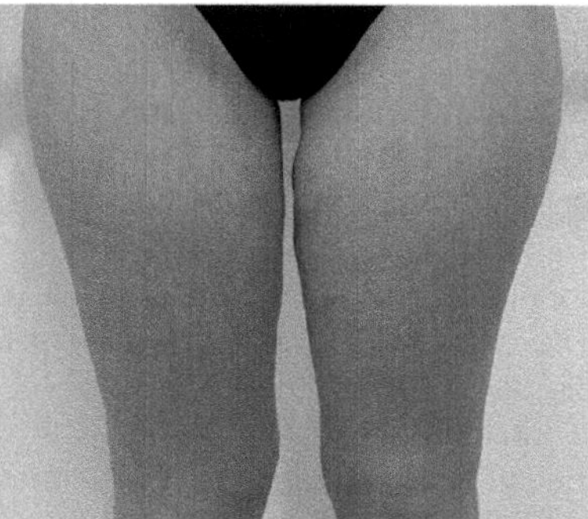

Fig. 11. Before and 6 months after. Patient with previous liposuction performed in another clinic, loose skin and irregularities, who does not wish to have a postoperative scar. 6 months after BodyTite 20W cannula with 1 sensor/40 power/40 external cut -off/8-10 kJ energy per 10 cm^2 of treated area + Morpheus8 Body–7-5-3 mm mode depth with 30 kJ, 30% to 40% overlapping, 3 stacks per place. One can notice the tightening effect on the skin and the still-present unevenness from the previous procedure on the left. The patient is satisfied with the result, given her knowledge that it is impossible to correct the unevenness without excision.

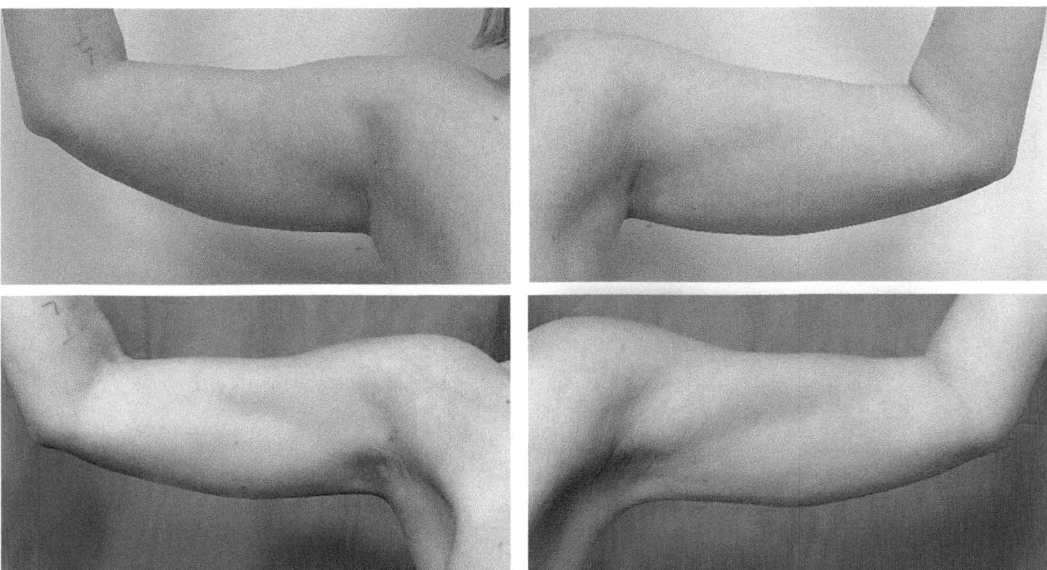

Fig. 12. Before and 6 months after. BodyTite with vibration-assisted liposuction–20W cannula/70 internal cut-off/40 external cut-off/10 kJ energy per side, it was worked at a depth of 2 cm. The work techniques are lining (tightening the skin by reaching 40°C external cut-off) and stamping (melting the fat cells by reaching 70°C internal cut-off). The procedure ended with lipoaspiration of liquefied subcutaneous fat using a 4 mm long curved cannula –120 mL lipoaspirate per side.

procedure ends with lipoaspiration of liquefied adipose (**Fig. 14**)

- AccuTite: use in neighboring area with the aim of overall improvement of the upper limb; use in combination with all options of brachioplasty; the parameters are: AccuTite handpiece/70 internal cut-off/40 external cut-off to achieve 6-8 kJ energy (see **Fig. 14**)
- Morpheus8 Body: at the end of the operation, extensive bipolar radiofrequency microneedling improves skin elasticity of the surrounding skin (see **Fig. 14**); set 7-5-3 mm burst mode depth with 30 kJ, 3 punches per site, (30% to 40% overlapping when without excision of skin and no overlapping when close to the excision side–stay at least 1.5 cm away),

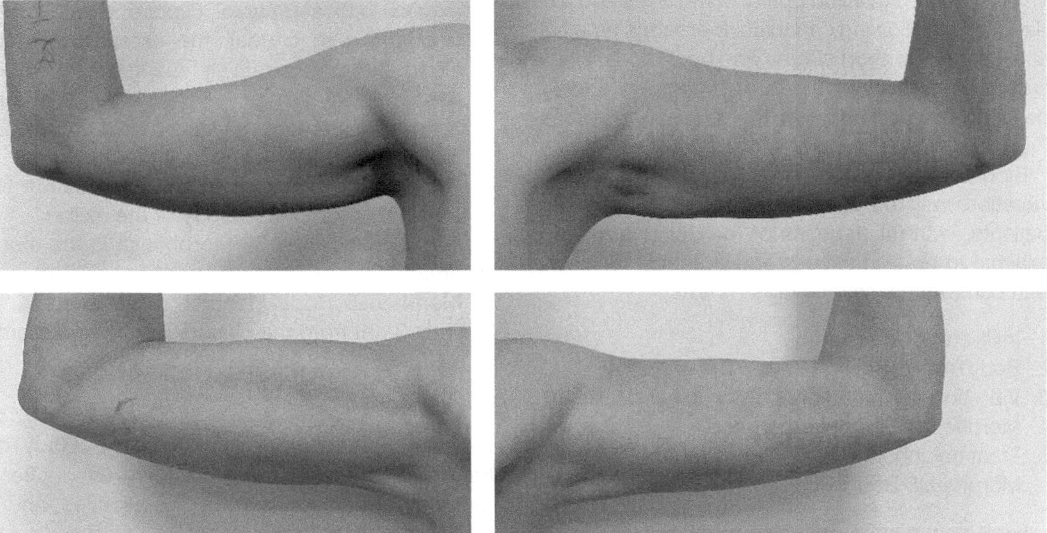

Fig. 13. Before and 6 months after. BodyTite- 20W cannula with one sensor/40 power/40 external cut-iff/10 kJ energy per side, working at a depth of 2 cm. The work technique is lining (tightening the skin by reaching 40°C external cut-off).

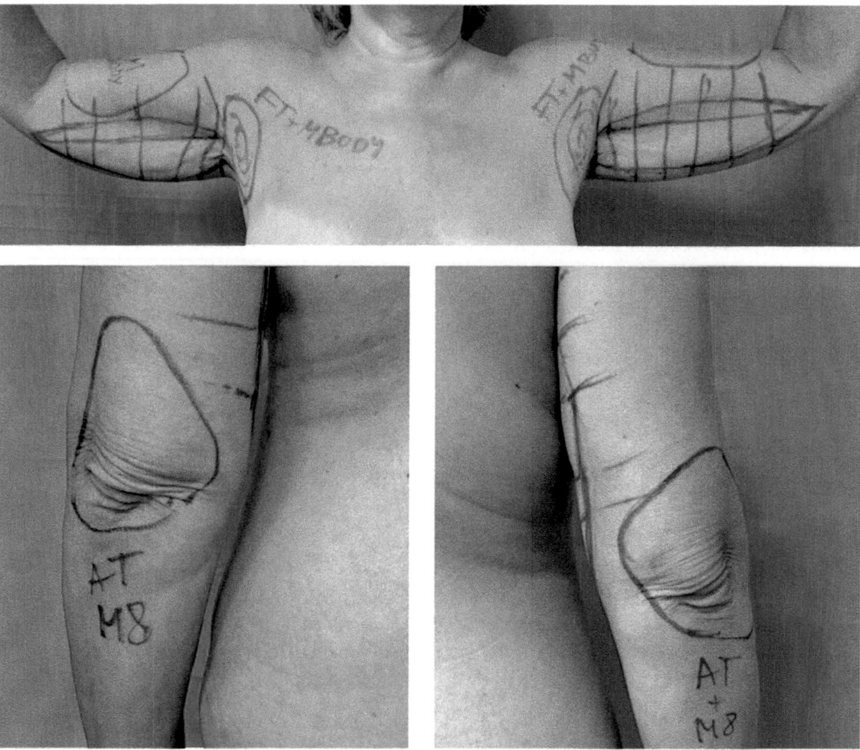

Fig. 14. Preoperative marking in a patient with brachioplasty in combination with vibration-assisted liposuction in the upper arm area; FaceTite with vibration-assisted liposuction and Morpheus8 Body in the armpit area (area marked with FT + MBODY); AccuTite in combination with Morpheus8 (area marked with AT + M8) for tightening and improving skin quality in the elbow area; Morpheus8 Body (area marked with MBODY in the armpit area) circularly in the upper arm area.

and the procedure can be repeated on 45th and 90th postoperative day

VASERLipo removes adiposity of the arms and axilla. Use the following cannulas: Mercedes type N3 and 4, long and short curved and bent types. Liposuction in combination with brachioplasty should be performed primarily in the excision site (see **Fig. 14**)

Bipolar radiofrequency may be combined with vibration-assisted liposuction. For normal weight patients, with fat deposits of the upper arm with minimal to no skin excess and potential for good skin contraction, several options exist:

1. Infiltrate Klein solution
2. BodyTite
3. Vibration-assisted liposuction as needed
4. Morpheus8 Body in burst mode
5. Treat neighboring areas FaceTite, AccuTite and Morpheus8 Body

Excisional surgery includes brachioplasty combined with vibration-assisted liposuction and bipolar radiofrequency of both upper arms and in neighboring areas (see **Fig. 14**; **Fig. 15**):

1. Infiltrate Klein solution
2. Vibration-assisted liposuction of excision site
3. Excision of the cutaneous-subcutaneous excess with segmental closure skin excision from distal to caudal; the excision is made along the preoperatively marked internal ellipse. Undermining the posterior flap and advancing it anteriorly with subsequent fixation to Lockwood fascia and layered closure
4. FaceTite with vibration assisted liposuction, followed by Morpheus8 Body of the axillas
5. AccuTite followed by Morpheus8 in the elbow area
6. Morpheus8 Body in burst mode of axilla, at least 2 cm from the closure for the upper arm

Secondary Surgery

Radiofrequency procedures include BodyTite, FaceTite, and AccuTite, which are used after 6 months to correct contour irregularities and/or additionally tighten the skin. Use the specified tip depending on the size of the surgical defect and reach 70°C for destruction of subcutaneous fat deposits and 40°C for additional tightening of the skin;

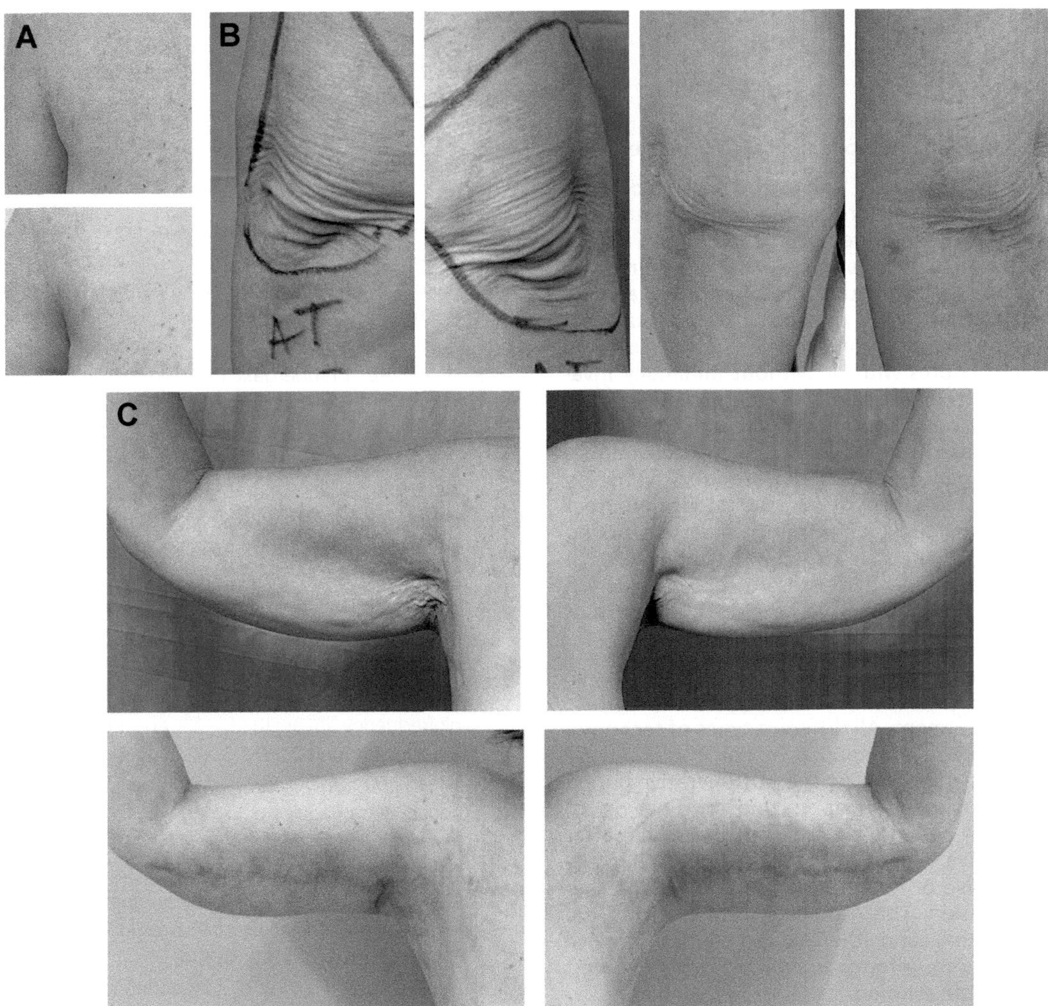

Fig. 15. (*A*) 1 year after brachioplasty in combination with vibration-assisted liposuction in the upper arm area; FaceTite with vibration-assisted liposuction and Morpheus8 Body in the armpit area; AccuTite in combination with Morpheus8 for tightening and improving skin quality in the elbow area; Morpheus8 Body (circularly in the upper arm area). The combination provides removal of excess skin and fat deposits in the armpit area + tightening and improvement of skin quality with removal of excess fat in the armpit area + tightening and improvement of skin quality in the elbow area + tightening and improvement of skin quality circularly in the armpit area. (*B*) 1 year after FaceTite with vibration-assisted liposuction and Morpheus8 Body in the armpit area (area marked with FT + MBODY). (*C*) 1 year after AccuTite in combination with Morpheus8 (area marked with AT + M8) for tightening and improving skin quality in the elbow area.

in each case, the goal is to achieve 8 to 10 kJ of energy per 10 cm^2 of treated area. Morpheus8 Body can be repeated after the 45th postoperative day.

SUMMARY & KEY POINTS

Using minimally invasive and noninvasive techniques alone or combined with excisional procedures leads to better aesthetic results in body contouring:

- Bipolar radiofrequency BodyTite, FaceTite, and AccuTite improve skin elasticity in areas neighboring the excision.
- Bipolar radiofrequency Morpheus8 Body improves skin elasticity not only in neighboring areas, but also about the excision.
- VASERlipo allows not only contouring, but definition of the muscle groups in treated areas and in neighboring areas when combined with excisional procedures.
- Noninvasive radiofrequency and electrostimulation procedures –EVOLVE X and trueSculptfleX – applied during the postoperative period expedite the recovery and optimize aesthetics.

CLINICS CARE POINTS

Based on the author's clinical experience

- In obese type of patients, there could be an improvement through noninvasive interventions (radiofrequency, ultrasound, and muscle electrical stimulation devices) or minimally invasive techniques (radiofrequency and ultrasound types of liposuction, vibrational type of liposuction), and/or surgical excisional procedures with or without minimally invasive techniques in the treated area and/or other neighboring body areas. In those type of patients, if minimally invasive techniques are applied as isolated procedure, overdoing the area could often lead to irregularities and sagging skin. Having said that, asking the patient to reach optimal body weight could lead to better results, but if surgery is the choice made, then excisional procedures should be included in the surgical plan.
- In massive weight loss patients, surgical excisional procedures are always the first choice of treatment. All different types of technologies could be applied in neighboring body areas and/or during the postoperative period with the aim of optimizing the final result. Often patients visit the author's clinic after massive weight loss, asking for a minimally invasive or noninvasive solution for the sagging skin. This should be avoided from the surgeon, and the patient should receive adequate information on which is the best possible solution for his or her problem.
- Combination of radiofrequency, ultrasound procedures, vibrational type of liposuction, excisional surgical procedures should be done with precision and adequacy regarding what, when, and where to combine. Based on the author's practical experience, excisional procedures could be combined with ultrasound definition in the same stage of treatment because of the vessel-sparing nature of the ultrasound-based liposuction procedures. When performing excisional procedures, radiofrequency techniques could be used in neighboring areas, considering the ablative effect of radiofrequency-based liposuction devices, thus eliminating possible wound healing problems at the incision site. Combination in 1 body area from above is possible, but when the radiofrequency procedure is less invasive, meaning Morpheus 8, and Morpheus 8 Body. When combining ultrasound for definition with radiofrequency for tightening, the surgeon should be careful regarding possible overheating and thermal injury of the skin, and/or undesirable fibrosis.

DISCLOSURE

International trainer for INMODE radiofrequency-based procedures.

REFERENCES

1. Sharkov E. Body contouring surgery – the role of non-invasive, minimal invasive and surgical technologies. Heidelberg, New York, Dordrecht, London: Springer; 2023. Manuscript submitted for publication.
2. Hoyos AE, Prendergast PM. High definition body sculpting. Heidelberg New York Dordrecht London: Springer; 2014. p. 73–80.
3. Villegas FJ. A novel approach to abdominoplasty: TULUA modifications (transverse plication, no undermining, full liposuction, neoumbilicoplasty, and low transverse abdominal scar). Aesthetic Plast Surg 2014;38:511–20.
4. Mulholland RS. 2th edition. The BodyTite book, 261. Barbados, WI: BoomerangFX International SRL; 2021. p. 734–50.
5. Dayan E, Burns AJ, Rohrich RJ, et al. The use of radiofrequency in aesthetic surgery. Plast Reconstr Surg Glob Open 2020;8(8):e2861.
6. Theodorou SJ, Del Vecchio D, Chia CT. Soft tissue contraction in body contouring with radiofrequency-assisted liposuction: a treatment gap solution. Aesthetic Surg J 2018;38:S74–83.
7. Mulholland RS. Radiofrequency energy for non-invasive and minimally invasive skin tightening. Clin Plast Surg 2011;38:437–48.
8. Cimino WW. History of ultrasound-assisted lipoplasty. In: Shiffman MA, Di Giuseppe A,, editors. Body contouring: art, science, and clinical practice. Berlin: : Springer; 2010. p. 399.
9. Cimino WW. The physics of soft tissue fragmentation using ultrasonic frequency vibrations of metal probes. Clin Plast Surg 1999;26:447–61.
10. Ogawa T, Hattori R, Yamamoto T, et al. Safe use of ultrasonically activated devices based on current studies. Expert Rev Med Devices 2011;8(3):319–24.
11. Scuderi N, Devita R, D'Andrea F, et al. Nuove prospettive nella liposuzione la lipoemulsificazone. Giorn Chir Plast Ricostr ed Estetica 1987;2(1):33–9.
12. Zocchi ML. Clinical aspects of ultrasonic liposculpture. Perspect Plast Surg 1993;7:153–74.
13. Zocchi ML. Ultrasonic assisted lipoplasty. Clin Plast Surg 1996;23(4):575–98.
14. Troilius C. Ultrasound-assisted lipoplasty: is it really safe? Aesthetic Plast Surg 1999;23(5):307–11.
15. Baxter RA. Histologic effects of ultrasound-assisted lipoplasty. Aesthetic Surg J 1999;19:109–14.
16. Cimino WW. Ultrasonic surgery: power quantification and efficiency optimization. Aesthetic Surg J 2001; 21(3):233–40.

17. Cimino WW. Ultrasound-assisted lipoplasty: basic physics, tissue interactions, and related results/ complications. In: Shiffman MA, Di Giuseppe A,, editors. Body contouring: art, science, and clinical practice. Berlin: : Springer; 2010.. p. 392.
18. Cimino WW. VASER-assisted lipoplasty: technology and technique. In: Shiffman MA, Di Giuseppe A,, editors. Liposuction principles and practice. Heidelberg: Springer-Verlag Berlin; 2006. p. 239–44.
19. Jewell ML, Fodor PB, de Souza Pinto EB, et al. Clinical application of VASER–assisted lipoplasty: a pilot clinical study. Aesthetic Surg J 2002;22(2):131–46.
20. Illouz YG. Surgical remodeling of the silhouette by aspiration lipolysis or selective lipectomy. Aesthetic Plast Surg 1985;9(1):7–21.
21. Hoyos A, Perez M. Dynamic-definition male pectoral reshaping and enhancement in slim, athletic, obese, and gynecomastic patients through selective fat removal and grafting. Aesthetic Plast Surg 2012; 36(5):1066–77.
22. Hoyos AE. High definition liposculpture. Paper presented at the XIII International Course of Plastic Surgery, Bucaramanga, Colombia; 2003.
23. Ersek RA, Salisbury AV. Abdominal etching. Aesthetic Plast Surg 1997;21(5):328–31.
24. Hoyos AE, Perez ME, Domínguez-Millán R. Variable sculpting in dynamic definition body contouring: procedure selection and management algorithm. Aesthetic Surg J 2021;41(3):318–32.
25. Hoyos AE, Millard JA. VASER-assisted high-definition liposculpture. Aesthetic Surg J 2007; 27(6):594–604.
26. Hurwitz DJ. Approach to the medial thigh lift after weight loss. In: Rubin PJ, Matarraso A, editors. Aesthetic Surgery after weight loss. Philadelphia: Saunders Elsevier; 2007. p. 113–30.
27. Rubin P, Jellew ML, Richter DF, et al. Body contouring and liposuction. Philadelphia: Saunders Elsevier; 2013. p. 353–74.
28. Aly AS. Body contouring after massive weight loss. St Louis (MO): Quality Medical Publishing; 2006. p. 213–36.
29. Hurwitz DJ. Comprehensive body contouring. theory and practice. Springer; 2016. p. 170–4.
30. Hurwitz DJ, Holland SW. The L Brachioplasty: an innovative approach to correct excess tissue of the upper arm, axilla and lateral chest. Plast Reconstr Surg 2006;117:403–11.
31. Al S. Aly body contouring after massive weight loss. St Louis, MO: Quality Medical Publishing, Inc; 2006. p. 312–7.
32. Rubin P, Jellew ML, Richter DF, et al. Body contouring and liposuction. Philadelphia, PA: Saunders Elsevier; 2013. p. 19–24.

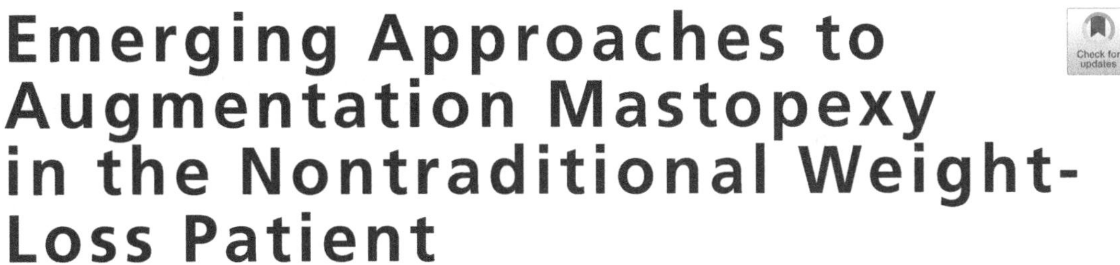

Emerging Approaches to Augmentation Mastopexy in the Nontraditional Weight-Loss Patient

Armando A. Davila, MD[a,b,*]

KEYWORDS

- Subfascial breast augmentation • Suspension mastopexy • Fat grafting • Breast mesh
- Breast reconstruction • Composite augmentation

KEY POINTS

- New types of weight-loss patients are presenting for body contouring owing to increased accessibility to surgical and nonsurgical options for weight loss (see Jennifer Capla and Steven A. Hanna's article, "Patient Evaluation and Surgical Staging," in this issue).
- The subfascial plane provides a more versatile, modern, and comprehensive approach to breast augmentation, translating the advantages of prepectoral breast reconstruction to aesthetic breast surgery.
- Composite breast augmentations harness the power of fat grafting to correct asymmetries and breast irregularities while producing a resilient breast to weight changes.
- Breast shaping via parenchymal manipulation and suspensory cerclage sutures fuses the dynamics of the breast soft tissue envelope and footprint to create a more natural breast.
- The evolution of mesh techniques and available materials allows for precise control of the breast boundaries, avoiding difficult-to-manage implant malposition.

 **Video content accompanies this article at http://www.plasticsurgery.theclinics.com.**

INTRODUCTION/HISTORY/DEFINITIONS/ BACKGROUND

The use of autologous tissue for autoaugmentation of the breast with parenchymal reshaping has been a favored technique. Parenchymal reshaping in the context of breast ptosis has been described for nearly 50 years, with gold-standard descriptions from Biggs, Graf, Lassus, Lejour, and Hall-Findlay, among others.[1] Despite years of comparative analysis and early approaches at augmenting soft tissue support with implanted materials, long-term outcomes remained similar regardless of technique and approach.[2]

The increase of gastric bypass in the 1990s and the appearance of the "massive weight loss" (MWL) patient presented a new challenge in breast contouring, with the appearance of classic weight-loss deformities in the breast: lateral breast roll with loss of lateral breast shadow, loss of skin elasticity with striae, severe parenchymal volume loss, and medialization of the nipple areolar complex (NAC) complex. Previous techniques, which approached the breast from central, superior, or superomedial pedicles, struggled against the NAC malposition and the relative soft tissue excess of the lateral chest. The late 1990s were plagued with high rates

[a] Pittsburgh Center for Plastic Surgery, 3109 Forbes Avenue #500, Pittsburgh, PA 15213, USA; [b] University of Pittsburgh, Pittsburgh, PA, USA
* Pittsburgh Center for Plastic Surgery, 3109 Forbes Avenue #500, Pittsburgh, PA 15213.
E-mail address: drdavila@pghplasticsurgery.com

Clin Plastic Surg 51 (2024) 161–171
https://doi.org/10.1016/j.cps.2023.07.008

of wound complications and poor long-term aesthetic results.

One of the earliest modern descriptions of MWL breast reshaping by Hurwitz and Agha-Mohammadi[3] via the "spiral flap" set a new standard approach to autoaugmentation of the breast, with techniques and modifications described by Rubin, Losken, Colwell, and Blondeel over the subsequent decade. The often-cited DSPRM (Dermal Suspension, Parenchymal Reshaping Mastopexy) by Rubin and colleagues,[4] a complex, highly undermining shaping technique, demonstrates the fundamental concepts in the MWL patient of volumization via excess lateral chest tissue (Spiral, Intercostal Artery Perforator, Lateral Thoracic flaps), shaping the tissue to increase projection, and improving parenchymal support via suture suspension.

Long-term outcomes are predictable; although traditional lift approaches presented with "bottoming out" because of parenchymal stress on a weakened lower pole, MWL glandular reshaping frequently presents with early NAC ptosis (unpredictable elongation of Sternal Notch [SN]:NAC rather than NAC: Inframmammary Fold [IMF]) from stretch of the upper chest tissues, and lateral migration of the parenchyma back into the heavily dissected lateral chest. The upper breast border as described by Hall-Findlay,[5,6] is predictability never raised in any form of parenchymal reshaping, and MWL patients frequently present with a significantly low upper breast border. Without the addition of structured volume via implant placement or focused fat grafting, the ideal result can be out of reach. As MWL skin envelopes make for poor brassieres to support the weight of the implant, complications are high. Staging implants or grafting to improve predictability can be tedious or cost prohibitive, and fat grafting donor sites can be elusive. The complexity of these cases has expanded as the scope of "massive weight loss" patient has grown. This article seeks to establish emerging techniques for these new dilemmas.

CASE 1: MESH-SUPPORTED BREAST AUGMENTATION IN THE THIN PATIENT WITH MASSIVE WEIGHT LOSS

A 46-year-old, 1.75m, G2P2, 57 kg (body mass index [BMI 18]), previously 195 pounds (BMI 29), woman presents for breast augmentation (**Fig.** 1A, C). Despite an average BMI, the patient underwent a laparoscopic gastric bypass losing 70 pounds. The patient is an active nicotine user and desires around 650-cc implants and a "fake," high-riding look. She presents with a low-set breast footprint and SN:NAC distance of 23 cm. A short NAC:IMF of 4 cm readily expands to 7 to 8 cm on stretch. Pinch is 0.5 to 1 cm, and striae are present throughout the breast. Extremely prominent central thoracic ribs and pectus carinatum are present. Surgical discussion involves preoperative counseling regarding smoking cessation, poor soft tissue quality, and the need for mesh support. One-year postoperatively, photographs demonstrate excellent control of the lower pole (**Fig.** 1B, D). The patient does not desire raising the slightly low-set NAC complex from 23 cm to 21 cm, which would be appropriate for her frame, as she wishes to avoid scars. The implants are mobile and soft, despite some lack of close cleavage owing to her pectus.

SURGICAL TECHNIQUE

Preoperative planning and measurements are completed. The pectus carinatum portends a wide base width of 13 cm, and a moderate plus profile 630-cc implant is selected to maximize central cleavage despite the curvature of the chest. With the history of smoking, multiple pregnancies, and thin pinch, a submuscular dual plane approach is planned, with avoidance of a periareolar mastopexy, to be added in the second stage if the patient desires. The patient is extremely high risk for implant malposition, bottoming out, and lateralization. Mesh chosen is GalaFLEX 3DR (P4HB; MonoMax; Tepha, Inc, Lexington, MA, USA) for ease of deployment, longevity, and strength. After local administration, a generous 5- to 6-cm IMF incision is made, and a dual-plane subpectoral pocket developed after subfascial release of approximately the lower third of the breast parenchyma. The muscle is allowed to window shade, and saline sizer is placed. After confirming pocket dimensions and sizer, the position of the mesh is marked. Care is taken to ensure sufficient room along the IMF for the mesh and no damage to the serratus fascia for strong suture placement. The sizer is removed, and the mesh is prepared on the back table, by removing the tabs and washing in antibiotic irrigation. The mesh is folded and inserted into the pocket and allowed to spring open with rim support (Video 1). A central suture is placed with 2-0 PDS that is lined up with the externally marked location, and then the 2 limb ends are secured at the natural curvature of the mesh and reconciled with the sizer markings. The sizer is replaced, and any areas where the mesh lifts from the chest wall is resecured with additional suture. A stay stitch with 3-0 Vicryl or PDS is placed at the cephalad portion of the mesh. The upper rim is partially exposed and trimmed to avoid palpability. The final implant

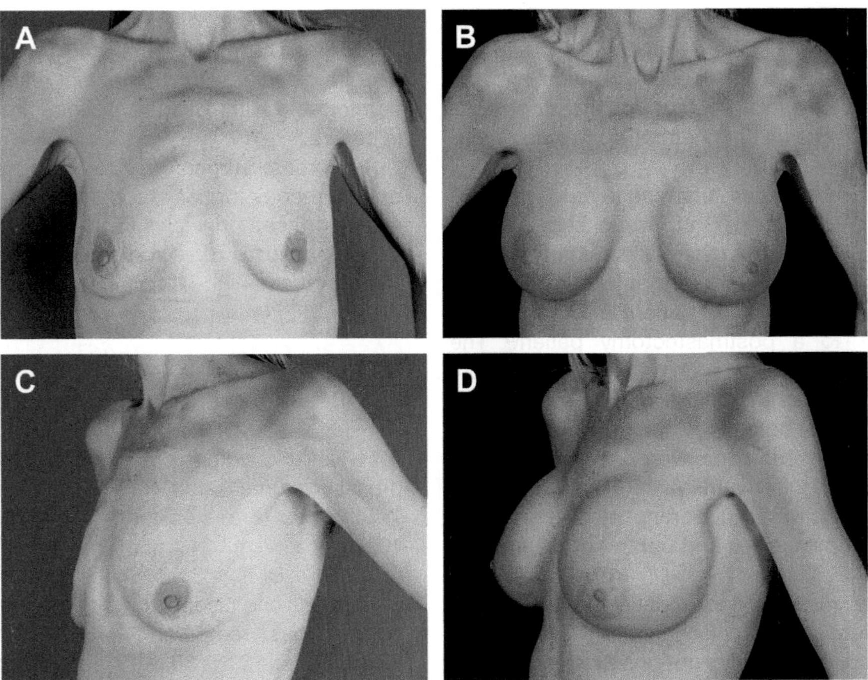

Fig. 1. Case 1. Before and after anterior (*A*, *B*), and left anterior oblique views (*C*, *D*): Severe hypomastia with laxity and striae (*A*). Prominence of sternum and pectus carinatum with ptosis (*B*). Well-supported, 630-cc implant despite visible implant borders due to lack of subcutaneous fat (*B*, *D*).

is placed with no-touch technique and Keller funnel. The suture is used to keep the mesh flattened during the insertion of the implant and then drawn upward to smooth the mesh over the implant. A single, clean gloved finger is inserted to smooth the mesh and avoid excess contact with the implant (see Video 1). The mesh is not sutured to the muscle. The breast is closed in multiple layers after sitting the patient to confirm positioning.

DISCUSSION

The extremely thin post–weight loss patient presents with a set of common deformities pertinent to augmentation of the breast. Starting from inside to out, deformations of the bony skeleton are particularly notable. The excess weight on the torso produces barreling of the chest, with prominence of the sternum, heavily angled at the sternal manubrial junction. The resulting movement curves the costocartilagious thorax. The resulting chest remains wider than expected for the weight and height of the patient. The costosternal junction appears widened, and bony prominence of the third to fifth ribs is accentuated. The nipple areolar complex does not follow suit and generally remains medialized with a wide areola. Tissue laxity laterally produces a “wide” breast base width. The IMF position is poorly defined, low on the chest, and can be readily slid or lifted off the chest wall. Breast volume is nonexistent, and the breast may be minimally ptotic.

The approach of parenchymal reshaping is not an option for these patients, as they present with almost no functional volume. Conservative fat grafting plays a role in contouring a final result, but they rarely have sufficient volume elsewhere to produce an adequate breast mound. Breast augmentation with an implant as the only viable option is fraught with complexity.

The excess curvature of the chest and “wide” base width complicate implant selection. Patients who choose modest implant sizes must opt for lower-profile implants to accommodate these abnormal dimensions. The result can be underwhelming, with poor projection, higher rates of rippling/visibility, and minimal correction of ptosis without significant mastopexy. The subfascial or submuscular pocket needs to accommodate the wide implant and portends overdissection of the pocket with subsequent implant malposition and lateralization. The savvy surgeon then opts for a larger implant to recruit the excess skin, maintain a narrower pocket, and improve projection. The resulting IMF migration, bottoming out, and “stargazing” NAC complex feels defeating (**Fig. 2**).

Controlling implant descent would require near complete submuscular coverage, and the mismatch between the muscle position and the breast envelope rarely allows for that control as evidenced by years of unnatural-appearing reconstructive breast surgery.

The answer then lies in turning to reconstructive surgery for solutions. Soft tissue support with mesh has evolved exponentially since the introduction of acellular dermal matrices. The breast of a thin post–weight-loss patient is fundamentally equivalent to a postmastectomy patient. The attenuated suspensory ligaments do not function, and weight gain and loss have violated the anatomic breast borders as if it had been surgical. Applying these reconstructive principles suddenly becomes straightforward. A minimum of inferior third coverage with supporting mesh can allow for larger implant sizes and control of the implant pocket.

Acellular matrices lack financial flexibility for most patients, even when animal-based dermal matrices are used. Newer options for mesh include absorbable products, including Durasorb (PDS) and GalaFLEX. P4HB is poly-4-hydroxybutyrate, a fully resorbable, biologically produced, and biocompatible mesh. It is produced via recombinant fermentation of *Escherichia coli* K12 and is a polymer of 4-hydroxybutyrate (4-HB), a natural human metabolite. The breakdown of the polymer to 4-HB occurs via hydrolysis in a slow 12- to 18-month degradation profile. 4-HB then is quickly broken down to co_2 and water via the Krebs cycle with a half-life of about 30 minutes. There are no metal catalysts used in its manufacturing that can result in contaminants, or intermediary byproducts during its disappearance, which gives patients piece of mind when it is used. Internally it behaves like a temporary texturing for the implant, having a Velcro-like surface, holding its position with minimal suturing. It leaves behind a slightly thickened capsule in its wake, providing longer-term support along its placement path. Early studies seem to indicate possible reduction of capsular contracture rates. Negatively, it is relatively inflexible, and unforgiving if placed incorrectly. It is possible to intervene early and move the mesh around for 6 months, as it is embedded in the capsule during that time, and capsule manipulation maneuvers can be applied to reposition the mesh while still holding strength. The 12- to 18-month degradation profile is long, but the increasing tensile strength of the capsule as it forms and the collagen remodels take around 6 months to maximally occur, and the next shortest product is PDS mesh, clocking in at less than 3 months, insufficient for full capsule strength. Functionally, the difference between PDS or P4HB mesh may be minimal, and it is up to the surgeon to decide which material they are most comfortable with. Biologic options are discussed in case 2.

Any breast surgeon familiar with mesh use in breast reconstruction should have no problem applying those principles to this new class of soft tissue support and will improve the longevity of results for these high-risk patients.

CASE 2: COMPOSITE BREAST AUGMENTATION IN THE OVERWEIGHT-WEIGHT-LOSS PATIENT

A 44-year-old woman presents for improvement in breast volume after GLP-1 agonist–induced weight loss (**Fig. 3**). Starting at a BMI of 37.4, 102kg at a height of 1.65m, the patient lost 16kg to reach a BMI of 31.6. She is satisfied with her weight loss and disappointed at the relative breast volume loss compared with other areas. Her SN:NAC distance is 30, with grade 3 breast ptosis, evidence of both moderate vertical and mild horizontal parenchymal construction with moderate pseudoherniation best appreciated on the three-quarter view. The horizontal constriction on left is greater than the right, with a widened overall torso from high BMI. Striae present throughout the breast indicate the potential for poor soft tissue support. Breast implants were sized at around 550 to 600 cc, so surgical discussion involves the need for mesh support. A moderate- to high-profile implant is selected to maximize coverage of the wide breast base. A subfascial approach is planned. Intraoperatively, 120 cc of fat is injected into each breast, primarily in the upper and medial poles. Postoperative photographs at 9 months demonstrate excellent upper pole retention, implant position, and breast shape. The NAC:IMF limb is slightly long, as only vertical mastopexy is performed, and patient is offered a small corrective J extension of the incision to correct mild glandular ptosis off the implant.

SURGICAL TECHNIQUE

The breast is approached using tuberous breast principles. The short scar, vertical mastopexy is incised within the mastopexy pattern, and the pectoralis is encountered in the lower third of the muscle. A subfascial pocket is developed. In IMF cases without mesh, an important stair step incision into the fascia is preferable. This allows for a small fascial flap at the IMF for secure closure and to lock the IMF more effectively. In cases with mesh, this is less critical, as the mesh will

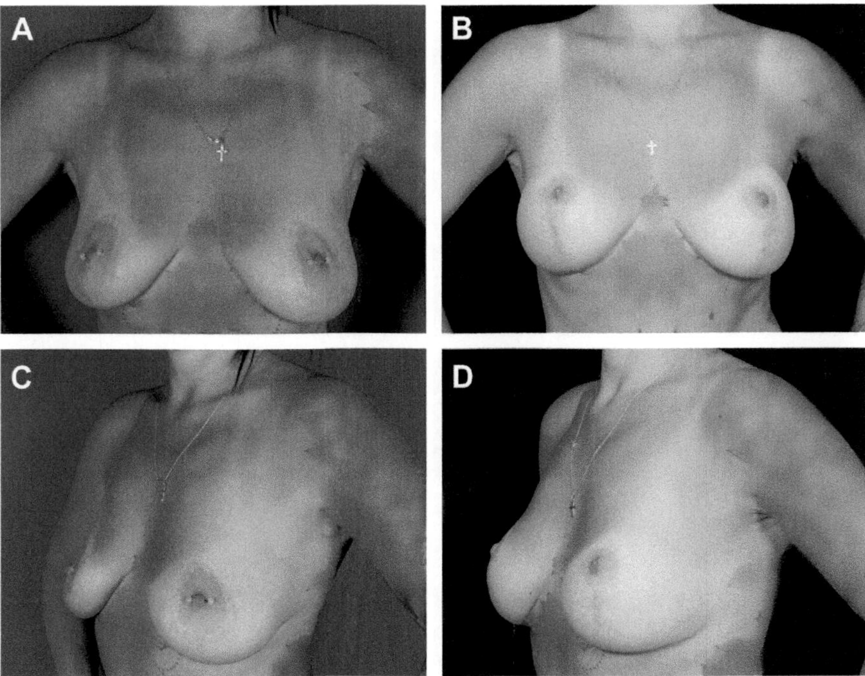

Fig. 2. Before and after anterior (*A, B*), and left anterior oblique views (*C, D*): Patient with hypomastia, striae, and periareolar lift to attempt to correct tissue laxity. (*A, C*) Patient presents desiring volume and declines internal mesh despite recommendations. Placed were 350-cc implants, and NAC was not raised, only reduced in size and converted to wise mastopexy. Despite patient satisfaction and volume correction, note bottoming out of implants and migration of the IMF scar onto the lower breast, despite wise mastopexy techniques to tighten envelope (*B, D*).

serve as the IMF restraint mechanism. The fascial elevation is performed meticulously with low-power coagulation electrocautery, using cut sparingly to avoid rents in the fascia. The muscular surface should be bare as the dissection proceeds with the longitudinal fibers visible. Bleeding should be minimal in the correct plane; excessive bleeding indicates too deep of a dissection, but too superficial, and parenchyma will herniate through the fascia. Blunt dissection of the upper pole is not possible as with submuscular augmentation, and the surgeon should continue a few centimeters higher than expected in the upper pole. A sizer is placed in the pocket, and the mastopexy is tailor tacked. After confirming the pocket and implant position, the edges of the sizer are marked for mesh placement. As in case 1, the mesh is prepared on the back table and placed in the pocket and is similarly secured with 2-0 PDS along the sizer markings and stay stitch. Final implant is once again placed with no-touch technique and Keller funnel. After mesh smoothing, the stay stitch is secured to the fascia edge to avoid collapse of the mesh during the mastopexy adjustments. A standard lollipop-style mastopexy is performed using closure with 3-0 PDO Quill sutures.

Before performing the mastopexy, fat harvest from the abdomen had been performed. The LipoGrafter system (MTF Biologics, Edison, NJ, USA) is used for both its simplicity and convenience. The completely on-field collection system can be easily attached to MicroAire power-assisted liposuction cannulas. The 12-track, Del Vecchio style cannula produces small globules ideal for breast grafting that does not require additional manipulation of the fat or filtration. Superwet technique is used, and then the harvesting bags are decanted on the back table. The multiuse bags can quickly be decanted and combined for a total of 1000 cc of fat immediately available during grafting without having to pause to harvest to empty canisters. The fat is delivered "wet," which this author prefers, allowing for better dispersal of the fat and less risk of cysts from lumpy depots of fat that drier processing techniques can produce. Overcorrection by about one-fourth of the total volume expected will account for volume lost owing to absorption of the remaining infranatant.

In cases of significant asymmetry or high-volume grafting, the fat is placed before insertion of the implant. This allows for more accurate placement and direct visual confirmation that the

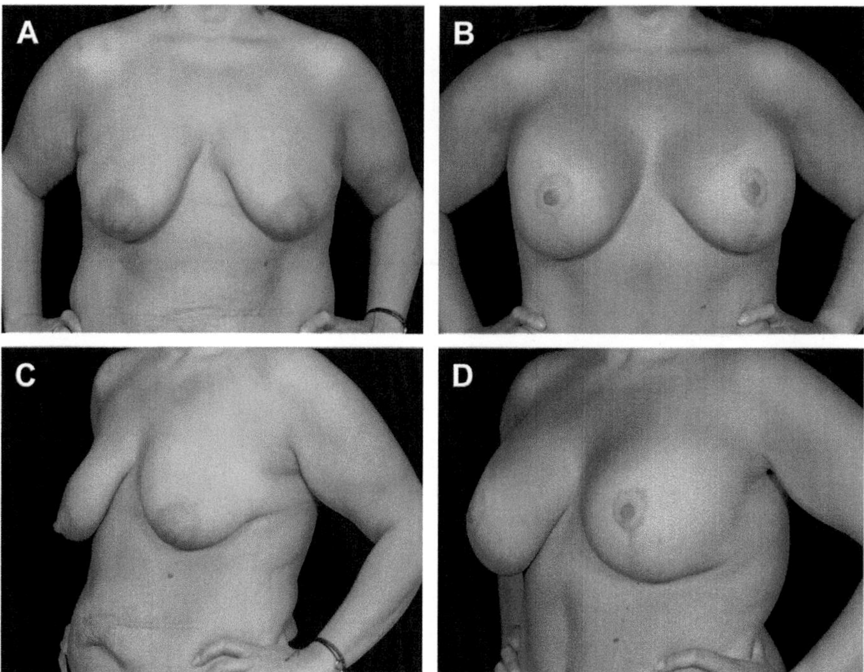

Fig. 3. Case 2. Before and after anterior (*A, B*), and left anterior oblique views (*C, D*): Striae and ptosis with relative hypomastia to overall habitus (*A*). Tuberous type breast deformity most notable on the oblique view with short distance between the upper breast border and IMF (*C*). After composite augmentation and vertical mastopexy, with appropriate NAC position and upper pole fullness (*D*). Slight glandular ptosis from long NAC:IMF from missing horizontal limb to mastopexy (*B*).

pectoral fascia is not violated with the injection cannula, minimizing spillage and contamination of the pocket with fat. Once the asymmetry appears visually corrected or the volume desired is reached, the implant is then placed, and then mastopexy is remarked and performed. For cases of only minor contour correction, particularly for correction of the upper and medial poles of the breast, fat is added after implant placement and mastopexy with careful technique to avoid damage to the implant.

DISCUSSION

The overweight-weight-loss patient has presented new challenges in body contouring. The emergence of this class of patient stems from greater availability of both surgical and nonsurgical techniques for weight loss and the continued trends of increasing obesity in the United States. Patients can lose significant amounts of weight that lead to traditional weight-loss deformities, but continued adiposity produces different challenges. These patients psychologically tend to compare themselves with traditional weight-loss patients but are often more demanding about results. The expectation is frequently that they have done the initial work of early weight loss, and then body contouring will help them “finish losing weight” after they plateau. They seek surgical intervention early when a particular body subunit (see chapter 11) starts to look poor, rather than waiting for the completion of weight loss and then seeking complete contouring. The breast is frequently this first subunit group, as the volume loss in the breast is disproportionate to their incomplete weight loss. It is important when evaluating this type of patient to carefully discuss the implications of further weight loss on the breast surgery, particularly as it pertains to implant sizing and mastopexies.

Composite breast augmentation has emerged from the extensive use of fat grafting in breast cancer reconstruction over the last 2 decades. Single-stage, high-volume grafting is now possible with advanced techniques and technologies. In the overweight-weight-loss patient, composite augmentation allows for the breast to adjust to continued weight changes, if both the patient loses weight, shrinking the breast volume proportionally, or increasing the breast volume if the patient regains the weight. In some cases, composite augmentation allows the surgeon to downsize the implant, particularly in cases of compromised skin quality.

Using 3D imaging (Vectra, Canfield, NJ, USA), preoperative volume assessments can provide guidance on single-stage grafting expectations. The author's expectation is that a "doubling" of volume can be injected in a single stage; that is, if the software parenchymal volume reads at 300 mL, then the same volume of wet fat can be injected safely into the breast in a single stage without risking over-fat necrosis.[7] Practically, never more than 500 mL of wet fat, or 2 full Lipo-Grafter bags, is injected into the breast in a single stage, even if the volumetric measurements are higher than that. Composite augmentations are also flexible in allowing for correction of asymmetry via fat rather than disparate sized implants, and it also allows for specific contouring of areas such as in tuberous deformities. Although slight differences in implants are acceptable, having implants greater than 50 to 75 cc in volume difference can have long-term unintended consequences. Their dimensions and/or profiles will be different and therefore will behave differently in the respective pockets. Adding 75 to 100 mL of fat to the smaller breast is reliable and future proofs the operation, allowing for easier implant exchanges even with patient variations in weight.

Mesh use is also featured in this case, but in a different surgical plane. In cases with sufficient upper pole pinch, even as low as 1 to 1.5 cm, it is preferred to use the subfascial approach. Further study of the subfascial approach has demonstrated indistinguishable long-term outcomes, similar capsular contracture rates, and patient satisfaction.[8,9] The subfascial approach completely eliminates concerns of muscle spasms, animation deformity, and chronic pain that result from muscle transection. The gold standard of reconstructive breast work has moved definitively to the prepectoral space, highlighting the regressive approach of submuscular cosmetic breast augmentation. In breast reconstruction, the prepectoral approach relies on acellular dermis to support the implant, and this was previously financially inaccessible to the cosmetic surgeon. However, safe, effective, and cost-efficient options are now available, and so the aesthetic surgeon now has the tools necessary to take on more complex cases where the breast lacks intrinsic support without heightened fear of malposition.

Although this case used GalaFLEX, discussed in case 1, an alternative mesh is discussed here. Meso Biomatrix (MTF Biologics) is in the acellular matrix family and can be used analogously to prepectoral methods with acellular dermal matricies (ADMs). Made from porcine peritoneum, it is thin, readily incorporated with less seroma risk, and mildly less flexible than dermal matrices. Behaving more like the less flexible absorbable meshes, it provides excellent support of implants at a fraction of the cost. Placement of this product can be more challenging than the easily deployed GalaFLEX, and so a periareolar or vertical mastopexy incision is preferred. This allows for complete deployment of the mesh after the implant is in place; securing the entire mesh pieces around the periphery, akin to prepectoral ADMs though a radial/periareolar mastectomy incision. The newer GalaFLEX Lite scaffold also behaves and can be deployed similarly.

The addition of these techniques to the surgeon's arsenal is essential for managing the high expectations of the complex deformities found in this new class of weight-loss patient, producing results that will be long lasting, even if unpredictable weight changes occur in the postoperative period.

CASE 3: MANAGING PROJECTION WITH SUSPENSORY CERCLAGE AFTER IMPLANT REMOVAL IN THE PATIENT WITH BREAST IMPLANT ILLNESS

A 52-year-old female patient presents with desire for implant removal (**Fig. 4**A, C). She has 20-year-old, smooth, round, saline implants, located in the subglandular position, approximately 325 cc in size. She reports improvements in her lifestyle with a focus on weight loss and health. She has lost some weight and feels that her breasts are now too large. She also reports that since contracting COVID-19, she has persistent left breast pain with normal breast ultrasounds and normal autoimmune panels. 3D volumetric analysis demonstrates approximately 700 to 800 cc of total breast volume, including implants. Preoperative discussion involves the possibility of replacing some of the lost volume with autologous fat, with an expected 150 to 200 mL of retention in a single stage. She does not desire that additional volume and wishes to be smaller. A Wise pattern, parenchymal reshaping mastopexy is planned, with implant and partial capsular removal. The patient requests capsules be sent. Careful discussion regarding the amount of capsule removal is essential. She agrees to subtotal removal. A cerclage suspension stitch is placed. Post-operatively, at 8 months, she demonstrates smaller, pleasing, and natural lifted breasts, strong breast projection, and restoration of her lateral breast margins (**Fig. 4**B, D). She is pain free and satisfied with her size.

SURGICAL TECHNIQUE

Mastopexy markings are approached via breast reduction techniques using the size of the implant

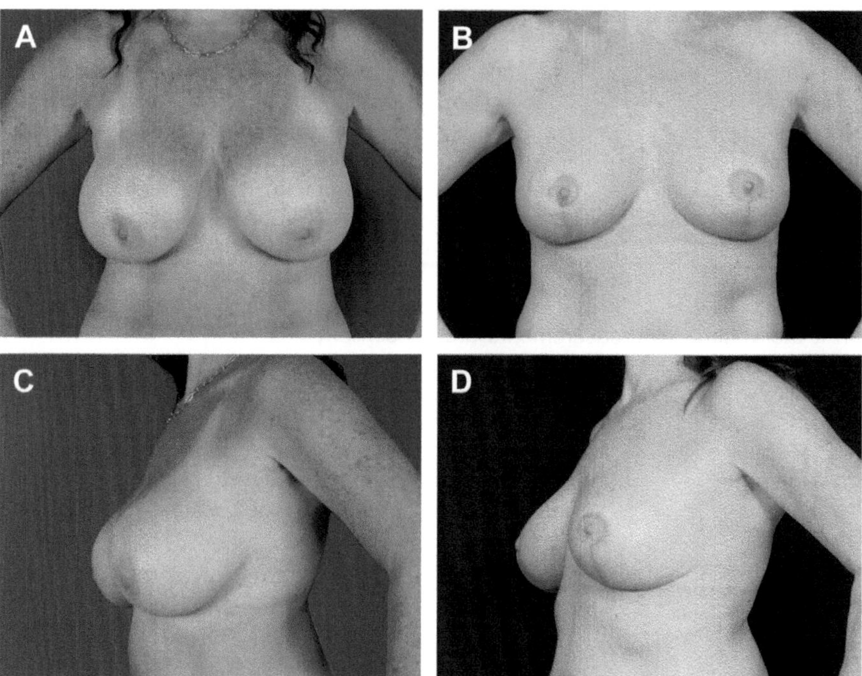

Fig. 4. Case 3. Before and after anterior (*A, B*), and left anterior oblique views (*C, D*): Large breasts with ptosis preoperatively (*A*). The dissected and mobile lateral chest from implant movement is difficult to appreciate in the standing position (*C*). After removal of the implant and cerclage (*B*). The lateral chest is adherent without drain use and maintains strong projection of the breast in combination with parenchymal reshaping (*D*).

as an estimated reduction volume. Superior or superomedial pedicle techniques are the cornerstone for the surgical approach with a generous IMF incision. The larger than normal IMF incision allows for improved access for capsule manipulation. Although a personal discussion with each patient, the preference is subtotal capsular removal in cases of breast implant illness (BII) to avoid patient complaints postoperatively. Extracapsular dissection is focused on for the first one-third to one-half of the implant. Then the implant is removed, and an additional, easily removed capsule is taken. An extremely adherent normal capsule is left in situ unless the patient has explicitly requested and accepted those additional risks. Any remaining capsule is scored or roughed to improve adherence. In BII cases that have implant rupture, best efforts are made to perform total periprosthetic capsulectomy without entering the capsule for contamination reasons.

After implant and capsular removal, the preference is to reattach the pectoralis if possible in subpectoral augmentations. A Kelly clamp is used to bring the muscle under stretch with assistance, and then 2-0 Ethibond is used as figure-of-eight sutures to the nearest rib periosteum. Then, a number 1 PDO barbed quill is used to overrun the muscle edge the full length of the IMF and along the lateral serratus attachments. The technique discussed in case 2, autologous fat augmentation, can be performed in this step under direct visualization. In cases where implants are subglandular, the surgeon will need to discuss with the patient leaving more of the anterior capsule to maximize fat retention in the breast tissue. Once any additional volume has been added, the mastopexy pattern is confirmed and de-epithelialized. An additional option, parenchymal reshaping techniques for volumization via local flaps, is reviewed in detail in chapter 11.

In the standard implant removal case, however, the goal is to re-create the regional breast adherences that are often dissected during formation of the pocket or that occur with implant malposition over time (**Fig. 5**). A suture cerclage suspension based on the principles of the reverse abdominoplasty with fat transfer (RAFT) suture technique is therefore used.[10] A number 2 PDO quill suture on a large CTX needle is used. The needle is partially straightened to better mimic the natural curvature of the breast. Starting at the midpoint of the IMF, the 2 limbs of the suture are run at the dermal/subdermal interface of the skin, meeting moderate resistance as the blunt needle

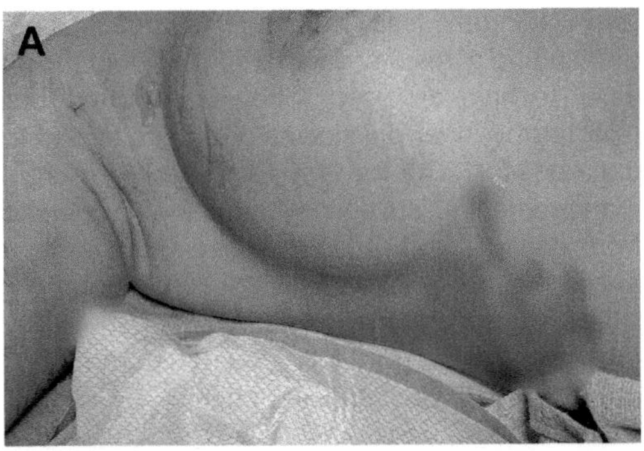

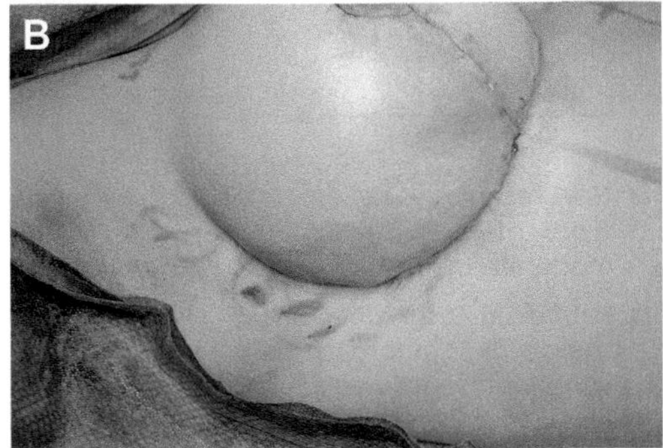

Fig. 5. Intraoperative views of a breast naturally augmented with autologous fat (A), and parenchymal reshaping mastopexy (B). Note the natural shadowing of the lateral breast border extending to the transition of the pectoralis (A). The reconstructed lateral breast border with cerclage suture (B). Placement of the suture is nonincisional; the highly indented shadow relaxes as the suture dissolves.

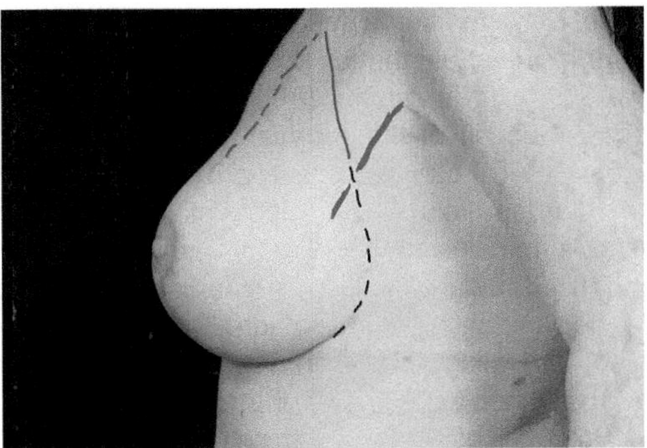

Fig. 6. Case 3. Postoperative left lateral demonstrating the path of the cerclage suture. Visible are the 3 exit and entry sites of the needle. The dotted black path shows the subdermal path of the suture during surgery. The solid blue represents the transition from subdermal to intramuscular at the pectoralis edge (red). The dotted blue represents the medial limb traveling intramuscular to the same periclavicular site.

is passed through the tissues. If too superficial, the needle will be impossible to pass; too deep and it will tear out of the loose underlying fat. These ends are run to the ends of the mastopexy. On the lateral limb, the lateral breast shadow is marked, and 2 to 3 percutaneous stabs are made with a 14-gauge needle (**Fig. 6**). Then, passing the suture at the same depth as in the IMF, the marked curvature is followed, exiting at the percutaneous stabs and reentering avoiding catching excess dermis. At the most superior point of the lateral breast shadow, where the shadow transitions to the retropectoral portion of the axilla, the suture is then plunged subcutaneously. Using a lighted retractor, it is directly visualized in the breast pocket and then driven underneath the pectoralis to deepen that anatomic interface. The barbed suture is then passed through the muscle 3 times without looping, and then is brought out through the skin. The medial limb is immediately run into the pectoralis muscle along the curvature of the medial cleavage, 3 passes through the muscle, and then is brought out through the skin adjacent to the other suture. The pathway emulates the underwire and strap of a brassiere. The sutures are then gradually cinched to provide the desired effect and projection. Care is taken to not overpull; the barbed suture will not release easily if overdone. A demonstration video on a breast reduction with J-torsoplasty highlights the technique with a wide exposure case. The video demonstrates the incisional approach laterally with the J-torsoplasty; typically, the suture is passed percutaneously (Video 2). The remainder of the mastopexy is completed via standard techniques. Once closed, the cerclage suture is trimmed by pressing down on the skin at the exit site, trimming the suture at its shortest possible length, and then pulling the skin out to release the barbs from the subcutaneous tissue. Narrowing the breast footprint via this method obviates drain placement (**Fig. 5**).

DISCUSSION

Breast deformities after implant removal share many characteristics with the MWL breast. Deflated parenchyma, thinned skin, and overly mobile or undefined breast borders are difficult to manage without the addition of new volume. Once relegated to elderly patients seeking terminal removal of their implants, removal of implants for health concerns in the young patient now represents a reconstructive dilemma. The emergence of entities like breast implant–associated anaplastic large cell lymphoma and squamous cell carcinoma , and the less well-defined BII, has promulgated increased request for elective and aesthetic implant removal without replacement. Unlike the elderly, terminal implant removal case, however, these patients still wish to maintain strong breast aesthetics postoperatively.

Autologous fat grafting (AFT) plays a strong role in the correction of these patients. As discussed in case 2, AFT can replace approximately 50% to 60% of lost volume in a single stage, depending on the remaining parenchymal estimate.[8,11] It is theorized implants provide internal tissue expansion to the parenchymal tissue much like external expansion, providing increased vascularity and delay phenomenon to the tissue, improving graft take.[12]

The focus of this case is the cerclage suspension stitch. Inspired by Dr Roger Khouri's RAFT technique,[10] its role is to reduce the total base surface area of the breast footprint, thus allowing the same breast volume to appear more projected. Analogous to moving from a moderate-profile to high-profile implant of same volume, the reduced base width means that the volume can only be accommodated in the anterior-posterior dimension. The RAFT technique goes further by releasing tissue connections in the lateral torso and upper abdomen to recruit that additional tissue to the breast alongside a permanent suture. A similar technique but with PDS suture has also been described as "Hamdi's Hammock."[12] Although elegant, the learning curve is high and does not build on techniques surgeons are already familiar with. The cerclage adapts this technique and fuses it with already established concepts; the reverse abdominoplasty, the J-torsoplasty, parenchymal reshaping. Similar to the RAFT suture, more tissue can be recruited into the breast by deepithelializing the tissue resection from a reverse abdominoplasty, or the J-torsoplasty, and incorporating it into breast via spiral techniques (see chapter 11). The cerclage then is brought in to narrow the breast footprint, which is then the lateral chest, and IMF are re-created and secured via the usual techniques for those surgeries.

Fundamentally, the cerclage acts like a brassiere underwire and exits the chest at the expected position of the brassiere strap, providing the same fundamental support. The suture is PDS and unfortunately can fail prematurely, as the suture is broken down, and adherences are not fully developed. This technique is used in breast reductions, and breasts that remain very large generally snap the suture around 6 to 8 weeks. Permanent suture is available in the Quill format, but if placed incorrectly, can be difficult to remove because of the barbs. The hope is that P4HB suture will expand further into the market with its acquisition by BD Medical with the potential for barbed iterations.

The BII population remains a growing challenge for surgeons. These patients are highly informed (even if from less reputable sources), highly demanding of results, and particular about the surgical techniques used. They have often been rejected by other physicians or surgeons and feel uncared for. Controversy surrounding surgical management exists even within our own societies, from capsule and muscle management to insurance coverage. Nevertheless, when encountering a patient practitioner who presents novel approaches, these patients can be some of the most satisfied postsurgical patients.

CLINICS CARE POINTS

- New techniques are emerging to handle new types of weight-loss patients, such as the moderate medication-assisted patient.
- Subfascial techniques are quickly becoming the de facto approach to breast augmentation, as advancements allow for comparable rates of contracture, implant stability, and natural appearance, all while avoiding animation and chronic pain.
- Fat grafting is a safe and versatile procedure that can complement nearly any breast augmentation technique and is important for the competent breast surgeon to have in their armamentarium.
- Parenchymal manipulation and advanced suture techniques continue to play an important role in shaping the deflated breast. The cerclage suture technique plays a reconstructive role in re-creating attachments lost to previous surgery or weight gain.
- Mesh materials have entered the mainstream and cannot be ignored. Deployed for the appropriate patient, their impact in supporting the soft tissues and implant is essential.

DISCLOSURE

The author has nothing to disclose.

SUPPLEMENTARY DATA

Supplementary data related to this article can be found online at https://doi.org/10.1016/j.cps.2023.07.008.

REFERENCES

1. Graf R, Biggs TM. In search of better shape in mastopexy and reduction mammoplasty. Plast Reconstr Surg 2002;110(1):309–22.

2. di Summa PG, Oranges CM, Watfa W, et al. Systematic review of outcomes and complications in nonimplant-based mastopexy surgery [published correction appears in J Plast Reconstr Aesthet Surg. 2019 Jun;72(6): 1049]. J Plast Reconstr Aesthet Surg 2019;72(2):243–72.
3. Hurwitz DJ. Agha-mohammadi S, post Bariatric surgery breast reshaping: the spiral flap. Ann Plast Surg 2006;56(5):481–6.
4. Rubin JP, Gusenoff JA, Coon D. Dermal suspension and parenchymal reshaping mastopexy after massive weight loss: statistical analysis with concomitant procedures from a prospective registry. Plast Reconstr Surg 2009;123(3):782–9.
5. Hall-Findlay EJ. The three breast dimensions: analysis and effecting change. Plast Reconstr Surg 2010;125(6):1632–42.
6. Bolletta E, Mcgoldrick C, Hall-Findlay E. Aesthetic breast surgery: what do the measurements reveal? Aesthet Surg J 2020;40(7):742–52.
7. Largo RD, Tchang LA, Mele V, et al. Efficacy, safety and complications of autologous fat grafting to healthy breast tissue: a systematic review. J Plast Reconstr Aesthet Surg 2014;67(4):437–48.
8. Graf RM, Junior IM, de Paula DR, et al. Subfascial versus subglandular breast augmentation: a Randomized prospective evaluation Considering a 5-year follow-up. Plast Reconstr Surg 2021;148(4): 760–70.
9. Gould DJ, Shauly O, Ohanissian L, et al. Subfascial breast augmentation: a systematic review and Meta-analysis of capsular contracture. Aesthet Surg J Open Forum 2020;2(1):ojaa006.
10. Khouri RK, Cardoso E, Rotemberg SC. The reverse abdominoplasty and fat transfer (RAFT) procedure: a minimally invasive, autologous breast reconstruction alternative. Isle of Ischia, Italy: Presented at the 25th Meeting of the European Assiciation of Plastic Surgeons (EURAPS); 2014.
11. Strong AL, Cederna PS, Rubin JP, et al. The Current state of fat grafting: a review of harvesting, processing, and injection techniques. Plast Reconstr Surg 2015;136(4):897–912.
12. Ramaut L, Hamdi M. Optimizing aesthetic results in free flap breast reconstruction: fat grafting and Hamdi's Hammock. Ann Breast Surg 2020;4: 28.

Secondary Body Contouring

Milind D. Kachare, MD[a,*], Brooke E. Barrow, MD, MEng[b], Sadri Ozan Sozer, MD[a]

KEYWORDS

- Body contouring • Secondary body contouring • Abdominoplasty • Lipoabdominoplasty
- Liposuction

KEY POINTS

- Patient dissatisfaction is addressed through clear communication, understanding dissatisfaction sources, and aligning expectations.
- Secondary body contouring surgery often addresses issues like incorrect initial procedure, recurrence, and aggressive liposuction.
- Correcting a high-riding scar and umbilical complications involves secondary surgeries for scar relocation and umbilical repositioning.
- Extensive scarring, large wounds, and fascial dehiscence require a comprehensive approach, involving scar revision and wound management techniques.
- Successful secondary body contouring hinges on a thorough preoperative assessment and a patient-centered approach.

 **Video content accompanies this article at http://www.plasticsurgery.theclinics.com.**

INTRODUCTION

Abdominal body contouring continues to increase in popularity in the field of plastic surgery and remains among the top aesthetic procedures performed.[1,2] Through its myriad of techniques, body contouring is an essential tool in addressing patient issues ranging from postpartum to massive weight loss (MWL), often after bariatric surgery. These surgeries, however, are not devoid of potential complications, especially those performed on the MWL population.[3] Complications range from infection, seroma, and wound dehiscence to more challenging situations, leading to suboptimal results from a host of factors, including inadequate preoperative planning, technical errors, or unpredictable tissue responses.[4,5]

These suboptimal results often pave the way for revisionary and secondary procedures, with the most common reasons for reoperation typically involving dissatisfaction with the initial aesthetic result, complications from the original surgery, or changes in the patient's body over time.[6,7] Secondary body contouring procedures are uniquely challenging, necessitating modification by the surgeon when caring for this subset of patients. This article outlines these challenges to help surgeons better understand and manage patients seeking secondary body contouring surgery.

PREOPERATIVE EVALUATION

The Disappointed Patient

Managing expectations and mitigating dissatisfaction are crucial aspects of secondary surgery. Unhappiness often stems from unmet expectations or misunderstandings about the initial surgical outcome.[8] Seek to understand the specific

[a] Private Practice, El Paso Cosmetic Surgery, 651 South Mesa Hills Drive, El Paso, TX 79912, USA; [b] Division of Plastic, Maxillofacial, and Oral Surgery, Department of Surgery, Duke University, 2301 Erwin Road, Durham, NC 2771, USA
* Corresponding author. 651 South Mesa Hills Drive, El Paso, TX 79912.
E-mail address: Milind.Kachare@gmail.com

Clin Plastic Surg 51 (2024) 173–190
https://doi.org/10.1016/j.cps.2023.09.003
0094-1298/24/

source of the patient's dissatisfaction, acknowledging their feelings and concerns. Assess the results of the initial surgery objectively and identify any actual complications or suboptimal outcomes. This evaluation serves not only to verify the patient's concerns but also to allow the surgeon to ascertain if a secondary surgical procedure or an additional surgical procedure is indeed necessary.

If secondary surgery is considered, ensure that the patient has a clear understanding of what can and cannot be achieved. This includes potential risks, benefits, and limitations. Use before-and-after pictures and plain language explanations to support your discussions.[8] This process can help realign the patient's expectations with the realistic outcomes of a secondary surgery. By involving the patient in each step of the decision-making process, you can encourage a sense of autonomy and partnership in the patient, fostering trust and satisfaction. You may also consider suggesting the patient seek a second opinion. This can validate your assessment and proposed treatment plan and further facilitate the patient's understanding and acceptance of the situation.

Even with the best surgical techniques and aesthetic judgment, you may encounter unhappy patients. The key is to remain calm and committed to a patient-centered approach, promoting open communication, setting realistic expectations, and providing comprehensive care. Managing unhappy patients before secondary surgery is not just about improving physical outcomes but also about fostering psychological well-being and patient satisfaction.[9]

Patient History

A comprehensive patient history is required before a secondary body contouring procedure. This should cover the patient's overall health and past medical issues with a particular emphasis on chronic conditions and nutrition. Obtain a complete list of medications and inquire about lifestyle aspects, like smoking, alcohol use, and exercise, which can greatly influence surgical results and recovery.[5,10,11]

In addition, dissatisfaction with body image can often signify underlying psychological conditions, like body dysmorphic disorder, mood disorders, or unattainable expectations, potentially requiring psychological assistance.[8,9]

Last, inquire about the initial body contouring procedure and the patient's level of satisfaction with their outcome.[12] It is worth emphasizing that maintaining professionalism and avoiding any disparaging remarks about the previous surgeon is good practice. The reality of surgical practice is such that no surgeon can accurately know their revision or secondary rate, as patients often prefer to consult a different surgeon for subsequent procedures.[13]

Patient Physical Examination

Begin with a general examination of the patient to assess their overall health status. Note the patient's body mass index (BMI), which may influence the decision for surgery and expected results. Several investigators have noted a BMI cutoff of 30 kg/m^2 because of the increased risk of complications and the need for reoperation.[3,5,11] In addition, the trajectory of weight change carries significant weight. For instance, a patient whose BMI elevates from 26 kg/m^2 to 30 kg/m^2 may present more surgical challenges than another whose BMI decreases from 34 kg/m^2 to 31 kg/m^2.

On examination, assess the skin quality, presence of scars from the previous surgery, asymmetry, contour irregularities, and degree of excess fat or skin. For each area, consider its characteristics and how it fits into the overall body proportion. Take a detailed account of the patient's scarring and healing from the previous surgery. Look for hypertrophic scars, keloids, or areas of poor wound healing.[7]

Photographs should be taken to document the preoperative state and for comparison in the future.[14,15] Obtaining photographs of the patient before their initial body contouring procedure may also be helpful.

While performing the physical examination, encourage the patient to express their concerns and goals. The physical examination is an opportunity to understand their anatomy, appreciate their concerns, and align your surgical plan with their goals.

PERIOPERATIVE EVALUATION

Like all surgeries, patient safety is paramount and involves several key aspects in the perioperative setting. One crucial aspect is the prevention of thrombotic events, including deep venous thrombosis and pulmonary embolism, with the appropriate use of mechanical and chemical prophylaxis.[16] In addition, proper patient positioning is key to the safety and accuracy during surgery, especially during lengthy or position-changing procedures. Incorrect positioning and padding may lead to injuries, as well as alter anatomy, which may lead to improper contouring.[17] Last, close communication with the anesthesia team is crucial to avoid complications.[10]

POSTOPERATIVE EVALUATION

A carefully devised and clearly articulated postoperative care strategy can significantly ease patient anxiety and augment their overall satisfaction. Diligent follow-up, vital for tracking recovery and swiftly addressing complications, is crucial. Considering the potential for increased anxiety or dissatisfaction stemming from previous surgery experiences, it is essential to manage expectations accurately and uphold transparent communication throughout this period. Consequently, through meticulous postoperative care, patient recovery can be optimized, and the likelihood of additional procedures can be minimized.

COMMON COMPLICATIONS LEADING TO SECONDARY SURGERY

Wrong Procedure or Insufficient Resection

Identification and prevention

For successful body contouring surgery, selection of the appropriate procedure is paramount. Sometimes, secondary surgery becomes necessary when the initially chosen procedure proves to be unsuitable. This may stem from misinterpretation of patient objectives, a lack of understanding of anatomic factors, or a mismatch between patient expectations and the results that can realistically be achieved with surgery.

Different body contouring procedures have unique indications. Rosenfield and Davis[11] presented a thorough outline and treatment algorithm for selecting the appropriate abdominoplasty procedure for each patient, ranging from liposuction only to fleur-de-lis and "corset" abdominoplasties, as well as panniculectomy or no surgery at all. Utilization of such algorithms can help guide management, but ultimately surgical judgment should be the final determinant of an individualized treatment plan. In many cases, particularly in MWL patients, a combination of procedures may be most appropriate to meet the patient's goals.[4,5,10,18,19]

Management

Managing a secondary body contouring surgery in patients who have previously undergone an unsuitable or insufficient procedure necessitates a comprehensive grasp of their current anatomic condition, the limitations of the prior operation, and their objectives for the revision surgery.

Based on the physical examination and discussion with the patient, a surgical plan tailored to the patient's needs should be designed. This might involve touch-ups, additional procedures, a different technique, or a completely different procedure than what was initially performed. For instance, if liposuction was done initially, but the patient has substantial skin laxity, an excisional procedure, such as an abdominoplasty or body lift, might be more appropriate. Moreover, a frequent mishap involves patients who have been treated with a mini or standard abdominoplasty, when they would have benefited more from an extended or circumferential approach.

Although choosing the appropriate procedure or procedures is important, careful preoperative and intraoperative decision making is necessary. The scar tissue from the initial procedure, altered anatomy, or compromised skin elasticity is among the reasons that secondary surgery is increasingly difficult. Surgical techniques may need to be adapted or modified accordingly, with a heightened focus on minimizing potential complications.

Matarasso and colleagues[7] presented a guideline for the management of secondary abdominal contour surgery, which included patients who had primary liposuction, modified abdominoplasty, or a full abdominoplasty and proceeded with either secondary liposuction or a full abdominoplasty. Other investigators have discussed the potential challenges that secondary abdominal contouring surgery may pose,[13,20,21] especially regarding tissue perfusion, including the senior author's review of 1000 consecutive cases of abdominoplasty with circumferential liposuction.[22] In this study, a delay-type effect was noted after the primary surgery, allowing for a safe readvancement of the abdominal flap.

Authors' experience

Several patients have sought help from a secondary surgeon because of a disparity between their expectations and the initial surgeon's perspective. The most frequent issue involved those who had undergone liposuction but suffered from poor skin elasticity and surplus skin. The corrective measure for these patients is often an excisional procedure, with abdominoplasty being the most common (**Fig. 1**).

However, a substantial number of patients were disappointed with the results because they were not adequately informed of the limitations and expected outcome. The authors typically encourage these patients to provide an image or an illustration that represents their anticipated postoperative appearance. This assists in accurate procedure selection to meet their desired outcome. As discussed earlier, a common scenario involves a patient who had a prior abdominoplasty but subsequently required an extended abdominoplasty. The main indication for this is lateral dog ears or excess lateral tissue causing bulging around the hips (**Fig. 2**). When undergoing secondary surgery, the surgeon should strategically evaluate the

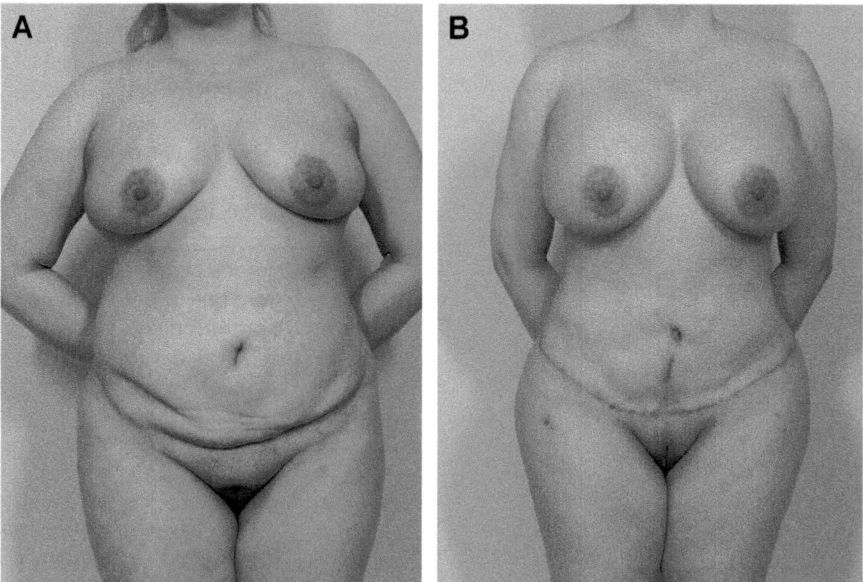

Fig. 1. (*A*) Preoperative anterior view of a patient who previously had liposuction, and (*B*) postoperative view following abdominoplasty with a vertical component from the previous umbilicus.

potential uses of the excess tissue, deciding whether it should be removed or transposed to enhance body contours (**Fig. 3**, Video 1).

Furthermore, several patients have needed additional procedures to achieve their ideal body contour. This can be facilitated through secondary liposuction, upper or lower body lifts, flankplasties, or buttock lifts. These additional procedures can supplement the primary abdominal procedure to deliver the desired aesthetic outcome (**Figs. 4** and **5**).

Last, particular attention is required when evaluating these additional procedures, notably buttock lifts. If performed accurately, they can significantly

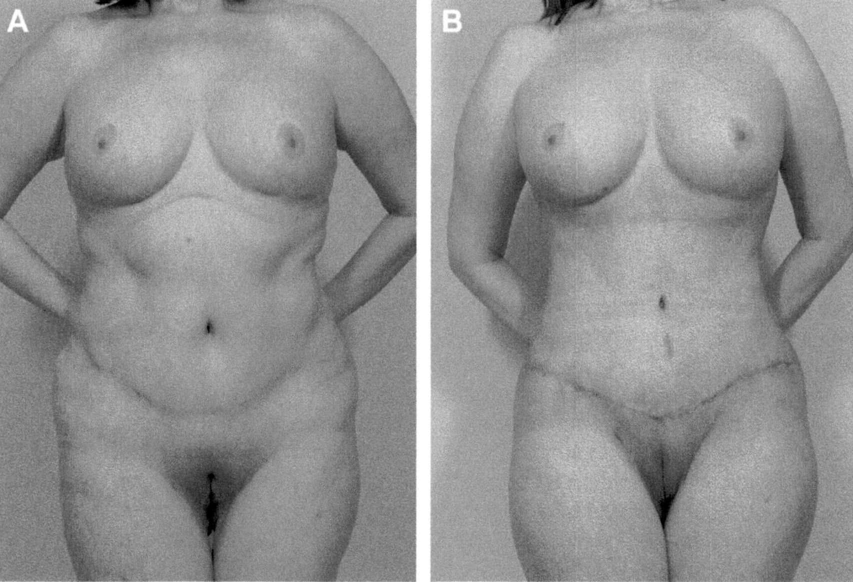

Fig. 2. (*A*) Preoperative anterior view of a patient who previously had an abdominoplasty, and (*B*) postoperative view following an extended abdominoplasty with a vertical component from the previous umbilicus and an upper back lift.

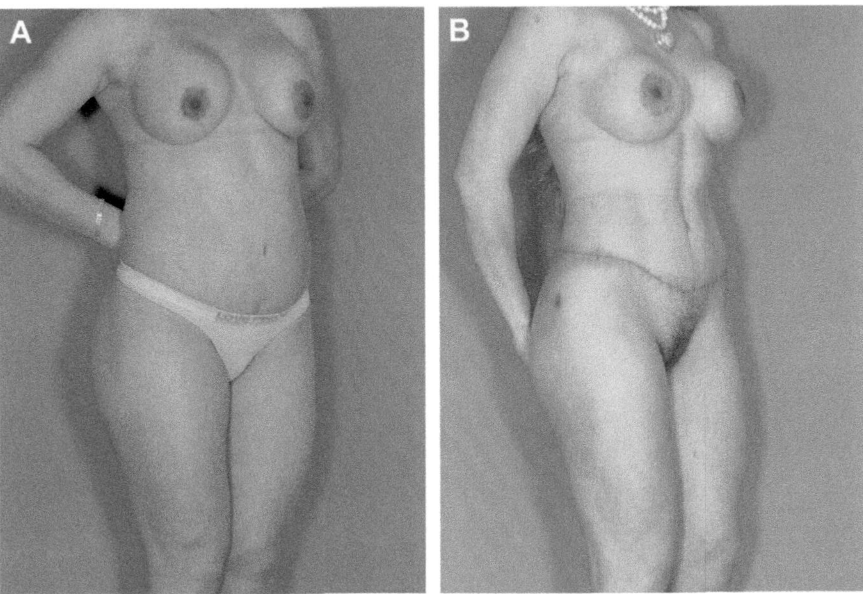

Fig. 3. (*A*) Preoperative oblique view of a patient who previously had an abdominoplasty, and (*B*) postoperative view following a lipoabdominoplasty with transposition of tissue along the lateral flank to the hip.

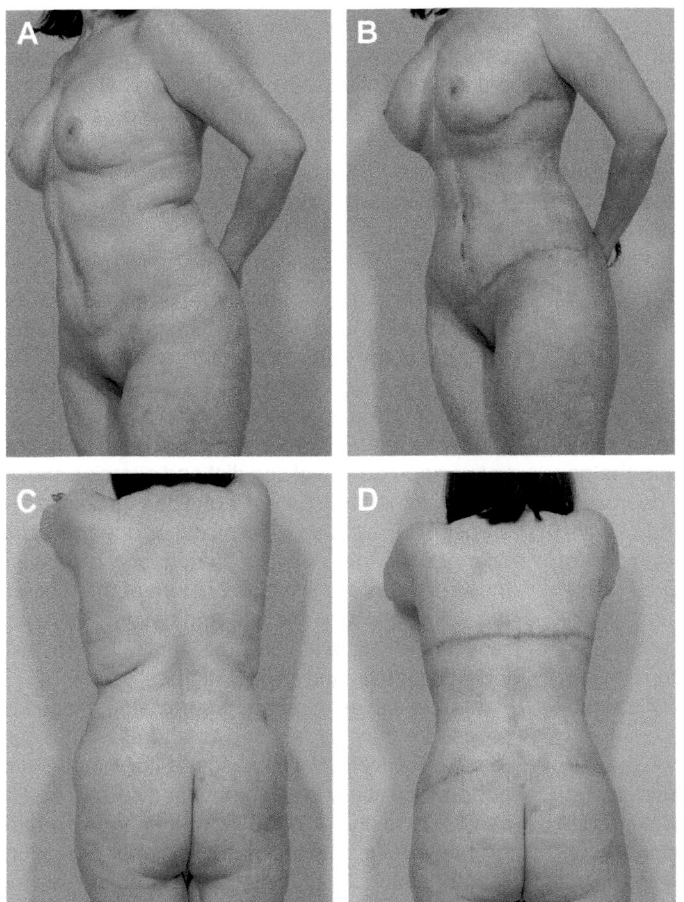

Fig. 4. (*A*, *C*) Preoperative oblique and posterior view of a patient who previously had an abdominoplasty, and (*B*, *D*) postoperative view following an extended lipoabdominoplasty and upper back lift.

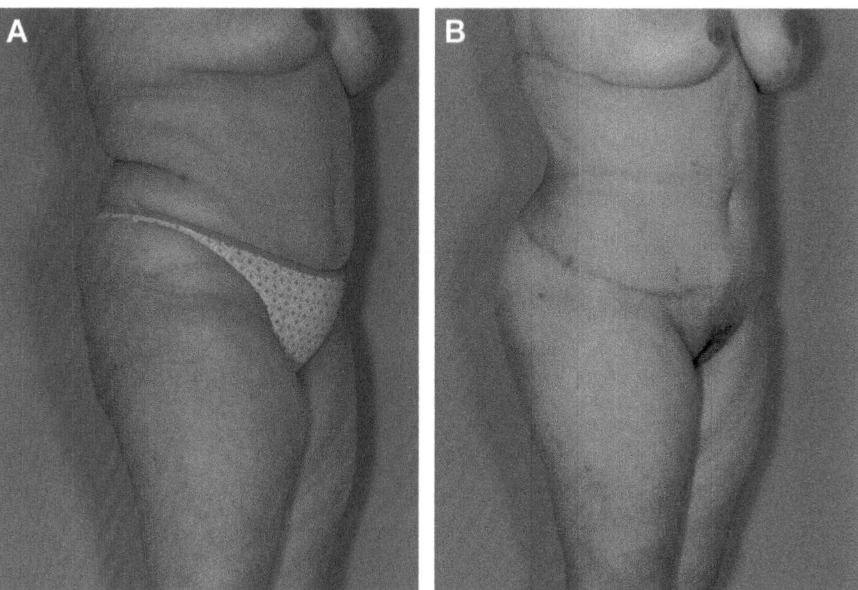

Fig. 5. (*A*) Preoperative oblique view of a patient who previously had an abdominoplasty, and (*B*) postoperative view following an upper back lift and buttock lift, without modification of the previous abdominoplasty.

enhance the overall result. However, deformities and irregularities are frequent, especially concerning complications arising from surgical tourism. The authors present a case of a patient who had industrial-grade oil injected for gluteal augmentation, which led to a necrotizing infection and severe contour deformities. The patient's situation was successfully managed using the senior author's well-established method of a split gluteal muscle flap for autologous buttock augmentation[23–25] (**Fig. 6**).

Recurrence

Identification and prevention

Recurrence in body contouring surgery is a challenging issue. The primary causes often include the natural aging process and changes in the patient's weight. With age, skin elasticity decreases from progressive loss of collagen and elastin, which can result in recurrent laxity or sagging of tissues, even after a successful procedure.[26] Similarly, weight fluctuations after surgery can significantly impact the longevity of body contouring results. Weight gain can lead to recurrence of localized fat deposits after liposuction or stretching of tightened skin.

Another key factor is the technique of the surgery itself. Inadequate resection of skin or fat, improper suturing, or insufficient muscle repair can lead to unsatisfactory results or early recurrence.[27] In addition, patients' individual biological factors, such as their healing capacity or collagen production, can also play a role in recurrence.[4]

Preexisting medical conditions, such as diabetes mellitus, or lifestyle habits, like smoking, can compromise wound healing and tissue regeneration, potentially affecting the surgical outcome. Last, the choice of an inappropriate procedure for the patient can result in recurrence, reinforcing the importance of a thorough preoperative evaluation and personalized surgical planning.

Management

A thorough evaluation of the recurrence is necessary to understand its cause. Discerning whether the recurrence is due to technical aspects of the initial surgery, changes in patient weight, aging, or other factors, guides the next steps.

If the recurrence is due to weight gain, a conservative approach involving diet and exercise should be recommended before considering secondary surgery. If the cause is technical or due to natural changes in the body, a secondary procedure may be indicated. The exact nature of the procedure will depend on the site and severity of recurrence, the patient's overall health, and their individual goals and expectations.

In some cases, a different surgical technique or procedure may be required to address the recurrence effectively. For instance, if liposuction was performed initially but the patient also has significant skin laxity, a more appropriate procedure for the revision might be an excisional procedure like abdominoplasty or body lift. Although several publications have demonstrated the safety of lipoabdominoplasty,[22,28] which is another option for

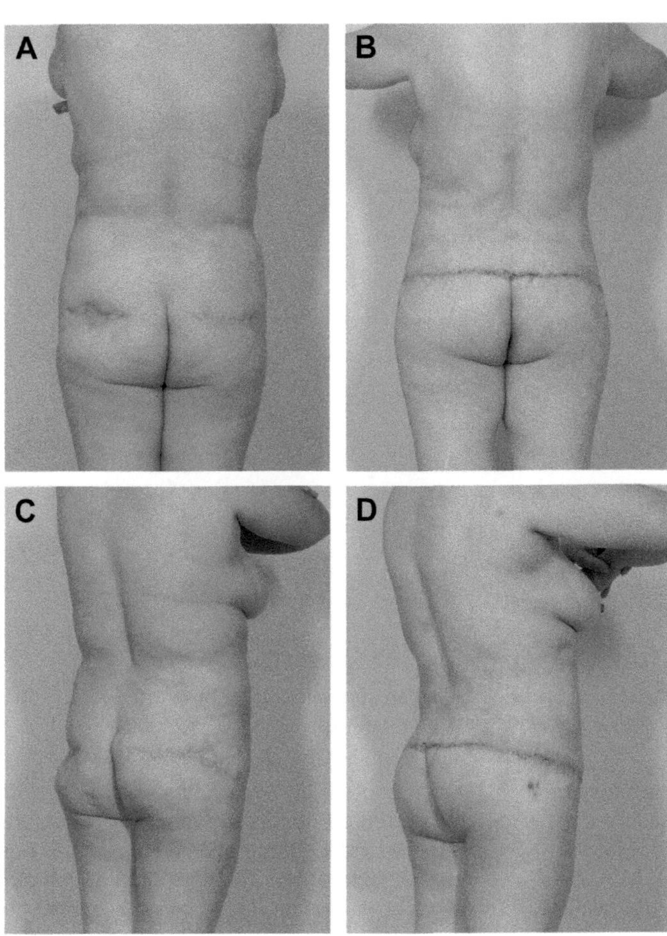

Fig. 6. (*A, C*) Preoperative posterior and oblique view of a patient who presented after having previously had industrial-grade oil injected bilaterally into her buttock in another country, which resulted in a necrotizing infection requiring several operative interventions. (*B, D*) Postoperative view following bilateral split gluteal muscle flaps for autologous buttock augmentation.

patients with recurrent skin laxity and soft tissue excess, this topic continues to be debated, and some patients may require secondary liposuction after their initial abdominoplasty.[29,30] It is imperative to understand the vascular anatomy or Huger zones of the abdominal wall, and areas to take caution during lipoabdominoplasty, such as the supraumbilical Huger zone 1. In addition, the incorporation of SAFE (Separation, Aspiration, and Fat Equalization) liposuction concepts as described by Wall and Lee[31] should be followed.

Reflecting on what might have led to the recurrence can help improve future surgical plans, both for the individual patient and for future patients. Through careful assessment, tailored surgical planning, and clear patient communication, recurrences in body contouring surgery can be effectively managed.

Authors' experience

Recurrences experienced by patients were typically due to weight fluctuations. These patients were treated as previously outlined, with a strategic plan implemented to minimize such weight fluctuations and allow for stability before undertaking secondary liposuction, readvancement of the abdominal flap, or a full secondary abdominoplasty. It has been demonstrated that all patients exhibit some degree of fascial separation or return of diastasis after surgery; therefore, a repeat plication should be performed in all cases of secondary abdominoplasty.[32] For certain patients, the issue extends beyond fascial laxity to include the weakening and laxity of the abdominal wall muscles. In such instances, these patients typically necessitate rectus muscle imbrication during the plication procedure (**Fig. 7**).

Aggressive Liposuction

Identification and prevention

Aggressive liposuction, characterized by the removal of a large volume of fat in a single procedure, can lead to a variety of issues that prompt patients to seek secondary body contouring surgery. Although liposuction is an effective tool for

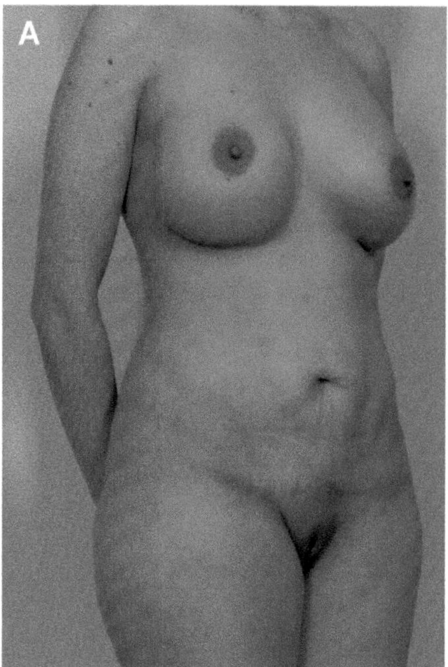

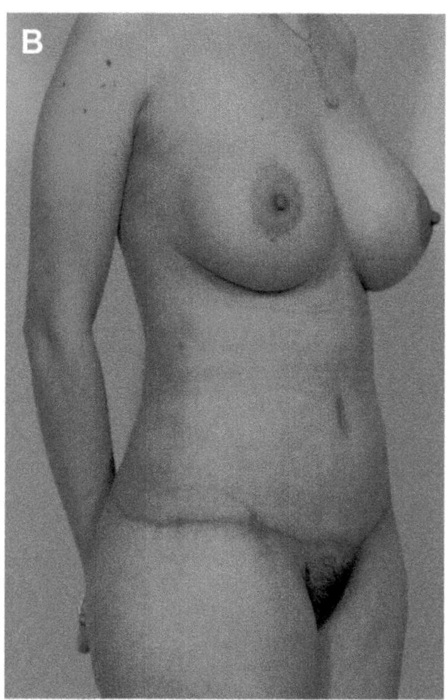

Fig. 7. (*A*) Preoperative oblique view of a patient who previously had an abdominoplasty, now with loose, redundant skin, and (*B*) postoperative view following an extended abdominoplasty.

addressing stubborn fat deposits and improving body contours, its aggressive application can result in unsatisfactory aesthetic outcomes or complications.[17]

One of the most common adverse outcomes is contour irregularities. Overaggressive liposuction can cause uneven fat removal, leading to a lumpy or wavy appearance of the skin.[17] Other irregularities include cannula line deformities from superficial liposuction and puckered scars at the incision site from failing to turn the suction off during insertion and removal of the cannula.[5] Patients with soft and loose fat are more prone to these irregularities, as this type of fat is easier to resect and susceptible to overresection.[17] Improper patient positioning can also contribute to these irregularities. This unevenness may not be immediately evident postoperatively and can become more apparent as swelling subsides.

Skin laxity is another problem associated with aggressive liposuction. When large volumes of fat are removed, the overlying skin may not retract adequately, particularly in older patients or those with poor skin elasticity. This can result in loose, sagging skin in the treated area.

Furthermore, aggressive liposuction can lead to complications, such as seromas, hematomas, or even more serious issues like damage to underlying structures or fat embolism. These complications may necessitate secondary interventions or surgeries for treatment.[4,5]

Finally, aggressive liposuction might lead to overly corrected areas, giving an unnatural appearance and leading patients to seek revision surgery for restoration of a more natural contour. Therefore, the desire for significant immediate change must be balanced with an understanding of the limitations and potential complications of the procedure.

Management

Surgically managing a patient who has undergone aggressive liposuction and now seeks secondary body contouring surgery presents unique challenges and requires a well-considered approach.

For patients presenting with contour irregularities, secondary liposuction might be used in adjacent areas to improve overall contour, whereas fat grafting can be used to correct depressions or divots. Careful and meticulous technique is essential to avoid overcorrection and to achieve a smooth and natural contour.[7,13,17] In the case of skin laxity following aggressive liposuction, excisional procedures might be required.[7,13]

In managing postoperative complications, such as seromas or hematomas, appropriate drainage or removal is necessary, potentially followed by supportive treatments to aid healing. Significant complications, such as damage to underlying structures, may require more complex reconstructive procedures and multidisciplinary approaches.

In all scenarios, a keen understanding of the patient's anatomy, the changes induced by the initial aggressive liposuction, and the patient's goals and expectations for revisionary surgery will guide the most appropriate strategy for surgical management. The overall aim is to restore a balanced, natural body contour, while ensuring patient safety and satisfaction.

Authors' experience

Numerous patients have sought help after undergoing liposuction, only to later require an excisional procedure, such as abdominoplasty. Nevertheless, a significant number of these patients had aggressive primary liposuction, resulting in pronounced contour abnormalities throughout the abdomen. These cases are particularly complicated; therefore, a staged approach tends to be most appropriate.

Initially, the patient should undergo area-specific rigotomies, along with secondary liposuction and fat grafting to help rectify the contour irregularities. After ample recovery time, allowing the fat graft to settle, the second stage consisting of an excisional procedure with advancement could be performed.

During this process, it is important to recognize that the presence of significant scar tissue from the previous surgery often limits the mobility of the abdominal flap. Scoring of the Scarpa fascia aids in advancing the flap, a notion also highlighted by Matarasso and colleagues[7] (**Fig. 8**, Video 2).

High-Riding Scar and Umbilicus

Identification and prevention

The placement of the incision and the umbilicus significantly influences the outcome of body contouring surgery.[5,33,34] These complications, often rooted in surgical technique, can have unsettling consequences.

Most commonly, a low transverse incision is preferred, with most describing a distance of 6 to 7 cm superior to the anterior vulvar commissure that proceeds laterally 1 to 2 cm above the inguinal crease, with the length depending on the type of abdominoplasty and amount of tissue excision planned.[35] Although variability exists for incision placement, an incision that is placed too high, causing a high-riding scar, can be very disconcerting to a patient.

In addition, an unnatural-appearing umbilicus, often characterized by improper size, shape, depth, or placement, is a common complication. It too can serve as an obvious indicator of an abdominoplasty, given the visibility of the surrounding scar.[36] Although aesthetics can vary, the most favored appearance involves a midline, vertically oriented, oval-shaped umbilicus, with superior hooding at the level of the iliac crests.[36,37] It typically has a mean depth of 1.16 cm and averages 0.6 to 3.0 cm in size.[38] Other possible complications involving the umbilicus include stenosis, closure, infection, or even necrosis, typically resulting from excessive dissection or compromised circulation.

Management

Dealing with a high-riding scar and umbilical complications after body contouring surgery necessitates a tailored approach, considering the specific nature and severity of each complication. Secondary surgery aims to reinstate an aesthetically appealing and natural-looking abdomen.

An unnatural appearance of the umbilicus owing to issues with its size, shape, depth, or position can be rectified by revisionary surgery that reshapes or resizes the umbilicus or relocates it to a more anatomically fitting location. It is a complex task, and a thorough understanding of the previous surgical approach is pivotal. Knowing whether the umbilicus retained its blood supply from the stalk, following a circumferential relocation, or from the subdermal plexus, following a float procedure, as well as the presence of a previous umbilical hernia, is crucial.[7,21,22,39] Notably, subsequent circumferential incisions after a float procedure, or vice versa, do not necessarily induce umbilical necrosis.[21,39] Still, an awareness of the perfusion-related risks and complications is imperative.

Patients must be apprised that when advancing the abdominal flap to manage a high-riding scar, special attention is required for the umbilicus. For minor superior displacements of the umbilicus accompanied by excess skin, an umbilical float procedure with supplementary advancement and excision of abdominal tissue to relocate the scar may suffice, bypassing the need for an additional scar. However, if the umbilicus is significantly malpositioned, patients should be prepared for another, likely vertical, scar.[7,21]

Although demonstrated to be safe, a concern remains for umbilical necrosis. Similar to infection, nonoperative management is initially appropriate and, depending on the extent of necrosis, it may be possible to salvage the umbilicus.

Stenosis of the umbilicus is a recognized complication, usually owing to the choice of a small circular scar shape, which increases the chances of a cicatricial event. Multiple stenting methods, including earplugs, have been described to maintain the umbilical opening without inducing pressure necrosis.[34]

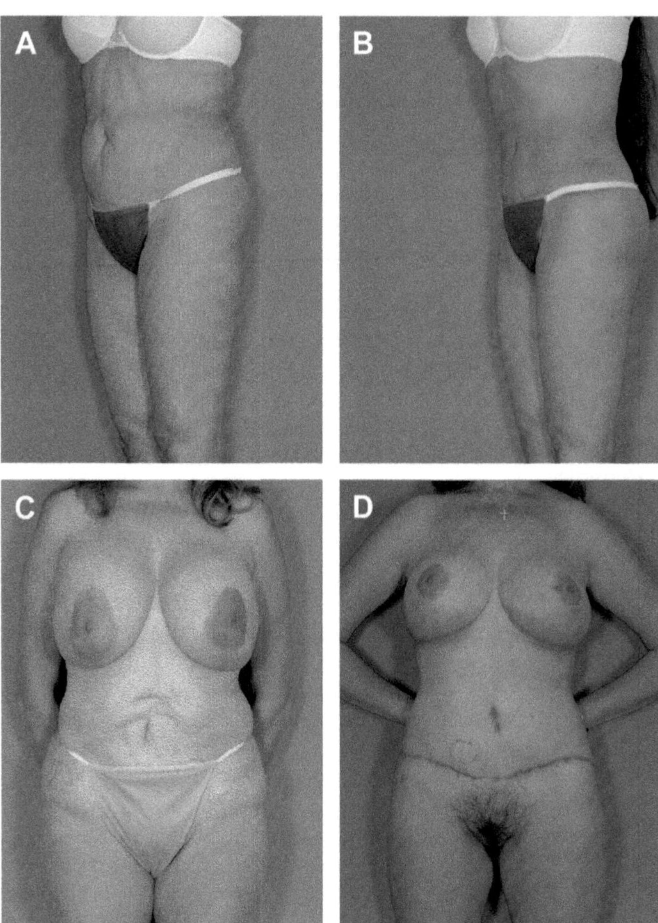

Fig. 8. (*A, C*) Preoperative view of 2 patients who previously had aggressive liposuction, and (*B, D*) postoperative view of the result after a staged approach with rigotomies, fat grafting, and eventual extended abdominoplasty.

Total umbilical loss or closure may call for neo-umbilicoplasty, because an absent umbilicus may appear abnormal. Various methods for umbilical reconstruction have been described,[40,41] including the use of abdominal flaps with or without external scars and graft utilization, as outlined comprehensively by Gardani and colleagues.[41]

With personalized surgical planning and diligent postoperative care, patients with high-riding scars are able to be repositioned with appropriate management of the umbilicus.

Authors' experience

Striving to retain the natural umbilicus is often advisable when possible. As demonstrated by Dean and colleagues,[21] the umbilicus can survive secondary procedures, even after previous severance of the stalk. Although various techniques exist for creating a new umbilicus, they often fall short in replicating the long-term aesthetic of a natural one. Therefore, attempts should be made to preserve the original.

During excisional procedures, the natural umbilicus can be preserved either by floating it downward or by relocating it through a different opening via a circumferential incision. If the umbilicus is high and aesthetically pleasing, it can be floated down. The umbilical stalk is divided at its base during the elevation of the detached abdominal flap, allowing for the exposure and repair of any existing umbilical hernia. After rectus fascial plication, the umbilicus is floated down and secured in its new location in 4 quadrants with interrupted 3-0 Polydioxanone (Ethicon, Inc, Somerville, NJ, USA) sutures. Caution should be taken to prevent an abnormally low repositioning (**Fig. 9**).

If the umbilicus is not high or shows visible scarring, a circular incision for relocation is preferred. Patients with existing scar tissue typically require a vertical scar component, and a delay procedure might be considered if a previous float procedure was performed[21,39] (**Fig. 10**).

For an entirely irreparable or previously removed umbilicus, reconstructive creation of a new one is

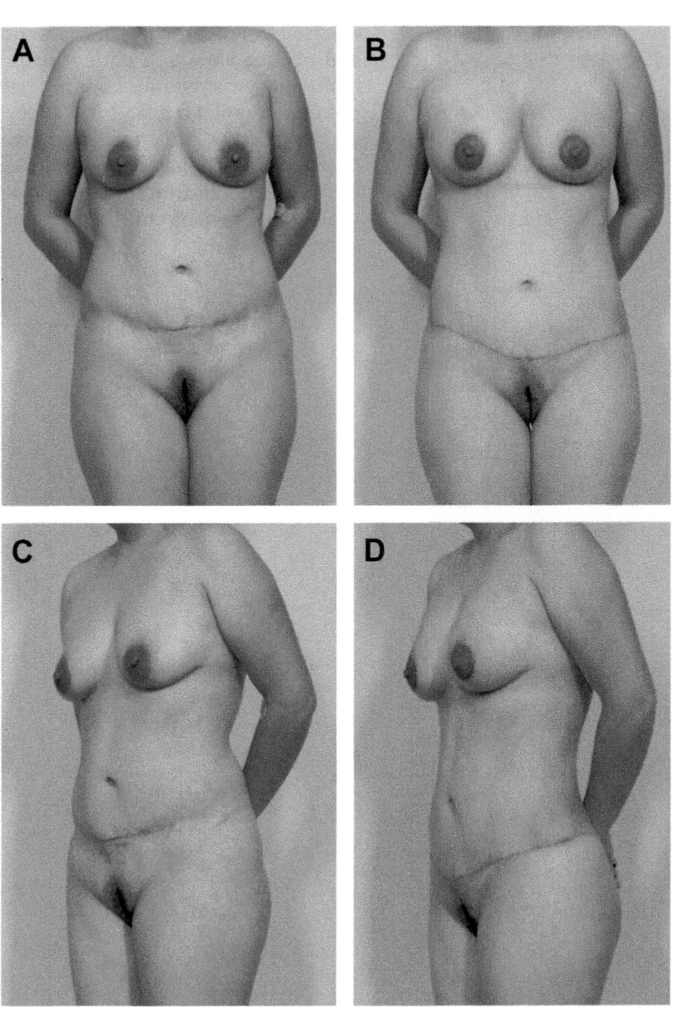

Fig. 9. (*A, B*) Preoperative anterior and oblique view of a patient with a high-riding scar and a minimal superiorly displaced umbilicus, and (*C, D*) postoperative views after readvancement of the abdominal flap with an umbilical float procedure.

necessary. This involves defatting a circular area in the midline of the detached abdominal flap and securing it to the rectus fascia with 4-0 Prolene (Ethicon, Inc) interrupted quilting or surgical net-like sutures. Typically, creating a depression similar to an umbilicus requires about 8 interrupted sutures, which should be left in place for 2 weeks. A common complication is a loss of depth, a shared issue among numerous techniques.[40,41] Despite best efforts, the reconstructed umbilicus often does not replicate the aesthetic of a natural one (**Figs. 11** and **12**, Video 3).

Extensive Scarring, Large Wounds, Fascial Dehiscence

Identification and prevention

Like any surgery, body contouring carries risks, with the specific issues of extensive scarring, large wounds, and fascial dehiscence often leading patients to consider a secondary procedure.[42]

Scarring is an inherent part of postoperative healing. Factors such as genetic predisposition, skin type, surgical technique, and postoperative care greatly influence the final scar quality. Scars may become hypertrophic or evolve into keloids, or present as wide, irregular, or misplaced, causing patient dissatisfaction and necessitating scar revision.[5,33]

Wound complications, such as infection, hematoma, or seroma, can negatively affect the healing process, leading to increased scarring or delayed healing. Contributing factors range from insufficient aseptic technique and suboptimal postoperative care to patient-specific conditions, like diabetes or smoking.[4,43] Large wounds or tissue necrosis may result from poor perfusion, attributable to either surgical technique or patient-related issues.

Fascial dehiscence, a separation at the fascial layer, is a more severe complication, typically owing to technical mishaps during closure,

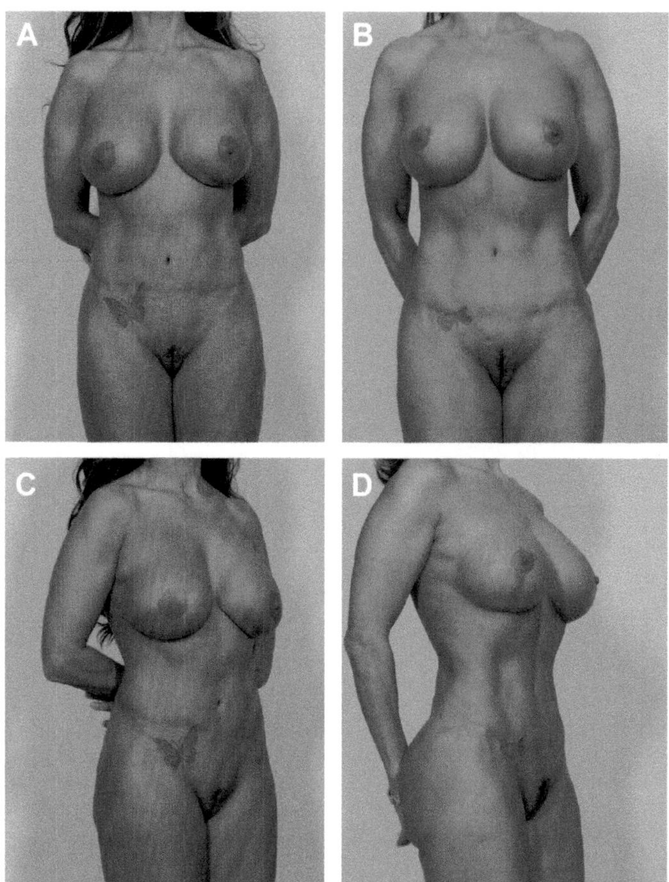

Fig. 10. (*A*, *B*) Preoperative anterior and oblique view of a patient with a high-riding scar and an appropriately positioned umbilicus, and (*C*, *D*) postoperative views after readvancement of the abdominal flap with repositioning of the umbilicus resulting in a vertical component from the previous umbilicus.

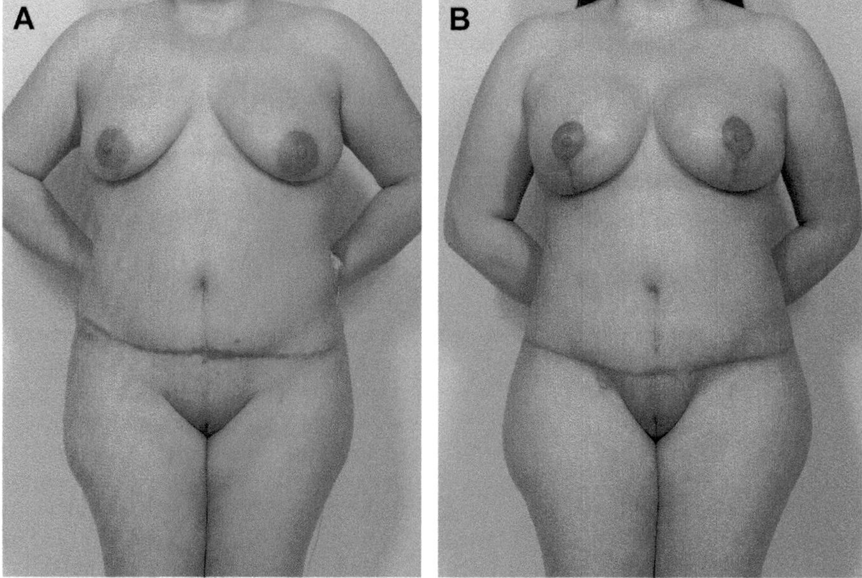

Fig. 11. (*A*) Preoperative anterior view of a patient who previously had an abdominoplasty, and (*B*) postoperative view following a secondary abdominoplasty and neo-umbilicoplasty.

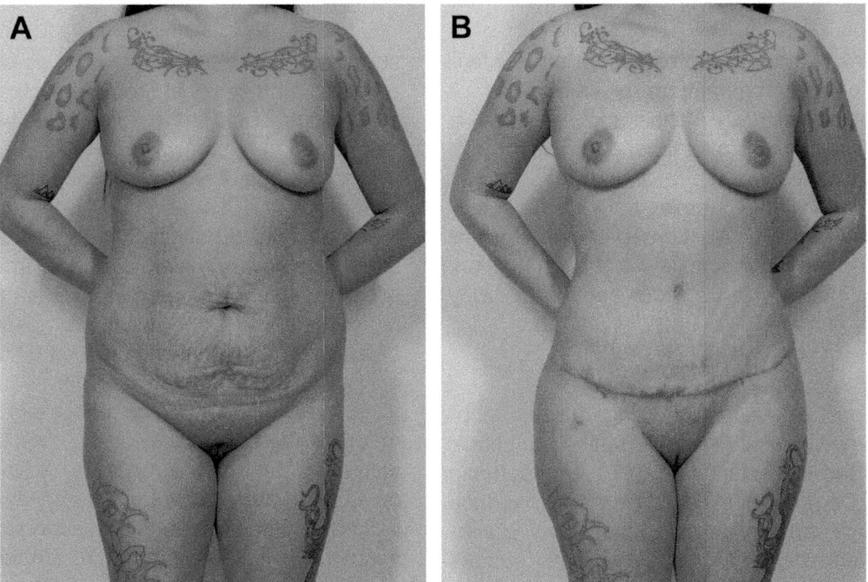

Fig. 12. (*A*) Preoperative anterior view of a patient who previously had liposuction, and (*B*) postoperative view following an abdominoplasty and neo-umbilicoplasty.

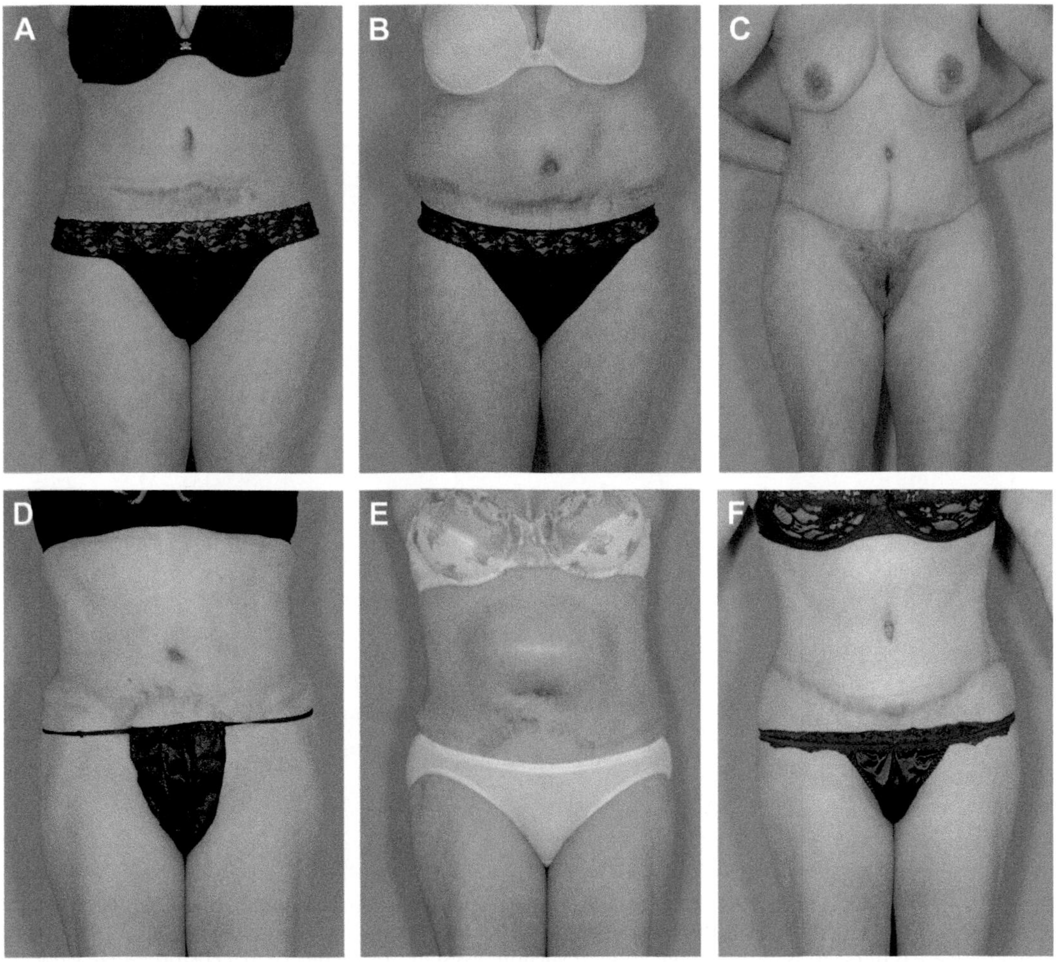

Fig. 13. (*A*, *D*) Preoperative anterior view of 2 patients with a high and wide scar, with minimal redundant skin following previous abdominoplasty. (*B*, *E*) Patients required tissue expansion to increase the available skin. (*C*, *F*) Postoperative views of the result after removal of the tissue expander and advancement of the newly expanded abdominal flap.

elevated intra-abdominal pressure, or patient factors, like obesity, malnutrition, or smoking.[7,27] A notable observation by Nahas and Ferreira[44] is the recurring diastasis over time, even with appropriate surgical technique.

Complications like these can detrimentally impact the aesthetic outcome, cause physical discomfort, and induce anxiety or dissatisfaction, prompting patients to consider secondary body contouring surgery.

Management

Scarring can be managed using various techniques, including scar revision surgery that entails removing the old scar and cautiously resuturing the site.[33] Considerations must be made to reduce unnecessary tension on the closure site, potentially implementing progressive tension sutures when the abdominal flap is reelevated to distribute the tension toward the fascial system, thereby reducing skin closure tension.[45] In addition, the advent of incisional dressings and tension-reducing devices may aid in scar quality improvement.[46,47] Depending on the individual case, supplementary treatments, such as silicone gels or sheets, intralesional steroid injections, or laser therapy, may be used to refine scar color, texture, and elevation.[5,48–50]

In the setting of wound complications, similar to infections, the cause must be identified and managed, which may involve the use of systemic antibiotics or surgical debridement for more extreme cases. Hematomas and seromas might necessitate surgical washout, aspiration, or drainage. If any skin irregularities or contour abnormalities persist after resolution, additional surgical intervention may be necessary, using the methods discussed previously.[4] Management of incisional dehiscence calls for diligent wound care, and potentially, surgical intervention. If the wound is clean, healing by secondary intention might be a suitable approach. Extensive dehiscence, however, may require surgical intervention, with a particular focus on minimizing tension on the wound edges to prevent recurrence. In situations where wounds cannot be closed primarily, consideration of other reconstructive methods may be necessary to ensure a closed, healed

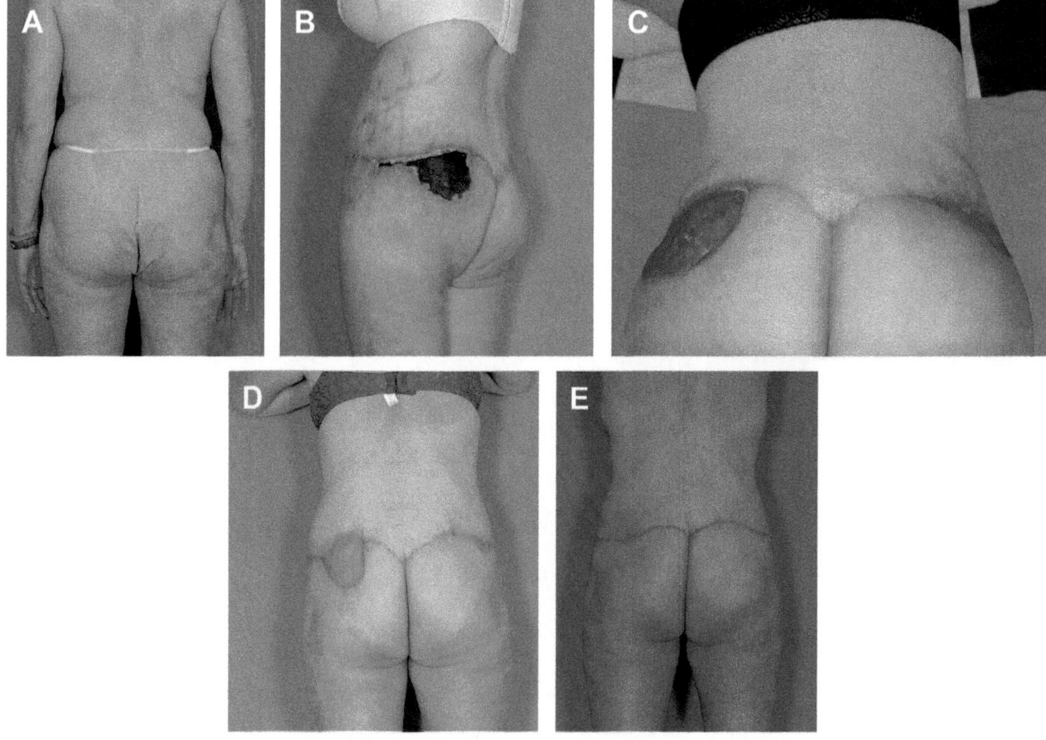

Fig. 14. (*A*) Preoperative posterior view of patient before circumferential abdominoplasty. (*B*) Postoperative oblique view of skin necrosis over the left posterior flank/buttock area. (*C*) On table view after debridement of bilateral areas of necrosis before application of vacuum-assisted closure device. (*D*) Postoperative view after skin graft of remaining wound, and (*E*) final result after serial excisions to revise the scar and remove the grafted area.

wound before embarking on any secondary body contouring procedures, as you may only have one chance to adequately repair the defect.

Fascial dehiscence, or recurrence, presents a great challenge in terms of management, often demanding surgical intervention for the rectification of fascial defects.[7,44] It is worth mentioning that the fascia tends to be weaker in subsequent operations, potentially requiring additional reinforcement, such as a mesh. Various techniques are available, each differing in their approach, sutures, and use of reinforcement.[27,32] Although common practice leans toward a one- or two-layered midline fascial closure using either absorbable or nonabsorbable sutures, there remains no universally recognized standard of care.[32]

In any case, secondary body contouring surgery must always be accompanied by meticulous postoperative care and follow-up to promote optimal healing and avert further complications.

Authors' experience

The senior author has encountered several complex cases that necessitated innovative solutions. For scar-related complications, when possible, an excisional procedure or readvancement was performed. Progressive tension sutures have been used during abdominoplasty procedures, yielding benefits such as enabling patients to stand immediately after surgery, reducing seroma formation, and aiding in the creation of more aesthetically pleasing skin closures. For extensive wounds, a sequential approach was adopted, focusing first on complete healing before proceeding with the required reconstruction. Fascial plication was repeated in all patients undergoing secondary surgery.

The presence of a high-riding scar was also a commonly observed complication, as described in a previous section. Addressing some of these, as well as scars from large wounds presented significant challenges, as the scar could not be eliminated through simple readvancement of the abdominal flap. Some patients required staged and serial excision and advancement, whereas others necessitated the use of skin grafts or tissue expanders to augment the available skin. This allowed for the excision of the old scar and the

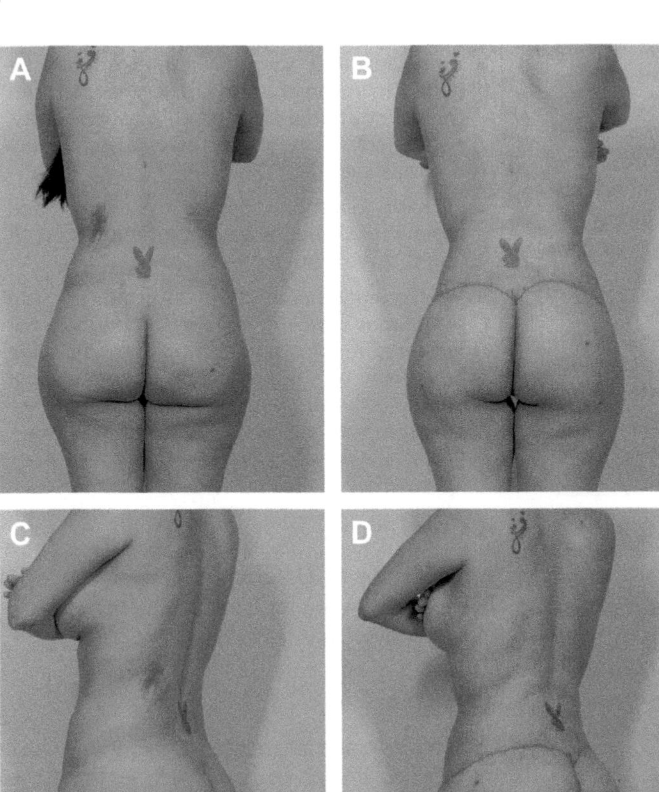

Fig. 15. (*A, B*) Preoperative posterior and oblique view of a patient who previously had bilateral gluteal augmentation with silicone implants and presented with malposition of her implants associated with pain. (*C, D*) Postoperative view after bilateral implant removal and split gluteal muscle flaps for autologous buttock augmentation.

repositioning and advancement of the skin to a more aesthetically pleasing location (**Figs. 13** and **14**).

Last, as previously mentioned, lower body lifts and gluteal augmentation procedures often come with their share of complications. The senior author has frequently dealt with complications arising from gluteal implants necessitating a secondary operation. Typically, this secondary procedure involves the removal of the implants, followed by a split gluteal muscle flap for autologous buttock augmentation[23–25] (**Fig. 15**).

AUTHORS' COMMON PRACTICE AND SURGICAL PEARLS FOR RISK REDUCTION

Seroma

The senior author previously reported a seroma rate of 19% in a series of 1000 consecutive cases.[22] However, with the subsequent introduction of progressive tension sutures in the practice, along with the elimination of drains, a notable reduction in the seroma rate has been observed, mirroring findings reported in recently published literature.[45]

Thromboembolism

The authors diligently assess all patients using the Caprini Risk Assessment Model to determine their susceptibility to thromboembolic incidents. The authors' protocols mandate maintaining adequate hydration before and during surgery. During the operation, they use mechanical prophylaxis with the use of sequential compression devices. After the procedure, the authors endorse early mobilization and provide a 3-week course of Xarelto (10 mg). In addition, they routinely perform conduct a Doppler ultrasound examination of both lower extremities on the seventh postoperative day.

Postoperative Garments

The authors instruct patients not to wear any postoperative garments during the initial 2 weeks following the procedure. These compression garments have been shown to increase lower-extremity venous stasis and recently have been demonstrated to have limited benefit in managing seroma and postoperative edema.[51,52]

SUMMARY

Body contouring operations, although frequently conducted, are not without complexities, especially because of the specific patient demographics. This leads to a notable frequency of revision and secondary body contouring procedures. Nevertheless, these secondary procedures can present unique challenges. It is essential to align patient expectations with achievable surgical possibilities, address any shortcomings thoughtfully, and strategize ways to optimize results. The aim with this article is to offer a comprehensive analysis of handling these intricate cases, thereby enriching the reader's armamentarium when embarking on secondary body contouring surgeries.

CLINICS CARE POINTS

- When dealing with secondary procedures, it is important to manage patients' expectations, continually reinforcing the notion that the best chance for optimal results was during the initial operation.
- Avoid getting distracted by the patient's complaints. As a plastic surgeon, you must evaluate the patient comprehensively, considering all angles in a 360° manner. For instance, a patient expressing dissatisfaction with a scar might also require additional liposuction, fat grafting, and excess skin removal along with the scar revision.
- Every aesthetic surgeon should initially be skilled in reconstructive surgery, as it forms the foundational basis of all plastic surgery, particularly when correcting secondary deformities.
- Exercise caution before excising and removing tissue; always contemplate if it might serve a purpose.
- Interestingly, secondary procedures can sometimes offer certain benefits. For instance, a prior abdominoplasty can serve as a delay of the detached abdominal flap, enabling the surgeon to take a more aggressive approach in the subsequent operation.

DISCLOSURE

The senior author, O. Sozer, is an investor in Brijjit. However, there are no financial interests or conflicts of interest in regards to this article.

SUPPLEMENTARY DATA

Supplementary data related to this article can be found online at https://doi.org/10.1016/j.cps.2023.09.003.

REFERENCES

1. American Society of Plastic Surgeons Plastic Surgery Statistics Report. ASPS National Clearinghouse

of Plastic Surgery Procedural Statistics, Available at: https://www.plasticsurgery.org/documents/News/Statistics/2020/plastic-surgery-statistics-full-report-2020.pdf. Accessed June 1, 2023.
2. The Aesthetic Society Aesthetic Plastic Surgery National Databank Statistics 2020–2021, Available at: https://cdn.theaestheticsociety.org/media/statistics/2021-TheAestheticSocietyStatistics.pdf. Accessed June 1, 2023.
3. Reischies FMJ, Tiefenbacher F, Holzer-Geissler JCJ, et al. BMI and revision surgery for abdominoplasties: complication Definitions Revisited using the Clavien-Dindo classification. Plast Reconstr Surg Glob Open 2023;11(2):e4411.
4. Matarasso A. Awareness and avoidance of abdominoplasty complications. Aesthet Surg J 1997;17(4): 256, 258-261.
5. Ferry AM, Chamata E, Dibbs RP, et al. Avoidance and correction of deformities in body contouring. Semin Plast Surg 2021;35(2):110–8.
6. Guest RA, Amar D, Czerniak S, et al. Heterogeneity in body contouring outcomes based Research: the Pittsburgh body contouring complication reporting system. Aesthet Surg J 2017; 38(1):60–70.
7. Matarasso A, Schneider LF, Barr J. The incidence and management of secondary abdominoplasty and secondary abdominal contour surgery. Plast Reconstr Surg 2014;133(1):40–50.
8. Desai V. Managing an unhappy patient. Indian J Plast Surg 2021;54(4):495–500.
9. Sykes J, Javidnia H. A contemporary review of the management of the difficult patient. JAMA Facial Plast Surg 2013;15(2):81–4.
10. Shrivastava P, Aggarwal A, Khazanchi RK. Body contouring surgery in a massive weight loss patient: an overview. Indian J Plast Surg 2008;41(Suppl): S114–29.
11. Rosenfield LK, Davis CR. Evidence-Based abdominoplasty review with body contouring algorithm. Aesthet Surg J 2019;39(6):643–61.
12. de Vries CEE, Klassen AF, Hoogbergen MM, et al. Measuring outcomes in Cosmetic abdominoplasty: the BODY-Q. Clin Plast Surg 2020;47(3):429–36.
13. Matarasso A, Wallach SG, Rankin M, et al. Secondary abdominal contour surgery: a review of early and late reoperative surgery. Plast Reconstr Surg 2005; 115(2):627–32.
14. Jabir S. A short introduction to Clinical photography for the plastic surgeon. World J Plast Surg 2016; 5(2):183–4.
15. Aveta A, Filoni A, Persichetti P. Digital photography in plastic surgery: the importance of standardization in the era of medicolegal issues. Plast Reconstr Surg 2012;130(3):490e–1e.
16. Kraft CT, Janis JE. Deep venous thrombosis prophylaxis. Clin Plast Surg 2020;47(3):409–14.
17. Dispaltro FL, Gingrass MK, Chang KN, et al. Correcting lipoplasty contour irregularities. Aesthet Surg J 2001;21(5):435–40.
18. Song AY, Jean RD, Hurwitz DJ, et al. A classification of contour deformities after bariatric weight loss: the Pittsburgh Rating Scale. Plast Reconstr Surg 2005; 116(5):1535–44 [discussion: 1545–6].
19. Shermak MA. Abdominoplasty with combined surgery. Clin Plast Surg 2020;47(3):365–77.
20. Samra S, Sawh-Martinez R, Barry O, et al. Complication rates of lipoabdominoplasty versus traditional abdominoplasty in high-risk patients. Plast Reconstr Surg 2010;125(2):683–90.
21. Dean RA, Dean JA, Matarasso A. Secondary abdominoplasty: management of the umbilicus after prior stalk Transection. Plast Reconstr Surg 2019; 143(4):729e–33e.
22. Sozer SO, Basaran K, Alim H. Abdominoplasty with circumferential liposuction: a review of 1000 consecutive cases. Plast Reconstr Surg 2018;142(4): 891–901.
23. Sozer SO, Erhan Eryilmaz O. Autologous flap gluteal augmentation: split gluteal flap technique. Clin Plast Surg 2018;45(2):269–75.
24. Sozer SO, Agullo FJ, Palladino H. Split gluteal muscle flap for autoprosthesis buttock augmentation. Plast Reconstr Surg 2012;129(3):766–76.
25. Sozer SO, Agullo FJ, Palladino H. Autologous augmentation gluteoplasty with a dermal fat flap. Aesthet Surg J 2008;28(1):70–6.
26. Lovell CR, Smolenski KA, Duance VC, et al. Type I and III collagen content and fibre distribution in normal human skin during ageing. Br J Dermatol 1987;117(4):419–28.
27. Gilbert MM, Anderson SR, Abtahi AR. Alternative abdominal wall plication techniques: a review of current literature. Aesthet Surg J 2023. https://doi.org/10.1093/asj/sjad112.
28. Farkas J, Roostaeian J, Barton F, et al. Abdominal Flap Perfusion in Abdominoplasty- Does Undermining Cause Any Untoward Effect?, Conference: The Aesthetic Meeting 2013 The American Society for Aesthetic Plastic Surgery.
29. Mendez BM, Coleman JE, Kenkel JM. Optimizing patient outcomes and safety with liposuction. Aesthet Surg J 2019;39(1):66–82.
30. Saldanha O, Ordenes AI, Goyeneche C, et al. Lipoabdominoplasty with anatomic Definition: an Evolution on Saldanha's technique. Clin Plast Surg 2020; 47(3):335–49.
31. Wall SH Jr, Lee MR. Separation, aspiration, and fat Equalization: SAFE liposuction concepts for comprehensive body contouring. Plast Reconstr Surg. Dec 2016;138(6):1192–201.
32. Nahas FX, Faustino LD, Ferreira LM. Abdominal wall plication and correction of deformities of the Myoaponeurotic layer: focusing on materials and techniques

used for Synthesis. Aesthet Surg J 2019;39(Suppl_2): S78–84.

33. Chambers A. Management of scarring following aesthetic surgery. In: Téot L, Mustoe TA, Middelkoop E, et al, editors. Textbook on scar management: state of the art management and emerging technologies. Cham, Switzerland: Springer Nature Switzerland AG; 2020. p. 385–95. The Author(s).
34. Kachare S, Kapsalis C, Kachare M, et al. Earplug umbilicoplasty: a simple method to prevent umbilical stenosis in a Tummy Tuck. Eplasty 2019;19:e12.
35. Rubin JP, Neligan PC. Plastic surgery - E-Book: volume 2: aesthetic surgery. Amsterdam, Netherlands: Elsevier Health Sciences; 2017.
36. Joseph WJ, Sinno S, Brownstone ND, et al. Creating the Perfect umbilicus: a systematic review of recent literature. Aesthetic Plast Surg 2016;40(3):372–9.
37. Ribeiro RC, Saltz R, Ramirez C, et al. Anatomical position of umbilicus in Latin-American patients. Eur J Plast Surg 2019;42(4):351–8.
38. Fell CK, Kachare MD, Moore A, et al. Does size really Matter? A review on how to determine the optimal umbilical size during an abdominoplasty. ePlasty 2023;23:e38.
39. Parsa FD, Cheng J, Hu MS, et al. The importance of umbilical blood supply and umbilical delay in secondary abdominoplasty: a case Report. Aesthet Surg J 2018;38(5):NP81–7.
40. Lee YT, Kwon C, Rhee SC, et al. Four flaps technique for neoumbilicoplasty. Arch Plast Surg 2015; 42(3):351–5.
41. Gardani M, Palli D, Simonacci F, et al. Umbilical reconstruction: different techniques, a single aim. Acta Biomed 2019;90(4):504–9.
42. Gusenoff JA. Prevention and management of complications in body contouring surgery. Clin Plast Surg 2014;41(4):805–18.
43. Kaoutzanis C, Gupta V, Winocour J, et al. Incidence and risk factors for Major surgical site infections in aesthetic surgery: analysis of 129,007 patients. Aesthet Surg J 2017;37(1):89–99.
44. Nahas FX, Ferreira LM. Concepts on correction of the musculoaponeurotic layer in abdominoplasty. Clin Plast Surg 2010;37(3):527–38.
45. Pollock TA, Pollock H. Drainless abdominoplasty using progressive tension sutures. Clin Plast Surg 2020;47(3):351–63.
46. Zwanenburg PR, Timmermans FW, Timmer AS, et al. A systematic review evaluating the influence of incisional Negative Pressure Wound Therapy on scarring. Wound Repair Regen 2021;29(1):8–19.
47. Eaves FF III. Commentary on: the Use of mean Gray Value (MGV) as a guide to tension-reducing Strategies in body contouring surgery reduces wound-related Morbidity. Aesthetic Surg J 2022;43(2): NP131–3.
48. Sidgwick GP, McGeorge D, Bayat A. A comprehensive evidence-based review on the role of topicals and dressings in the management of skin scarring. Arch Dermatol Res 2015;307(6): 461–77.
49. Commander SJ, Chamata E, Cox J, et al. Update on Postsurgical scar management. Semin Plast Surg 2016;30(3):122–8.
50. Monstrey S, Middelkoop E, Vranckx JJ, et al. Updated scar management practical guidelines: non-invasive and invasive measures. J Plast Reconstr Aesthet Surg 2014;67(8):1017–25.
51. Fontes de Moraes BZ, Ferreira LM, Martins MRC, et al. Do compression garments prevent Subcutaneous edema after abdominoplasty? Aesthetic Surg J 2022;43(3):329–36.
52. Keane AM, Keane GC, Tenenbaum MM. Commentary on: do compression garments prevent Subcutaneous edema after abdominoplasty? Aesthetic Surg J 2022;43(3):337–9.

Moving?

Make sure your subscription moves with you!

To notify us of your new address, find your **Clinics Account Number** (located on your mailing label above your name), and contact customer service at:

Email: journalscustomerservice-usa@elsevier.com

800-654-2452 **(subscribers in the U.S. & Canada)**
314-447-8871 **(subscribers outside of the U.S. & Canada)**

Fax number: 314-447-8029

Elsevier Health Sciences Division
Subscription Customer Service
3251 Riverport Lane
Maryland Heights, MO 63043

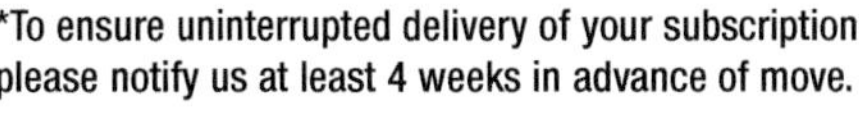

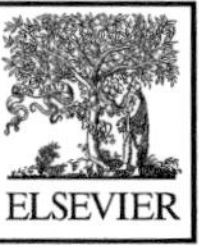

9780443130953